Edward Nettleship, William Thomson

Diseases of the Eye

Edward Nettleship, William Thomson

Diseases of the Eye

ISBN/EAN: 9783742809759

Manufactured in Europe, USA, Canada, Australia, Japa

Cover: Foto ©Lupo / pixelio.de

Manufactured and distributed by brebook publishing software
(www.brebook.com)

Edward Nettleship, William Thomson

Diseases of the Eye

DISEASES OF THE EYE.

BY

EDWARD NETTLESHIP, F.R.C.S.,

OPHTHALMIC SURGEON TO ST. THOMAS'S HOSPITAL; SURGEON TO THE ROYAL LONDON
(MOORFIELDS) OPHTHALMIC HOSPITAL; LATE OPHTHALMIC SURGEON TO
THE HOSPITAL FOR SICK CHILDREN, GREAT ORMOND STREET.

FOURTH AMERICAN

FROM THE

FIFTH ENGLISH EDITION.

WITH A CHAPTER ON

EXAMINATION FOR COLOR-PERCEPTION.

BY

WILLIAM THOMSON, M.D.,

PROFESSOR OF OPHTHALMOLOGY IN THE JEFFERSON MEDICAL COLLEGE OF PHILADELPHIA.

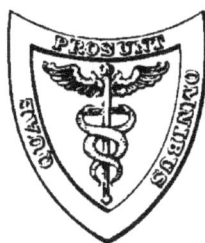

PHILADELPHIA:
LEA BROTHERS & CO.
1890.

DORNAN, PRINTER.

TO

JONATHAN HUTCHINSON, F.R.S.,

CONSULTING SURGEON TO THE MOORFIELDS OPHTHALMIC HOSPITAL
AND TO THE LONDON HOSPITAL, ETC.,

THIS

BOOK IS DEDICATED

IN GRATEFUL ADMIRATION OF HIS EMINENT QUALITIES AS A
CLINICAL TEACHER AND INVESTIGATOR.

AMERICAN PUBLISHERS' PREFACE.

In presenting to the medical profession the fourth American edition of Dr. Nettleship's work on "The Diseases of the Eye," the publishers desire to state that no pains have been spared to place it in every particular upon a level with the latest developments of the specialty of which it treats.

In addition to a most thorough and careful revision by the author, comprising many important changes and additions, there has been inserted as a supplement the chapter from the previous edition upon the Detection of Color-blindness, from the pen of Dr. William Thomson, whose painstaking investigations upon this subject are widely known, and his methods generally adopted for the examination of railroad employés.

Every care has been taken with the typography, and in all respects the publishers feel assured that the work will be found to merit in an increased degree the confidence awarded by the profession to the previous editions.

PHILADELPHIA, 1890.

PREFACE TO THE FIFTH EDITION.

THE general work of revision and of correction for the press for the present edition has been carried out with much pains by Mr. Holmes Spicer.

The bulk of the volume has been but little increased, though I have taken every care to include such new matter as seemed suitable for a book of this class, and considerable changes will be found, especially in the chapter on Operations. The number of illustrations is the same as in the last edition; but Figures 9, 50, 53, 95, and 131 have been replaced by new cuts; and for the colored papers of the former editions, there has been substituted, at the suggestion of the Publishers, a copy of Professor Holmgren's well-known plate, executed at Stockholm with the kind permission of the Professor.

September, 1890.

PREFACE TO THE FIRST EDITION.

THE aim of this little book is to supply students with the information they most need on diseases of the eye during their hospital course. It was apparent from the beginning that the task would be a difficult one, all the more as several excellent manuals, covering nearly the same ground, are already before the public. That not one of them singly appeared exactly to cover the ground most important for the first beginner in clinical ophthalmology encouraged me to attempt the present work.

The scope of the work has precluded frequent reference to authors, those named being chiefly such as have made recent additions to our knowledge in this country. I am greatly indebted to Dr. Gowers, Dr. Barlow, and other friends for much information, and for many valuable suggestions. My best thanks are due to Mr. A. D. Davidson for his kind assistance in reading the sheets for the press.

WIMPOLE STREET: *October*, 1890.

CONTENTS.

CHAPTER VII.

DISEASES OF THE CORNEA.

CHAPTER X.

INJURIES OF THE EYEBALL.

CHAPTER XI.

CATARACT.

CHAPTER XV.

AMBLYOPIA AND FUNCTIONAL DISORDERS OF SIGHT.

CHAPTER XVI.

DISEASES OF THE VITREOUS HUMOR.

CHAPTER XVII.

GLAUCOMA.

CHAPTER XVIII.

TUMORS AND NEW-GROWTHS.

CHAPTER XXI.

STRABISMUS AND PARALYSIS.

CHAPTER XXII.

OPERATIONS.

PART III.—DISEASES OF THE EYE IN RELA-TION TO GENERAL DISEASES.

CHAPTER XXIII.

A. GENERAL DISEASES.

B. LOCAL DISEASE AT A DISTANCE FROM THE EYE.

[SUPPLEMENT.

EXAMINATION FOR COLOR-PERCEPTION.

APPENDIX.

PART I.

MEANS OF DIAGNOSIS.

THE following abbreviations will be used in this work:

T.	Tension of the eyeball.	cm.	Centimetre.
E.	Emmetropia.	mm.	Millimetre.
M.	Myopia.	D.	Dioptre, the unit in the metrical system of measuring lenses; a lens whose focal length is 1 m.
H.	Hypermetropia.		
m. H.	Manifest hypermetropia.		
l. H.	Latent hypermetropia.		
Pr.	Presbyopia.	y. s.	Yellow spot of the retina.
As.	Astigmatism.	O. D.	Optic disc.
Acc.	Accommodation.	F.	Field of vision.
p.	Punctum proximum or near point.	V.	Visus, acuteness of sight, power of distinguishing form.
r.	Punctum remotissimum or far point.		
p. l.	Perception of light.	*Symbols.*	+ A convex, — a concave, lens. ' Foot, '' Inch, ''' Line.
P.	Pupil.		
m.	Metre.		

--

CHAPTER I.

OPTICAL OUTLINES.

1. RAYS of light are deviated or refracted when they pass from one transparent medium, *e. g.*, air, into another of different density, *e. g.*, water or glass.

2. If the deviation in passing from vacuum into air be represented by the number 1, that for crown-glass, of which ordinary lenses are made, is 1.5, and for rock crystal,

2

"pebble" of opticians, 1.66. Such a number is the "refractive index" of the substance. Every ray is refracted except the one which falls perpendicularly to the surface, Fig. 1, a.

FIG. 1.

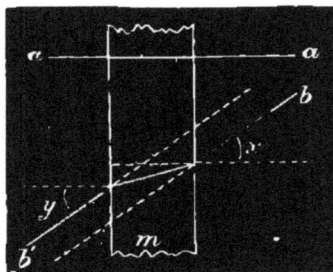

Refraction by a medium with parallel sides.

3. In passing from a less into a more refracting medium the deviation is always toward the perpendicular to the refracting surface; in passing from a more into a less refracting medium it is always, and to the same extent, away from the perpendicular, Fig. 1, b; i. e., the angle x in the figure = the angle y.

FIG. 2.

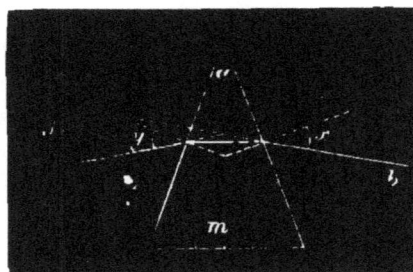

Refraction by a prism.

4. Hence, if the sides of the medium, Fig. 1, m, be parallel, the rays on emerging (b') are restored to their original

direction (*b*) and, if the medium be thin, very nearly to their original *path.*

5. But if, *as in a prism*, the sides of *m* form an angle, Fig. 2, *a*, the angles of incidence and emergence, *x* and *y*, still being equal, *b'* must also form an angle with *b*. The

Fig. 3.

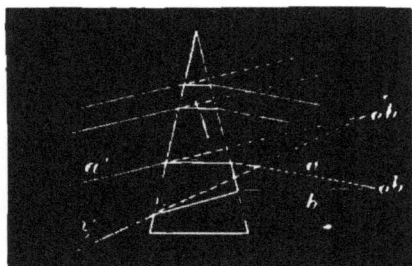

Apparent displacement of object by a prism.

angle *a* is the "refracting angle" or edge of the prism; the opposite side is the "base." The figure shows that light is always deviated *toward the base.* The deviation, shown by the angle *d*, is equal to about half the refracting

Fig. 4.

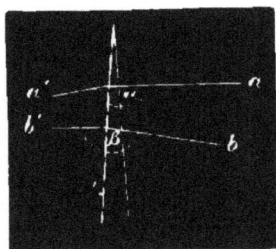

Refraction the same for different angles of incidence.

angle *a* if the prism be of crown-glass. The *relative* direction of the rays is not changed by a prism; if parallel or divergent before incidence, they are parallel or similarly divergent after emergence. Fig. 3.

6. An object seems to lie, or is "projected," in the direction which the rays have *as they enter the eye; ob*, Fig. 3, seen by an eye at a' or b', seems to be at $o'b$, where it would be if the rays a' b' had undergone no deviation.

7. For very thin *prisms* the deviation, a and β, Fig. 4, remains the same for varying angles of incidence. For thin *lenses* this is expressed by saying that the angle d, Fig. 5, is the same for the rays a a', b b', and c c', inci-

Fig. 5.

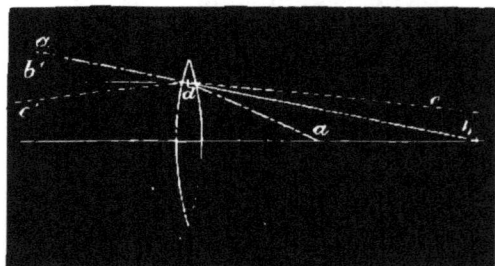

Refraction by a thin lens the same for all rays incident at the same distance from the axis.

dent at different angles, but at the *same distance from the axis.*

8. **An ordinary lens** is a segment of a sphere, plano-convex or plano-concave, or of two spheres whose centres are joined by the axis of the lens, biconvex or biconcave.

9. A lens is regarded as formed of an infinite number of minute prisms, each with a different refracting angle. Fig. 6 shows two such elements of a convex lens, the angle (a) of the prism at the edge of the lens being larger, and therefore, in accordance with § 5, refracting more, than β, the angle of the prism near the axis. If two parallel rays, a and b, traverse this system, a will be more refracted than b, and the rays will meet at f. Fig. 7 shows the cor-

responding facts for a concave lens, by which parallel rays
are made divergent.

Fig. 6.

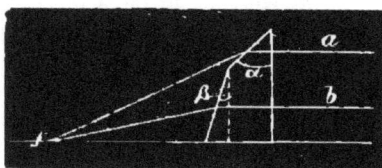

Prismatic elements of a convex lens.

Fig. 7.

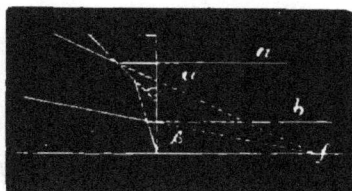

Prismatic elements of a concave lens.

10. The only ray not refracted by a lens is the one
passing through the centre of each surface; compare § 2,
which is the **principal axis**, *ax*, Fig. 8. *Secondary axes* are

Fig. 8.

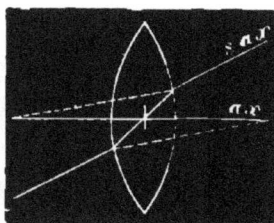

Axes of a lens.

rays, such as *s. ax*, entering and emerging at points on the
lens parallel to each other, and hence, see § 4, not altered
in direction: all rays which pass through the central

point of the lens are secondary axes, except the principal axis.

11. The **principal focus**, f, Fig. 10, of a lens is the point where the rays, $a\ a$, that were parallel before they traversed the lens meet, after they have passed through it; the deviation of each ray varying directly with its distance from the principal axis, Fig. 6.

But this is only approximately true. In an ordinary lens the rays, a, Fig. 9, which traverse the margin are refracted

FIG. 9.

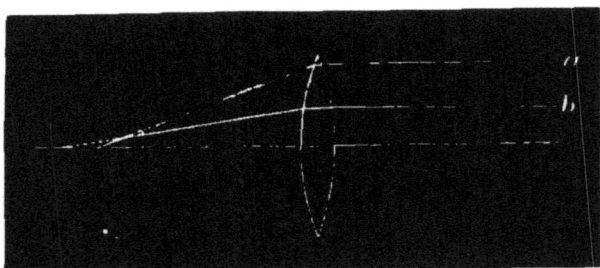

Spherical aberration.

more, and meet sooner, than the rays (b) which lie nearer the axis; and the result is, not one focus, but a number of foci.

FIG. 10.

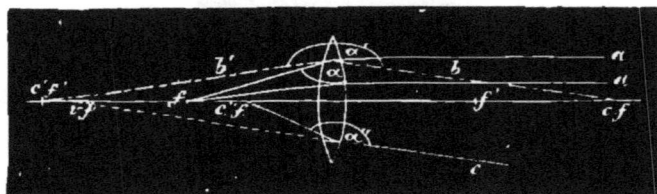

Foci of a convex lens.

"Spherical aberration" increases with the size of the lens. In the eye it is, to a great extent, prevented by the iris, which cuts off the light from the margin of the crystalline lens.

If parallel rays are incident from the side toward f, Fig.
10, they will be focussed at f', at the same distance from
the lens as f; hence every lens has two principal foci—
anterior and posterior.

12. The *path* of a ray passing from one point to another
is the same, whatever its *direction;* the path of the ray
$b\,b'$, Fig. 10, is the same, whether it pass from cf to $c'f'$, or
in the contrary direction.

13. From § 7 it follows that in Fig. 10 the angles a and
a' are equal, and hence the ray b, diverging from cf, will
not meet the axis at f, but at $c'f'$; cf and $c'f'$ are *conjugate points*, and each is the *conjugate focus* of the other.
The angle a or a' remaining the same, then if cf be further from the lens $c'f'$ will approach it.   A ray, c, directed
toward the axis will be focussed at $c''f''$, because the
angle $a''=a$; no real point conjugate to $c''f''$ exists: but
if the ray start from $c''f''$ it will, on taking the direction
c, appear to have come from vf, which consequently is the
virtual focus of $c''f''$, see § 6.

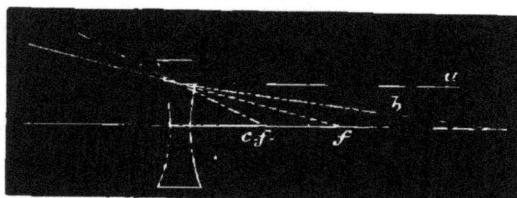

Foci of a concave lens.

14. All the foci of concave lenses are virtual. In Fig.
11, a, parallel to the axis, is made divergent, see Fig. 7,
its virtual focus being at f; similarly cf is the virtual conjugate focus of the point emitting the ray b.

15. In equally biconvex or biconcave lenses of crown-
glass *the principal focus, f,* is at the centre of curvature of

either surface of the lens, *i. e.*, $f = r$, the radius ; in plano-convex, or concave, lenses $f = 2r$.

16. **Images.**—The image formed by a lens consists of foci, each of which corresponds to a point on the object. Given the foci of the boundary points of an object, we have the position and size of its image.

In Fig. 12 the object *a b* lies beyond the focus *f*. From the terminal point *a* take two rays, **a** and **a**′, the former a secondary axis, and therefore unrefracted ; the latter par-

Fig. 12.

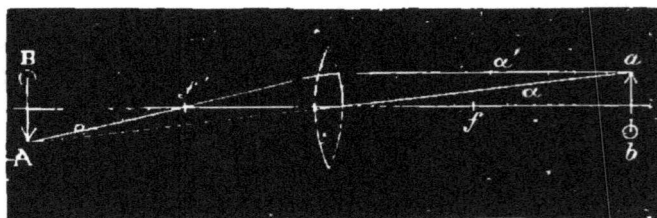

Real inverted image formed by a convex lens.

allel to the principal axis, and therefore passing after re-fraction through the principal focus *f*′. These two rays, and all others which pass through the lens from the point *a*, will meet at A the conjugate focus of *a*. Similarly the focus of the point *b* is found, and the real inverted conju-gate image of *a b* is formed at A B. The relative sizes of *a b* and A B vary as their distances from the lens.

If *a b* be so far off that its rays are virtually parallel on reaching the lens, its image A B will be at *f*′, and very small. If *a b* be at *f*, its rays will become parallel after refraction, §§ 11 and 12, and form no image. If *a b* lies between *f*, or *f*′, and the lens, the rays will diverge after refraction, and again will not form an image, see Fig. 10, *c*″*f*″.

But in the last two cases a virtual image is seen by an eye so placed as to receive the rays.   In Fig. 13 two rays from a take after refraction the course shown by a and a', virtually meeting at A. see Fig. 10, cf; and an observer at x will see at A B a virtual, magnified, erect image of $a\,b$.

FIG. 13.

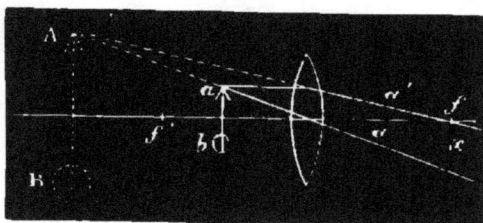

Virtual erect image formed by a convex lens.

The enlargement in Fig. 13 is greater the nearer $a\,b$ is to f', and greatest when it is at f'.   But as A B has no real existence, its apparent size varies with the known or estimated distance of the surface against which it is projected.   A uniform distance of projection of about 12″ (30 cm.) is taken in comparing the magnifying power of different lenses.

When $a\,b$ is at f', Fig. 13, we shall find on trial that the image A B can be seen well only by bringing the eye close up to the lens ; at a greater distance only part of the image will be seen, and this part will be less brightly lighted.   This is important in direct ophthalmoscopic examination.   Thus in Fig. 14 an observer placed anywhere between the lens and x, receiving rays from every part of $a\,b$, will see the whole image.   But if he withdraw to y, his eye will receive rays only from the central part of $a\,b$, and will therefore not see the ends of the object.

It is easily shown by similar constructions that the

images formed by concave lenses are always virtual, erect, and diminished, whatever the distance of the object, Fig. 15. *Compare* Fig. 11.

FIG. 14.

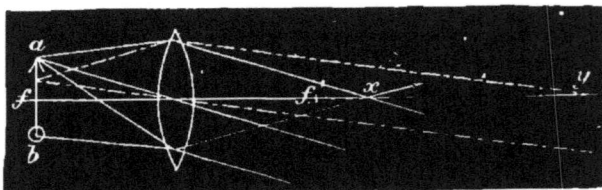

Virtual image : result of observer varying distance of his eye from the lens.

17. The size of the image, whether real or virtual, varies with (1) the focal length of the lens, and (2) the distance of the object from the principal focus.

(1) The shorter the focus of the lens, the greater is its effect, or the "stronger" it is ; *the refractive power of a lens varies inversely as its focal length.*

FIG. 15.

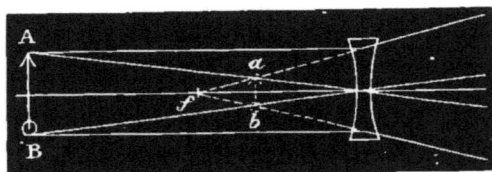

Image formed by a concave lens.

(2) For a *convex* lens, the image, whether real or virtual, is larger, *i. e.*, the effect greater, the nearer the object is to the principal focus, whether within or beyond it.

For a *concave* lens, the image is smaller, *i. e.*, the effect greater, the further the object is from the lens, whether within or beyond the focus.

18. **Prisms.**—Any object viewed through a prism seems displaced towards the edge of the prism, and the amount of the displacement varies directly as the size of the refracting angle, §§ 5 and 6. The eye is directed towards the position which the object now seems to take; and this

FIG. 16.

FIG. 17.

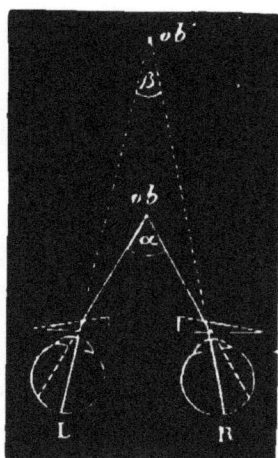

Effect of prisms in lessening convergence.

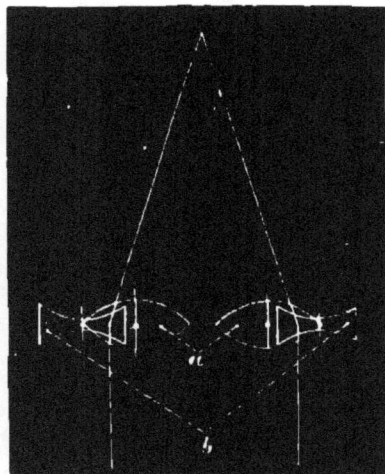

Lenses acting as prisms.

effect may be variously utilized: 1. *To lessen the convergence* of the visual lines without removing the object further from the eyes. In Fig. 16 the eyes, R and L, are looking at the object, *ob*, with a convergence of the visual lines represented by the angle α. If prisms be now added with their edges towards the temples, they deflect the light, so that it enters the eyes under the smaller angle β, as if it had come from *ob'*, and towards this point the eyes will be directed, though the object still remains at *ob*. The same effect is given by a single prism of twice the strength before one eye, though the actual movement is then limited to the eye in question. If spectacle lenses be placed so that the visual lines do not pass through their centres, they act as prisms; though the strength of the prismatic action varies with the power of the lens and the amount of this " decentration," see § 9, Figs. 6 and 7.

Table showing the Prismatic Effect of Decentering Lenses (Maddox).

Lens.	Amount of Decentration in Millimetres.		
	5 mm.	10 mm.	15 mm.
1 D . .	17'	35'	52'
2 D . .	35	1° 9	1° 43
3 D . .	52	1 43	2 34
4 D . .	1 - 10	2 18	3 26
6 D . .	1 43	6 26	5 9
8 D . .	2 18	4 35	6 50

In Fig. 17 the visual lines pass outside the centres of the convex lenses, *a*, and inside those of the concave lenses, *b*. Each pair therefore acts as a prism with its edge outwards. 2. To *remove double vision* caused by slight degrees of strabismus. The prism so alters the direction of the rays as to compensate for the abnormal direction of the visual line. In Fig. 18, R is directed towards *x* instead of towards *ob*, and two images of *ob* are seen, see Chapter XXI. The prism, *p*, deflects the rays to *y*, the yellow spots, and single binocular vision is the result. 3. *To test the strength of the ocular muscles.* In Fig. 19 the prism at first causes diplopia by displacing the rays from the yellow spot, *y*, of the eye R, see Chapter XXI. By a compensating rotation of the eye, cornea, outwards, shown in the figure by the change of the transverse axis from 1 to 2, *y* is brought inwards to the situation of *im*, the images are fused and single vision restored; the effect of the prism is overcome by the action of the external rectus. This "fusion power" of the several pairs of muscles may be expressed by the strongest prism that each pair can overcome. The fusion power of the two external recti is represented by a prism of about 8°; that of the two internals by 25° to 50° or more; that of the

FIG. 18.

FIG. 19.

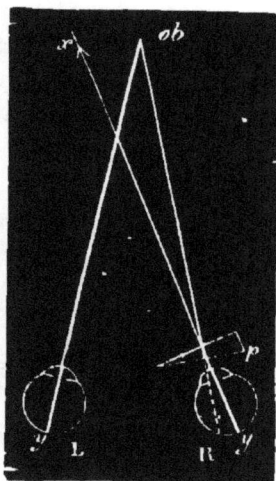

Diplopia removed by prism.

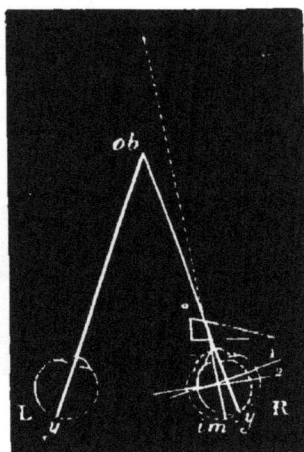

Prism used for testing strength of muscle.

superior and inferior recti, acting against each other, by only about 3°. 4. *Feigned blindness of one eye* may often be exposed by means of the diplopia, unexpected by the patient, produced by a prism. The prism should be stronger than can be overcome by any effort, e. g., 8° or 10°, base upwards or downwards. The patient is best thrown off his guard if the prism be held before the sound eye. If he now exclaims that he sees double, he must of course be seeing with both eyes.

19. **Refraction of the eye.**—The eye presents three refracting surfaces—the front of the cornea,[1] the front of the
lens, and the front of the vitreous; and in the normally
formed or emmetropic eye (E.), with the accommodation
relaxed, the principal focus, § 11, of these combined dioptric media falls exactly upon the layer of rods and cones
of the retina ; *i. e.*, the eye in a state of accommodative rest
is adapted for parallel rays The point at which the
secondary axial rays, see § 10, Fig. 8, cross, the " porterior
nodal point," *n*, Fig. 20, lies, in the normally formed eye,
at 15 mm. in front of the yellow spot of the retina, and

Fig. 20.

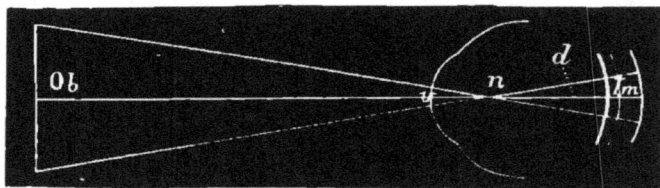

Visual angle and retinal image. *Ob*, object ; *v*, visual angle ; *n*, nodal
point where the axial rays cross ; *d*, distance from *n* to the retina.
The position of the retina in different states of refraction is shown by
the three curved lines to the right, H. being represented by the line
nearest to, and N. by the one furthest from, *n*, whilst the middle thin
line shows the retina in E.

very nearly coincides with the posterior pole of the crystalline lens.   The angle included between the lines joining
n with the extremities of the object, *ob*, is the *visual angle*, *v*.
If the distance, *d*, from *n* to the retina remain the same,
the size of any image, *Im*, on the retina will depend on the

---

[1] The posterior surface of the cornea being parallel with the anterior
causes no deviation, and the aqueous has the same refractive power as
the cornea. Hence the refractive effect of the cornea and aqueous together is the same as if the corneal tissue extended from the front of
the cornea to the front of the lens.

size of the angle v, and this again on the size and distance of *ob*. But if the distance, d, alters, the size of the image, *Im*, is altered without any change in v. Now the length of d varies with the length of the posterior segment of the eye; it is greater in myopia (M.) and less in hypermetropia (H.); and hence the retinal image of an object at a given distance is, as the figure shows, larger in myopia and smaller in hypermetropia than in the normally formed eye. The length of d also varies with the position of n, and this is influenced by the positions and curvatures of the several refractive surfaces. n is slightly advanced by the increased convexity of the lens during accommodation, and much more so if the same change of refraction be induced by a convex lens held in front of the cornea: hence convex lenses, by lengthening d, enlarge the retinal image. Concave lenses put n further back, and, by thus shortening d, lessen the image. If the lens which corrects any optical error of the eye be placed at the " anterior focus" of the eye,[1] 13 mm., or half an inch, in front of the cornea, n moves to its normal distance (15 mm.) from the retina, whatever the length of the eye, and the images are therefore reduced or enlarged to the same size as in the emmetropic eye. For definition of astigmatism see Chapter XX.

The length of the *visual axis*, a line drawn from the yellow spot to the cornea in the direction of the object looked at, is about 23 mm. The centre of rotation of the eye is rather behind the centre of this axis, and 6 mm. behind the back of the lens. The focal length of the cornea is 31 mm., and that of the crystalline lens varies from 43 mm. with accommodation relaxed, to 33 mm. during strong accommodation.

The **optical conditions of clear sight** are as follows:

(1) The image must be clearly focussed on the retina, *i. e.*, the retina must lie exactly at the focus of the rays

[1] The anterior focus is the point where rays which were parallel in the vitreous are focussed in front of the cornea.

which proceed from the object looked at: (2) it must be
formed at the centre of the yellow spot, Chapter II., § 11:
(3) it must have a certain size, and this is expressed by
the size of the corresponding visual angle, v, Fig. 20; with
good indoor light v must be equal to at least 5 minutes,
$\frac{1}{12}$th of a degree, in order that the form of the image may
be perceived; an object subtending any smaller angle,
down to about 1 minute, is still visible, though only as a
point of light:[1] (4) the cornea, lens, and vitreous must be
clear: (5) the illumination must be sufficient. *Influence
of the pupil:* Other things being equal, the larger the
pupil the worse is the sight, definition being lessened by
the spherical aberration caused by the marginal part of
the lens, Fig. 9. See Artificial Pupil.

The smaller the pupil, the less the spherical aberration (p.
30), and, *cæt. par.*, the better the V. Also, the smaller the
pupil the less is the accommodation needed for near vision.
If the pupil be so small as to subtend an angle, "angle of divergence," of not more than 5 minutes with any point on the
object, the object will be clearly seen without accommodation.
By calculation it appears that if the pupil had a diameter =
0.66 mm., it would subtend an angle of divergence of 5 minutes
at about 0.5 m. (18″); *i. e.*, with a pupil of 0.66 mm. print
should, in a good light, be clearly seen at 18″ without any
accommodation. That this is true may be proved by looking
at fine print through a hole of the above size in a thin card
held as close as possible to the eye.

Numeration of spectacle lenses.—Some system of num-
bering is required which shall indicate the refractive power
of the lenses used for spectacles. Two systems are current.
In the *first system*, which was till lately universal, the unit
of strength is a strong lens of 1″ focal length. As all the
lenses used are weaker than this, their relative strengths
can be expressed only by using fractions. Thus, a lens of

---

[1] In bright light, as in the open air, the minimum visual angle is
considerably less than 5 minutes.

2″ focus, being half as strong as the unit (§17, 1), is expressed as $\frac{1}{2}$; a lens of 10″ focus is $\frac{1}{10}$; of 20″ focus $\frac{1}{20}$; and so on. The objections are, that fractions are inconvenient in practice; that the intervals between the successive numbers are very unequal; and that the length of the inch is not the same in all countries, so that a glass of the same *number* has not quite the same focal length when made by the Paris, English, and German inches respectively.[1] In the *second system*, which has almost displaced the old one, the metrical scale is used, the unit is a weak lens of 1 metre (100 cm.) focal length, known as a dioptre (D), and the lenses differ by equal refractive intervals. A lens twice as strong as the unit, with a focal length of half a metre, 50 cm., is 2 dioptres (2 D), a lens of ten times the strength, or one-tenth of a metre focus, 10 cm., is 10 D, and so on. The weakest lenses are 0.25, 0.5, and 0.75 D, and numbers differing by 0.5 or 0.25 D are also introduced between the whole numbers. A slight inconvenience of the metrical dioptric system is that the number of the lens does not express its focal length. This, however, is obtained by dividing 100 by the number of the lens in D; thus the focal length of 4 D $= \frac{100}{4} = 25$ cm. If it be desired to convert one system into the other, this can be done, provided that we know what inch was used in making the lens whose equivalent is required in D. The metre is equal to about 37″ French and 39″ English or German; a lens of 36″ French (No. 36 or $\frac{1}{36}$ old scale), or of 40″ English or German (No. 40 or $\frac{1}{40}$), is very nearly the equivalent of 1 D. A lens of 6″ French ($\frac{1}{6} = \frac{6}{36}$) will therefore be equal to 6 D; a lens of 18″ French ($\frac{1}{18} = \frac{2}{36}$) = 2 D, etc.; a lens of 4 D $= \frac{4}{36} = \frac{1}{9}$, *i. e.*, a lens of 9″ French, etc.

The following lenses are used for spectacles, and are, therefore, necessary in a complete set of trial glasses. The

---

[1] 1″ English = 25.3 mm., 1″ French = 27 mm., 1″ Austrian = 26.3 mm., 1″ Prussian = 26.1 mm.

first column gives the number in D, the second the focal length in centimetres, the third the approximate numbers on the French inch scale, the denominator of each fraction showing the focal length in French inches. It will be seen that some metrical lenses have no exact equivalents on the inch system. In this table, and throughout the book, convex lenses are indicated, according to custom, by the $+$ sign; concave lenses by the $-$ sign.

Prisms are numbered by their angle of refraction, which is (p. 27) about double the angle of deviation; another method is to name the prism by the number of degrees of deviation which it produces; to indicate that degrees of deviation are meant the letter d should be used; thus prism $2°\,d$ indicates that the prism produces a deviation of $2°$ (Maddox).   Prisms cannot be used as spectacles of a greater strength than about $4°\,d$ in each eye on account of the dispersion of light which they produce.

1.	2.	3.	1.	2.	3.
D. (Dioptres.)	Focal Length in cm.	No. and Focal Length in Paris inches.	D. (Dioptres.)	Focal Length in cm.	No. and Focal Length in Paris inches.
0.25	400		5	20	$\frac{1}{7}$
0.5	200	$\frac{1}{72}$	5.5	18	
0.75	133	$\frac{1}{50}$	6	16	$\frac{1}{6}$
1	100	$\frac{1}{36}$	7	14	$\frac{1}{5}½$
1.25	80	$\frac{1}{30}$	8	12.5	$\frac{1}{4}$
1.5	66	$\frac{1}{24}$	9	11	$\frac{1}{4}$
1.75	57	$\frac{1}{22}$	10	10	$\frac{1}{3}½$
2	50	$\frac{1}{18}$	11	9	
2.25	44	$\frac{1}{16}$	12	8.3	$\frac{1}{3}$
2.5	40	$\frac{1}{14}$	13	7.7	
2.75	36	$\frac{1}{13}$	14	7	$\frac{1}{2}¾$
3	33	$\frac{1}{12}$	15	6.7	$\frac{1}{2}½$
3.5	28	$\frac{1}{10}$	16	6.2	$\frac{1}{2}¼$
4	25	$\frac{1}{9}$	18	5.5	$\frac{1}{2}$
4.5	22	$\frac{1}{8}$	20	5	

CHAPTER II.

(1) **To detect irregularity of the corneal surface,** the patient faces the window and follows with his eyes an object, *e. g.*, the uplifted finger, held about 18″ from him and moved slowly in different directions. The image of the window reflected from the cornea will become distorted or broken as it passes over any irregularity, such as an abrasion or ulcer.

(2) **To estimate the tension of the eyeball** (T.) : The patient looks steadily down and gently closes the eyelids; the observer then makes light pressure on the globe through the upper lid, alternately with a finger of each hand as in trying for fluctuation, but much more delicately. The finger-tips are placed very near together, and as far back over the sclerotic as possible, not over the cornea. The pressure must be gentle, and be directed vertically *downwards, not backwards.* It is best for each observer to keep to one pair of fingers, not to use the index at one time and the middle finger at another. Patient and observer should always be in the same relative position, and it is best for both to stand and face one another. Always compare the tension of the two eyes. Be sure that the eye does not roll upwards during examination, for if this occur a wrong estimate of the tension may be formed Some test both eyes at once with two fingers of each hand. Normal tension is expressed by T. n. Recognizable increase and decrease are indicated by the + or — sign, followed by the figure 1, 2, or 3. Thus T.+1 means decided increase ; T.+2, greater increase, but eye can still be indented ; T.+3, eye very hard, cannot be indented by

moderate pressure ; T.—1 —2 —3 indicate successive degrees of lowered tension. A note of interrogation (T.? + or ?—) for doubtful cases, and T. n. for normal, give nine degrees which may be usefully distinguished. Even good observers sometimes differ as to the minor changes of tension. Apart from variations in delicacy of touch, it is to be remembered that eyes deeply set in the orbits are more difficult to test, and that T. in a few cases really does change at short intervals, e. g., within half an hour. Increase in the rigidity of the sclerotic, which often occurs in old age ; or in its thickness, as the result of disease, may increase the apparent tension, though the internal pressure may be normal or even too low. When an eye contains bone it feels like wood covered with wash-leather.[1]

(3) **The field of vision** (F.), properly, *of indirect vision,* is the entire surface from which, at a given distance, light reaches the retina,[2] the eye being stationary, Fig. 21. If each part of the field be equidistant from the part of the retina to which it corresponds, the field will be hemispherical, with its inner or concave surface towards the eye ; it may, however, be projected on to a flat surface, and for many clinical purposes this is sufficient. For roughly testing the field, e. g., in a case of chronic glaucoma, or of atrophy of optic nerve, or of hemianopsia, the following is generally enough. Place the patient with his back to the window ; let him cover one eye, and look steadily at your eye or nose, as a centre, from a distance of 18″ or 2′. Then hold up your hands with your fingers spread out in a plane with your face, and ascertain the greatest distance from the central point at which they remain visible when moved

[1] Plates of bone, sometimes joined so as to form a cup, are not uncommonly found on the inner (retinal) surface of the choroid in eyes which have been long blind from irido-choroiditis.

[2] Strictly " the percipient part of the retina." It now seems established that the most peripheral zone of the retina is not sensitive to light. (Landolt.)

in various directions—up, down, in, out, and diagonally.
The patient must look steadily at the face, and *not allow
his eye to wander* after the moving fingers.

FIG. 21.

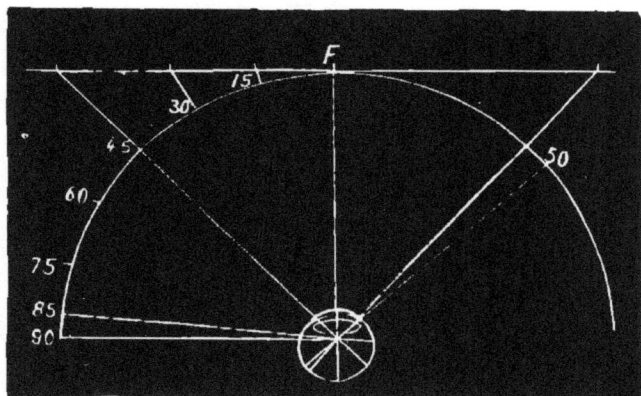

Field of vision with radius of 12″, projected up to 45° on to a flat surface
two feet square. F, fixation spot.

A more exact method is to make the patient gaze, with
one eye covered, at a white mark, the " fixation spot," on a
large blackboard at a distance of 12″ or 18″, and to move
a piece of white chalk set in a long black handle, from
various parts of the periphery towards the fixation spot,
until the patient exclaims that he sees something white.
If a mark be made on the board at about eight such peripheral points, a line joining them will give, with fair accuracy, the boundary of the visual field if this be not larger
than 45° in any direction; but beyond that angle the
object, if on a flat surface, will be much too far from the
eye to make the test accurate, see Fig. 21. A true map,
unless the field be much contracted, can be made only by
means of an instrument, the perimeter, which consists
essentially of an arc marked in degrees, and movable

around a central pivot on which the patient fixes his gaze. Thus measured the field covers a somewhat oval portion of the hemisphere, the smaller end being upwards and inwards, Fig. 22. From the fixation point it extends $90°$ or

FIG. 22.

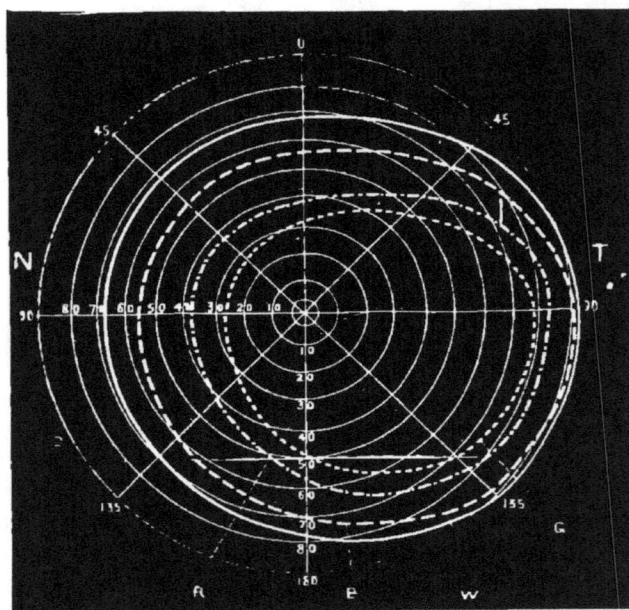

Field of vision of right eye as projected by the patient on the inner surface of a hemisphere, the pole of which forms the object of regard (half-diagrammatic). T. temporal, N, nasal side. w, boundary for white B, for blue ; R, for red ; G, for green. (Landolt.)

more in the outward direction, but only about $65°$ or rather less inwards, upwards, and downwards. The visual fields of the two eyes overlap only at their inner and central parts, so that binocular vision is impossible in the outer part of the field, Fig. 23.

(4) **Color-perception** is best expressed by the power

of discriminating between various colors without naming them. The best test-objects are a series of skeins of colored wool, or, for pocket use, smaller strips of colored paper, or colored stuffs A color-blind person will expose his defect by placing together, or "confusing" as similar, certain colors, usually mixed tints, which to the normal eye appear quite different. The set of wools now in common use was introduced by Professor Holmgren, of Upsala.[1]

FIG. 23.

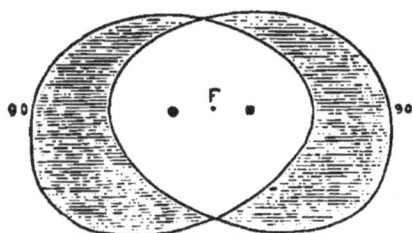

Binocular field of vision. The white part is the portion common to the two eyes, i. e , possessing binocular vision ; the shaded (temporal) part shows the portion in which binocular vision is wanting. F, fixation point. The two blind spots are marked by round spots. (Simplified, after Förster.)

See Appendix. Acquired color-blindness (from atrophy of the optic nerves) may often be detected quite well by asking the names, if the patient has been well trained in colors. But for the congenitally color-blind the "confusion test," without names, is far better : first, because such persons can often distinguish ordinary colored objects from one another by differences of *shade*, i. e., by differences in the quantity of white light which they reflect, and hence they escape detection unless tested with a large series of different colors in many shades, some of which shades, containing equal quantities of white, will look, to them, exactly

[1] De la Cécité des Couleurs, etc., 1877.

alike; and secondly, though such persons often use the names for colors freely, the words do not convey the same meaning to them as to those with normal color-sense, and hopeless confusion results from an examination so made. For details see Chapter XV. and Supplement.

(5) **Testing the acuteness of sight.**—By acuteness of sight (V. or S.) is meant the power of distinguishing *form*, and, as commonly used, the term refers only to the centre of the visual field, the peripheral part of the retina having a very imperfect power of distinguishing form and size. V. varies considerably in different persons whose eyes are normal. It is said to diminish somew¹at in old age, without disease of the eye (Donders)   The standard taken as normal is the power of distinguishing square letters that subtend a visual angle of 5 minutes, Fig. 20 and p. 40, the limbs of which are of uniform thickness, each limb subtending an angle of 1 minute (Snellen's Test-types). Rays forming so small an angle are very nearly parallel, and may be considered as coming from an object at an infinite distance. The types are made of various sizes, each being numbered according to the distance, in feet or metres, at which it subtends a visual angle of 5 minutes. Thus, No. 6 subtends this angle at 6 m., No. 3 at 3 m., No. 1 at 1 m., etc. Numerically, acuteness of vision is expressed by a fraction, of which the denominator is the number of the type D, and the numerator the greatest distance (d) at which it can be read, $V = \frac{d}{D}$: if No. 6 is read at 6 m. $\frac{d}{D} = \frac{6}{6}$ or 1, *i. e.*, V is normal; if only No. 18 can be read at 6 m. $\frac{d}{D} = \frac{6}{18}$; if only 60, then $\frac{d}{D} = \frac{6}{60}$. Any distance greater than about 3 m. may be selected for this test ; *i. e.*, No. 3 read at 3 m., or No. 5 at 5 m., generally shows the same acuteness as No. 6 read at 6 m. But at distances less than 3 m. the accommodation comes into play, and the illumination is often brighter; hence No 1 at 1 m. (¹) does

not necessarily show the same state of sight as No. 6 at 6 m. ($\frac{6}{6}$). It is therefore best, by recording the fractions unreduced, to indicate the distance at which the test was used. For testing near vision, Snellen's types are thought by some to be practically inferior to those of Jaeger and others, in which the letters have the form and proportions found in ordinary type. See Appendix. If V. be very bad, less than $\frac{6}{60}$ or $\frac{1}{15}$, it may be expressed accurately enough by noting the distance at which the outspread fingers can be counted when exposed to a good light and against a dark background. Below this point we can still distinguish good from bad, or uncertain, perception of light and shade (*p. l.*), by alternately exposing and shading the eye with the hand, without touching the face.

(6) **Accommodation** (*Acc.*) is tested clinically by measuring the nearest point (*punctum proximum*, *p.*) at which the smallest readable type (Snellen's 0.5 or Jaeger's 1) can be clearly seen. The *region* of accommodation is the space

FIG. 24.

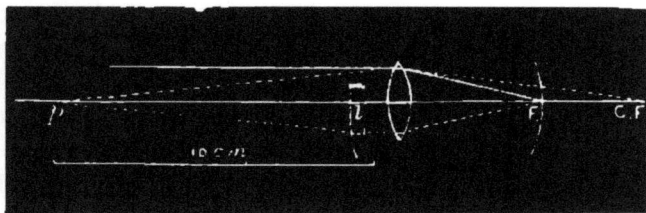

Accommodation represented by a convex lens.

in which it is available (see Presbyopia). The *amplitude*, *power*, or *range* of Acc. is expressed in terms of the convex lens whose focal length = the distance from the cornea[1] to *p.*, this being the lens which adapts V. in an eye with-

---

[1] Strictly, from a point about $\frac{1}{3}''$ in front of the cornea, since the glass cannot be placed upon the eyeball.

out Acc. from the farthest point of distinct vision (*punctum remotissimum, r.*) to p. Thus in Fig. 24 let p be at 10 cm.: if Acc. be then relaxed, *i. e.*, the eye be adapted for parallel rays, the rays from p will be focussed at c. F., behind the retina; but V. will again be clear at 10 cm. if a lens, l, of 10 cm. focus ($= 10$ D., see p. 41) be held close to the cornea; because rays from p will be made parallel by l before entering the eye (Chapter I., §§ 11 and 12) and will therefore be focussed on the retina.

Convergence of the visual axes upon a point at any given distance is usually associated with accommodation for the same distance. The two functions can, however, be somewhat dissociated to an extent that varies with age and in different persons; *i. e.*, Acc. can be either relaxed a little or increased a little, without changing any given degree of convergence; this independent portion is known as the *relative accommodation*.

(7) **The pupils** are to be examined as to their equality, size in ordinary light, mobility, and form. The pupils are often large and inactive, and sometimes oval, in amaurotic patients, in glaucoma, and in paralysis of the circular fibres of the iris, supplied by the third nerve. They may be too large, though active, in myopia and in conditions of defective nerve tone. Wide, recent dilatation of one pupil or both, with dimness of sight but without ophthalmoscopic signs of disease, is usually traceable to atropine or belladonna, used by accident or design. When very small the pupil is seldom quite round.

The centre of the pupil usually lies a little to the nasal side of the corneal centre.[1] The pupils should be round and, when equally lighted, equal in size. When one eye is shaded its pupil should dilate considerably, and on

[1] This eccentricity varies in degree and exact position in different persons. Compare Irregular Astigmatism.

exposure contract quickly to its former size, "*direct reflex action;*" during this trial the other pupil will act, but to a much less extent, "*indirect reflex action.*" The pupils contract when the gaze is directed to a near object, say 6″ distant, *i. e.*, during accommodation and convergence, and dilate in looking at a distant object; but the range of this "*associated action*" is much less than that of the reflex action. The pupil dilates when painful impressions are made on the sensory nerves of the skin, *e. g.*, by the faradaic brush or by pricking with a pin. The pupils may be motionless to light and shade from iritic adhesions (Chapter VIII.) or from atrophy of the iris in glaucoma or other local disease ; such conditions should be carefully noted or excluded. Reflex action is lost when the eyes are blind from disease of the optic nerves or retinæ; if only one eye be blind, the direct action of the pupil is lost in that eye, but (unless there be disease of the third nerve) its indirect action is much increased. When one eye is blind the pupil is often rather larger than that of the other. Reflex action may also be lost without any affection of sight, and *without loss of associated action.* Chapters XXI. and XXIII.

Permanent inequality of the pupils without disease, either of eyes or of nervous system, is rare, but temporary dilatation of one pupil is not uncommon. When very active pupils are suddenly exposed after being shaded they often oscillate for a few seconds before settling, and finally remain a little larger than at the first moment of exposure. Considerable differences in the action of the pupils, both in *range* and *rapidity,* are compatible with health ; in general, however, the pupils become smaller and lose both in range and rapidity of action with advancing years: atropine also often causes only partial dilatation in old people. Marked inactivity, with small size, should excite suspicion of spinal or cerebral disease (Chapter XXIII.). The pupils are smaller whenever the iris is congested, whether this be a

merely local condition, e. g., in abrasion of cornea, or form
part of a more general congestion, as in typhus fever[1] and
in plethoric states, or be caused by venous obstruction, as
in mitral regurgitation and bronchitis.   They are large in
anæmia, in conditions, such as aortic insufficiency,[2] where
the systemic arteries are badly filled, and during rigors;
irritation of the sympathetic nerve in the neck is an occasional cause of mydriasis.[3]   Chapter XXI.

(8) **Note the color of the iris,** and compare it with that
of the fellow-eye.   Occasionally the two irides, although
healthy, differ in color, one being blue or gray, the other
brown or greenish ; more frequently a large sector-shaped
patch of dark color occupies part of the iris of one eye.
Small pigmented spots are often seen on the iris.   If the
iris of an inflamed eye look greenish, that of its fellow
being blue, we should suspect iritis; and if the iris of a
defective eye be different from its fellow, some morbid
change should be suspected.   Chapter VIII.

(9) **Information derived from the bloodvessels visible
on the surface of the eyeball.**—Three systems of vessels
have to be considered in disease ; but most of them are too
small to be easily seen in health.   (1) The vessels proper
to the conjunctiva, *posterior conjunctival vessels,* in which it
is not important to distinguish between arteries and veins,
Fig. 25, *Post. Conj.,* and Fig. 26.   (2) The *anterior ciliary
vessels,* lying in the subconjunctival tissue; their perforating
arterial branches supply the sclerotic, iris, and ciliary body,
their veins receive blood from Schlemm's canal and the
ciliary body.   The perforating branches of the *arteries,*

[1] The small pupil of typhus and the frequently large pupil of typhoid
are ascribed by Murchison to the differences in the vascularity of the
iris in these diseases.   Continued Fevers, p. 541.

[2] Medical Examiner, March 2, 1879.

[3] This condition seems to be rare ; I can hear but little of it in the
experience of my medical friends.

Fig. 25, A, are seen in health as several comparatively large tortuous vessels which stop short about $\frac{1}{12}''$ or $\frac{1}{8}''$ from the corneal margin, Fig. 27 ; their very numerous, small, non-

FIG. 25.

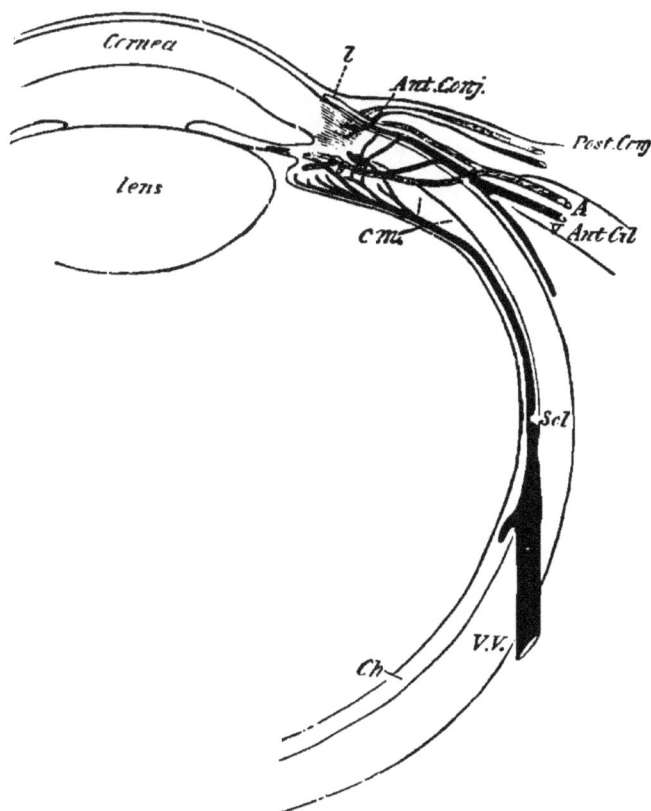

Vessels of the front of the eyeball. *c.m.* Ciliary muscle. *Ch.* Choroid. *Scl.* Sclerotic. *V. V.* Vena vorticosa. *l.* Marginal loop-plexus of cornea. *Ant.* and *Post. Conj.* Anterior and posterior conjunctival vessels. *Ant. Cil. A.* and *V.* Anterior ciliary arteries and veins. (Simplified and altered from Leber.)

perforating (episcleral) branches are invisible in health, but form, when distended, a pink zone of fine, nearly straight, very closely-set vessels round the cornea, Fig. 25, A, and Fig. 28, "ciliary congestion," "circumcorneal zone," see Iritis and Diseases of Cornea; the perforating *veins* are very small, but more numerous than the perforating arte-

FIG. 26.

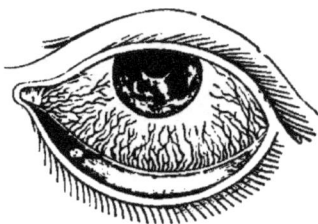

Conjunctival congestion, engorgement of the posterior conjunctival arteries and veins.   (After Guthrie.)

FIG. 27.

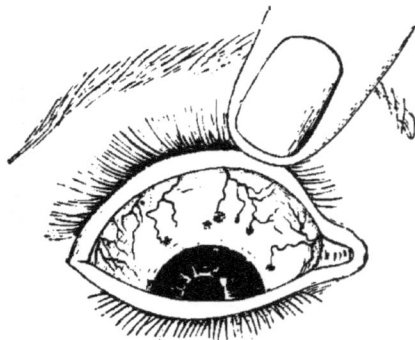

Congestion of the perforating branches of the anterior ciliary arteries. (Dalrymple.) The dusky spots at the seats of perforation are often seen in dark-complexioned persons.

ries, Fig. 25, v, and their episcleral twigs form a closely-meshed network, Fig. 29.   (3) The vessels proper to the margin of the cornea and immediately adjacent zone of conjunctiva, *anterior conjunctival vessels*, and their *loop plexus on the corneal border*, Fig. 25, *l*, and Fig. 53; by these numerous minute branches, which are offshoots of the anterior ciliary vessels, Systems 1 and 2 anastomose.

Speaking generally, congestion composed of (1) tortuous, bright-red (brick-red) vessels (System 1) moving with the

FIG. 28.   FIG. 29.

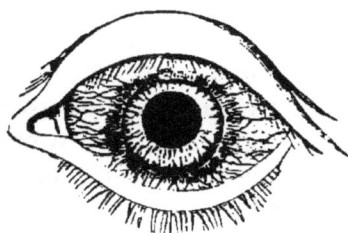

" Ciliary congestion," engorgement of episcleral twigs of anterior ciliary arteries. (After Dalrymple.)

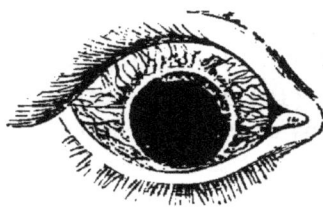

Congestion of anterior ciliary
veins, episcleral venous plexus.
(After Dalrymple.)

conjunctiva when it is slid over the globe, and least intense just around the cornea, Fig. 26, indicates a pure conjuncti-vitis (ophthalmia), and is usually accompanied by muco-purulent or purulent discharge. (2) A zone of pink con-gestion surrounding the cornea, and formed by small, straight, parallel vessels, closely set, radiating from the cornea, and not moving with the conjunctiva, anterior ciliary *arterial* twigs, Fig. 28, points to irritation or in-flammation of the cornea, or iris. A more scanty zone of dark or dusky color, Fig. 29, which, when severe, is finely reticulated, *episcleral venous plexus*, often points to glau-coma, but may accompany other diseases, especially in old people. Congestion in the same region, more deeply seated, and of a peculiar lilac tint, especially if unequal in different parts of the zone, shows cyclitis or deep scleritis. (3) Con-gestion in the same zone, and also composed of small vessels, but superficially placed, bright red, and often en-

croaching a little on the cornea, *anterior conjunctival ves-*
sels and *loop plexus of cornea*, Fig. 53, shows a tendency
to irritable but often superficial corneal inflammation.
Localized or fasciculated congestion generally points to
phlyctenular disease, Figs. 45 and 46. Although in the
severe forms of all acute diseases of the front of the eye
these types of congestion are usually mixed and but imperfectly distinguishable, much information may often be
derived from attention to the leading forms described.

(10) **The mobility of the eyeball** may be impaired in
any or every direction, and in any degree. Commonly only
one eye is affected. First, to test the lateral and vertical
movements, direct the patient with both eyes open to look
successively towards, or follow a pencil or finger moved in,
each of the four directions, up, down, right, and left; next,
to test the convergence power, he looks at the object held
vertically in the middle line, rather below the horizontal,
and gradually approached from 2′ to about 6″. In each
position we must notice both eyes; thus, when the patient
looks to his right we have to note the outward movement of
his right and the inward movement of his left. The fixed
marks for the inward and outward movements are the inner
and outer canthi, and as the apparent range of movement
judged in this way varies a little in different people, the
corresponding movements of the two eyes should always be
compared. In looking strongly outwards the corneal margin
does not in all persons quite reach the outer canthus, but it
should always reach the inner canthus during inward rotation. In children and stupid people the movements are often
defective from inattention. In very myopic eyes the movements are somewhat defective in all directions. The vertical
movements are best shown by noting the position of the cornea in relation to the border of the lower lid; the border of
the upper lid is less trustworthy, since there may be some
ptosis or other cause of inequality between the two sides.

The range of movement of the eye, "field of fixation," or "field of direct vision," can be measured on the perimeter in the same way as the ordinary field of "indirect vision." The test-object, e. g., a word of small print, moved along the various meridians from the centre towards the periphery, is followed by the eye under examination until it can no longer be read, i. e., until the visual axis can no longer be directed to it. A coarse test-object would be recognized by parts of the retina away from the yellow spot, and must, therefore, not be used. In this way it is found that the normal range of movement of the eye extends through about 45° in each direction from the centre. The state of mobility of the eye, and the progress, in cases of ocular paralysis, may be accurately recorded in this way.[1]

(11) **Squint or strabismus** exists if the visual axes are not both directed to the same object. A squint may be the result either of over-action, or of weakness or paralysis, of a muscle. The internal recti, by excessive contraction, often cause convergent squint; but most other forms of strabismus result from actual defect of nervous or muscular power.

When a squint is well marked there is no difficulty in identifying the squinting eye as the one which is misdirected when an object is held up to the patient's attention; in most cases the patient always squints with the same eye, but a few persons can squint with either indifferently, *alternating squint.* Nor is there often any doubt as to whether the squint is internal, convergent, or external, divergent, i. e., whether the axis of the squinting eye crosses that of its fellow between the patient and the object he looks at, or crosses it beyond this object, or even positively diverges from it; upward or downward squint, though less common, is almost as evident. But to prove beyond doubt which is the squinting eye, direct the patient

[1] For further details consult a paper by Landolt in Trans. Internat. Med. Congress, 1881, vol. iii. p. 25 (London).

to look at a pencil held up in the middle line at about 18″ from his face, and with a card or piece of ground-glass cover the apparently sound, or " working" eye, the squinting eye will at once move so as to look at, or " fix" the pencil, proving that it had previously been misdirected. If the sound eye be watched behind the screen, it will be seen to squint as soon as the affected eye " fixes" the object ; this is known as the *secondary squint*, and its direction is the same as that of the original or *primary squint*. Thus, if the primary squint be convergent, the secondary will also be convergent.   In squint from over-action, or from mere disuse, of one muscle, the secondary and primary deviations are equal, but in paralytic squint the secondary often exceeds the primary.   If the squinting eye retain full range of movement, *i. e.*, move in companionship with its fellow in all directions, the squint is termed *concomitant*, in contradistinction to *paralytic;* hence in every case of squint it is necessary to test the mobility of the eyes.   It is also important to note whether the squint is constant or only occasional (*periodic*).[1]

It was, until lately, usual to measure the squint (when necessary) by means of a scale placed on the lower lid and graduated in such a way as to indicate in lines (or mm.) the amount of deviation.   The centre of this scale, marked zero, is placed over the centre of the lid, and therefore cor-

---

[1] We sometimes meet with an *apparent squint*, either external or internal.   The *optic* axis of the eye passes from a point rather to the inner side of the y. s. through the centre of the cornea, and forms a small angle ("angle *a*") with the *visual* axis, the line which joins the y. s. to the object looked at and which commonly cuts the cornea rather within its centre.   As we judge of the apparent direction of a person's eyes by the centres of his corneæ, *i. e.*, by the *optic* axes, a slight apparent outward squint will be produced if the angle, *a*, be, as in many hypermetropic eyes, larger than usual, and an apparent convergent squint if, as in myopia, it be smaller.   Apparent squint is always slight, and the screen test described in the text gives a negative result.

responding to the centre of the pupil if there be no squint; the number which corresponds to the centre of the pupil of the squinting eye gives the linear measurement of the deviation. A more accurate and more rational method, introduced by Landolt, gives the deviation in terms of the angle, d, Fig. 30, formed by the visual axis of the squinting eye where it cuts that of the working eye. In Fig. 30, L is the squinting left eye of the patient placed at the

FIG. 30.

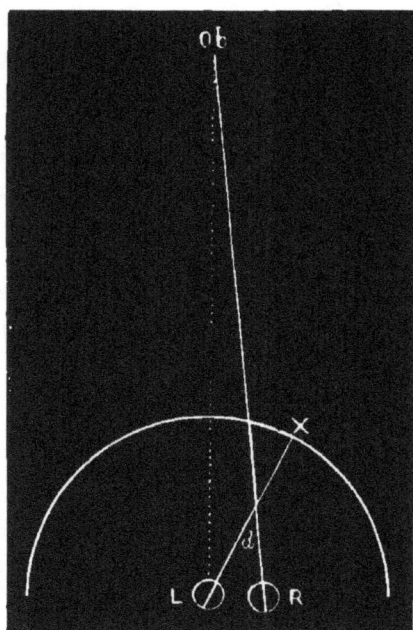

Angular measurement of squint. (After Landolt.)

centre of a perimeter; L ×, the direction of its visual axis; L Ob, the direction its visual axis should have; Ob, an object, as far off as possible, at which the patient is to look; × a small candle-flame which the observer, stationed close behind the perimeter, moves along the arc until he sees its image reflected from the centre of the squinting cornea; the size of the angle × L Ob, read off on the perimeter, is nearly[1] the same as that of the angle of deviation d.

(12) **Diplopia (double sight)** is almost always a result of squint, and is usually most troublesome when the deviation is so slight as to be hardly perceptible. Diplopia caused by squint is, of course, binocular, and disappears when one eye is covered. Uniocular diplopia (double sight with one eye), however, often occurs in commencing cataract, and sometimes in healthy but astigmatic eyes; it has also been met with in some cases of cerebral tumor. In the former cases it has a physical cause in the crystalline lens (see Cataract); in the latter it must depend upon some psychical change.

To find out what defect of movement is causing binocular diplopia, darken the room, and ask the patient to follow with his eyes a lighted candle, held about 6' from him, moved successively into different positions, and to describe the relative places of the double images in each position. Ascertain which of the two images belongs to each eye by placing before one eye a strongly-colored glass, or by covering one eye and asking which image disappears. In many cases the image formed in the squinting eye (the "false" image) is less bright or distinct, and this difference gives a valuable means of distinguishing the sound from the affected eye; but the patient does not always notice a difference between the two images, and there may then be difficulty in proving which eye is at fault. The patient's replies may be recorded on such a diagram as Fig. 123; other radii may of course be added for intermediate positions; the false image is marked by the dotted line, the true one by the unbroken line. With this graphic representation of the candle as it appears to the patient, we can

---

[1] The angles × L Ob and d would be exactly equal if Ob were far enough away to make L Ob and R Ob parallel.

deduce from the apparent position of the false image what movements of the corresponding eye are at fault, and consequently which muscle or muscles are defective. It is *essential that the patient should not move his head* during the examination, and that he remain throughout at the same distance from the candle. Remember that, in the extreme lateral movements, the nose eclipses one image. When the double images are very wide apart, *i e.*, when there is much squint, the patient often fails to notice the false image.

For the diagnosis of a case of diplopia it is often sufficient to ask in which directions the double sight is most troublesome, and how the images appear in respect to height, lateral separation, and apparent distance from the patient. Chapter XXI.

(13) **The apparent size** of an object depends, in the first place, on the size of its *retinal image*, and this, as already shown, § 19, p. 38, depends upon (*a*) the size of the visual angle, and (*b*) the distance of the retina from the nodal point. It is clear that in Fig. 20 a smaller object placed nearer to the eye or a larger one placed further off might subtend the same angle as Ob, and therefore have a retinal image of the same size. There are, however, other factors contributing to our estimate of the size of objects, especially contrast of size and shade, estimation of distance, and effort of accommodation.

A white object on a black ground looks larger than a black object of the same size on a white ground. The further off an object is judged to be, the larger does it look. The greater the accommodative *effort* used, whatever may be the distance of the object, the smaller does it appear; thus patients whose eyes are partly under the influence of

---

[1] Apparent distance is also influenced by the color of the object. The chromatic aberration of the eye is said to afford the explanation, rays of different refrangibilities being focussed on slightly different parts of the retina.

atropine, and presbyopic persons whose glasses are too weak complain that near objects, if looked at intently for a short time, become much smaller; whilst when one eye is under the action of eserine, causing spasm of the accommodation, objects appear larger than if held at the same distance from the other eye. Prisms with their bases towards the temples seem to diminish objects seen through them by necessitating excessive convergence of the eyes, the converse of Fig. 16.

(14) **Protrusion (proptosis) and enlargement of the eye.**—Unequal prominence of the two eyes is best ascertained by seating the patient in a chair, standing behind him, and comparing the summits of the two corneæ with each other, and with the bridge of the nose, or the line of the eyebrows. The appearance of prominence or recession, as seen from the front, depends very much on the quantity of sclerotic exposed ; thus, slight ptosis gives a sunken appearance to the eyes, and in slight cases of Graves's disease the proptosis seems to increase when the upper lids are spasmodically raised. It is to be remembered that real prominence of the eye may depend on enlargement of the eyeball, myopia, staphyloma, or intra-ocular tumor, as well as on its protrusion, and that if only one eye be myopic, the appearance will be unsymmetrical. Decided proptosis may follow tenotomy or paralysis of one or more ocular muscles. In hypermetropia, in which the eyeball is too short, and in the rare cases of paralysis of the cervical sympathetic, the eye often looks sunken.

(15) **The uses of prisms** have been explained at p. 35.

(16) **Examination by focal illumination** is described in Chapter III.

CHAPTER III.

THIS includes (1) examination by focal or oblique light ; (2) examination by the ophthalmoscope.

1. EXAMINATION BY FOCAL OR OBLIQUE LIGHT.

In using *focal, oblique,* or *lateral illumination* the anterior parts of the eye are examined with the light of a lamp concentrated by a convex lens. The method is used to detect or examine opacities of the cornea, changes in the appearance of the iris, alterations in the outline and area of the pupil from iritis, and opacities of the lens. Such an examination is to be made by routine in every case before using the ophthalmoscope. We require a somewhat darkened room, a convex lens of two or three inches focal length, one of the large ophthalmoscopic lenses, and a bright, naked lamp-flame.

The patient is seated with his face towards the light, which is about 2′ distance. The lens, held between the finger and thumb, is used like a burning-glass, being placed at about its own focal length from the patient's cornea, and in the line of the light, so as to throw a bright pencil of light on the front of the eye at an angle with the observer's line of sight. Thus all the superficial media and structures of the eye can be successively examined under strong illumination, the distance of the lens being varied a little according as its focus is required to fall on the cornea, the iris, or the anterior or posterior surface of the crystalline lens. Fig. 31. By varying the position of the light and

of the patient's eye, making him look up, down, and to
each side, we can examine all parts of the corneal surface,
of the iris, of the pupillary area, i. e., the anterior capsule
of the lens, and of the lens-substance. If the light be
thrown at a very acute angle on the cornea or lens, opacities are much more visible than if it fall
almost perpendicularly. By habitually
magnifying the illuminated parts by a
second lens held in the other hand, much
additional information can be gained.

For complete exploration of all parts
of the crystalline lens the pupil must be
dilated with atropine, but careful examination without atropine will generally
enable us to detect opacities lying in or
near the axis of the lens even if deeply
seated. In examining the posterior pole
of the lens the light
must be thrown almost
perpendicularly into
the pupil, and the ob-
server must place his
eye as nearly in the
same direction as is
possible without inter-
cepting the incident
light. Opacities of the
cornea and anterior

FIG. 31.

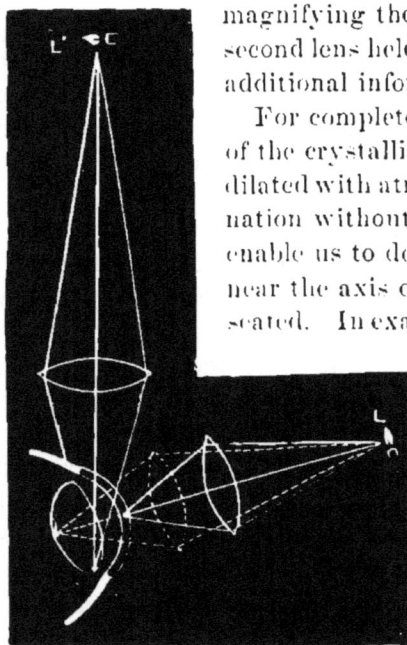

Focal illumination.

layers of the lens appear whitish, deep opacities in the lens,
especially in old people, look yellowish, by focal light.
Tumors, large opacities in the vitreous, and retinal detachments may be seen by this method if they lie close behind
the lens. Minute foreign bodies in the cornea will often
be seen by focal light when invisible, because covered by
hazy epithelium, in daylight.

2. OPHTHALMOSCOPIC EXAMINATION.

The ophthalmoscope enables us to see the parts of the eye behind the crystalline lens, by making the observer's eye virtually the source of illumination for the observed eye. Rays of light entering the pupil in a given direction are partly reflected back by the choroid and retina, and on emerging from the pupil take the same or very nearly the same course that they had on entering (§ 12, p. 31). Hence the eye of the observer, if so placed as to receive these returning rays, must also be so placed as to cut off the entering rays: as, therefore, no light can enter in the necessary direction, none can return to the observer's eye. This is why the pupil is usually black. Although with a large pupil, especially in a hypermetropic or myopic eye, the observer receives some of the returning rays, because he does not intercept all the entering light, and in this way sees the pupil of a fiery red instead of black, still for any useful examination the observer's eye must, as already stated, be in the central path of the entering, and emerging, rays. This end is gained by looking through a small hole in a mirror, by which light is reflected into the patient's pupil, and this perforated mirror is the ophthalmoscope. There are two ways of seeing the deep parts of the eyeball by this means.

A. **The indirect method** of examination, by which a clear, real, inverted image of the fundus, somewhat magnified, is formed in the air between the patient and the observer.

The following simple experiment will show how this is effected: Take two convex lenses of about 2″ focal length each; hold one in the left hand, at about 2″ from this print; take the other in the right hand, and, moving your head a few inches back, hold the second lens at about its focal length in front of the first; you will then see an inverted image of the print slightly magnified. *a.* Observe that in order to see this image clearly you have to make an effort, and that you cannot see both the image of the print and the print itself, clearly, at the same moment; this is because the eye of the observer (*obs*, Fig. 32) cannot be adjusted for the image (*im*) and the more distant object (*ob*) at the same time. The fundus of the eye seen on this principle is magnified about five diameters, if the eye be normal.

Fig. 32.

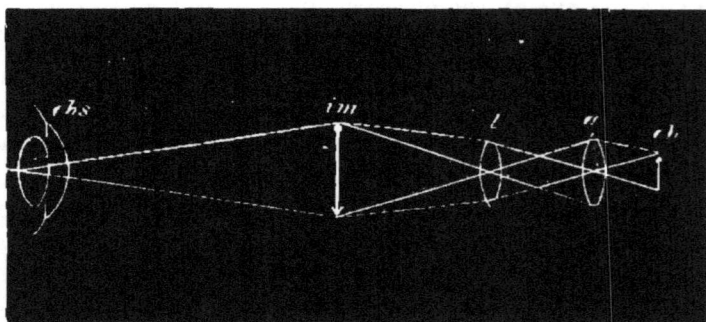

ob. The object. *a*. The first lens. *l*. The second lens. *im*. The magnified inverted image of *ob* viewed by the observer, *obs*.

The image is larger in II and smaller in M. *b*. Notice that if the observer's head be moved slightly from side to side, the image will appear to move in the opposite direction.

B. **The direct method** of examination, by which, except when the eye is myopic, a virtual, erect image is seen, more magnified than in the former method and situated behind the patient's eye.

The conditions are the same as those under which a magnified image of any object is seen through a convex lens, Fig. 13, as in the following experiment : Hold a convex lens of, say 3″ focal length, at any distance from this page not greater than 3″, and place your eye close to the lens.

The print will be magnified, and seen in its true position, i. e., "erect." a. The enlargement will be more the greater the distance of the lens from the page up to 3″ (§§ 16 and 17, p. 34). If the distance be further increased, the print will not be seen clearly. The image is a "virtual" one, because it is the image which would be formed if the rays which enter the eye in a diverging direction could be prolonged backwards until they met behind the lens, Figs. 13 and 35. b. If the lens be placed just at its focal length from the paper, the image will be seen clearly only if the accommodation be completely relaxed. c. If it be nearer to the page, more or less accommodation must be used, or else the observer must withdraw his head further from the lens. d. If, keeping the lens quite still, the observer withdraw his head, the field of view will be lessened, Fig. 14, whilst the image will appear to increase in size without really doing so, and these changes will be greater the nearer the lens is to its focal distance from the paper; if it be almost exactly at its principal focal distance, only a very small part of the print will be seen when the head is withdrawn. e. If the head be moved a little from side to side, the image will appear to move in the same direction.

The emmetropic eye, with the accommodation fully relaxed, is adjusted for distant objects, i. e., parallel rays, and receives a clear image of such objects on the layer of rods and cones of the retina, p. 38. A clear image of the *fundus of the eye*, i. e., the retina, optic disc, and choroid, can be obtained in such an eye, as in the experiment just described, where the distance of the lens from the paper was equal to or less than its focal length, on condition that the eyes, both of patient and observer, be adjusted for infinite distance, i. e., for parallel rays; in other words, that the accommodation of both be relaxed. The fundus so seen is magnified about 20 diameters.

In order to use the ophthalmoscope[1] it is first necessary
to learn to manage the mirror and light. (1) Seat the
patient in a darkened room and place a lamp with a large
steady, naked flame on a level with his eyes, a few inches
from his head, and about in a line with his ear. The lamp
may be on either side, but is usually placed on his left, and
it is better to keep to the same side until practice has given
steadiness to the various combined movements which are
necessary. (2) Sit down in front of the patient with his
face fronting your own, feature to feature. It is most convenient for the observer's face to be a little higher than
that of the patient. (3) Take the mirror of the ophthalmoscope, without any lens behind, and without the large
lens, in your left hand for examining the patient's left eye,
and *vice versâ* for his right eye, hold it, mirror toward the
patient, close to your own eye, and with the sight-hole
placed so that, with your other eye closed, you see the patient through it. Now rotate the mirror slightly toward
the lamp until the light reflected from the flame is thrown
into the patient's pupil, and open your other eye. (4) You
will so far have seen nothing except the front of the patient's eye, unless atropine have been used, for he will have
looked at the centre of the mirror, and his pupil, strongly
contracted, will look either black or very dull red. (5)
Now tell him to look steadily a little to one side, into va-
cancy, or at an object on the other side of the room. The
pupil will now become red—bright fiery red if it be rather
large, a duller red if it be small or the patient's complexion be dark. In one position, when the eye under examination looks a little inward, the red will change to a
yellowish or whitish color, and this indicates the position
of the optic disc. (6) Learn to keep the light steadily on
the pupil, during slow movements backward and forward

[1] For choice of instruments see Appendix.

and from side to side, taking care that the patient keeps his eye all the time in the same position, and does not follow the movements of the mirror; the test of steadiness will be that the pupil remains of a good red color in all positions. Up to this point the examination may be made without atropine; and so far only a uniform red glare will have been seen, no details of the fundus being visible, unless the patient be either myopic or considerably hypermetropic.

In order to see the details of the fundus it is best to begin by learning the *Indirect Method*, Fig. 33, for, though rather less easy, it is more generally useful than the direct.

Take the mirror without any lens behind it in one hand,[1] and one of the large convex "objective" lenses corresponding to *l* in Fig. 32 in the other. Always, if possible, have the pupil dilated with atropine, for by this means you learn to see the fundus much more quickly and easily. In examining the patient's right eye apply the mirror with your right hand to your right eye, holding the lens in your left hand; it is best to reverse everything for his left eye, but the position of the light need not be changed. The hand which carries the lens should be steadied by resting the little or ring-finger against the patient's brow or temple.

We usually begin by looking for the optic disc, which is one of the most important and easily seen parts. As the disc lies to the nasal side of the posterior pole of the eye, the cornea must be rotated a little inward, *i. e.*, the back of the eye outward, in order to bring the disc opposite the pupil, when the observer is immediately in front; the right eye, *e. g.*, must be directed to the observer's right ear, or to the uplifted little finger of his mirror hand. The patient

---

[1] But many learn to see the image more quickly and easily by placing a convex lens of 4 D. behind the mirror. If the observer wears glasses for reading, he should wear them, or put a lens of the same strength behind the mirror, for the indirect examination.

FIG. 33.

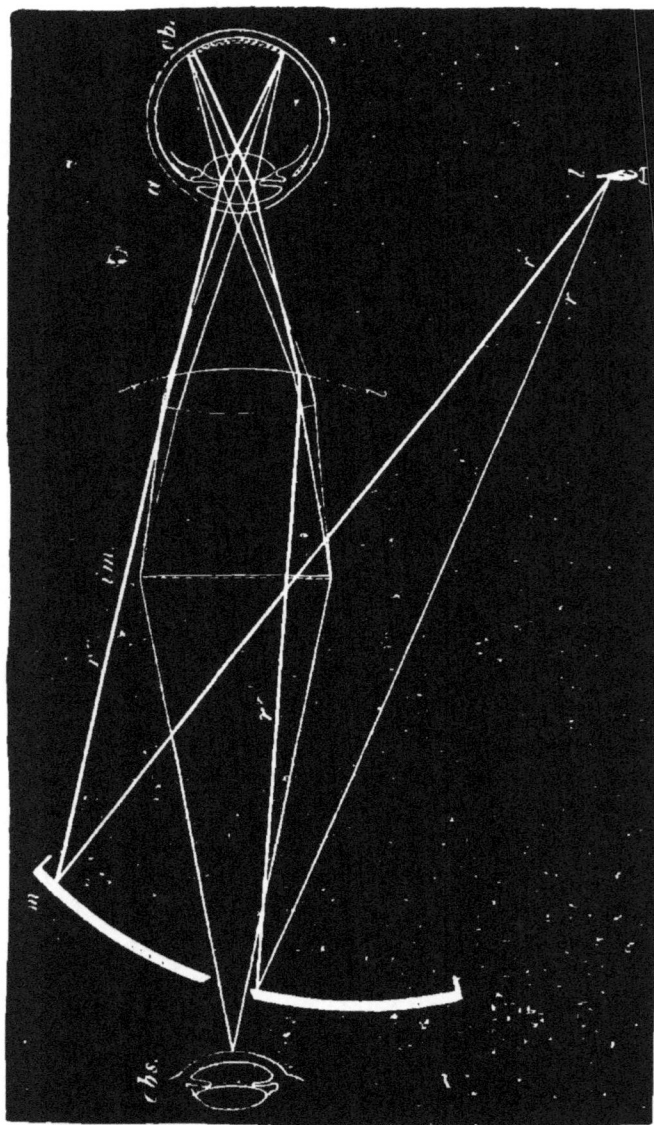

Ophthalmoscopic examination by the "indirect method." Lettering as for Fig. 32. In addition, the thick lines, *r' r'*, rays from the lamp, are reflected from the mirror *m*, in the directions *r' r'*, traverse the lens *l*, and are focussed in front of the retina *ob*, on which they therefore throw a diffused light. From the fundus thus lighted, pencils of rays (shown by thin lines) are given off, which emerge from the eye parallel and form a clear inverted image, *im*, at the focus of the lens *l*; this image is viewed through the sight-hole by the observer *obs*. The distance between *obs* and *m* is about 10″, and from *im* to *a* about 5″.

must turn his eye, not his head, in the required direction. The lens should be held about 2″–3″, and the observer's eye be about 15″, from the patient's eye; the image of the fundus being formed in the air 2″ or 3″ in front of the lens, will thus be situated about 10″ from the observer.

The bright-red glare, from the *choroid*, will be obvious enough; but most beginners find some difficulty in avoiding the reflection of the mirror from the patient's cornea, and in adjusting the accommodation and the distance of the head, so as to see the image clearly. The head must be slowly moved a little further from or nearer to the patient, and at the same time an attempt made to adjust the eyes, both being kept open, for a point between the observer and the lens. As a rule, the disc and retinal vessels are seen clearly at the first sitting.

The optic disc—the ending of the optic nerve in the eye above the lamina cribrosa, *optic papilla*, Figs. 34 and 36—is round, well defined. much lighter in color than the fiery red of the surrounding fundus, and numerous blood-vessels are seen to radiate from its centre, chiefly upward and downward. As soon as the disc can be easily seen the student must pass on to the study of the most important details of this part itself, and of the other parts of the fundus. Some of these will be described here, and others in the chapters on the Diseases of the Choroid and Retina, and on the Errors of Refraction.

The disc, as a whole, is grayish-pink in color with an admixture of yellow. It is nearly circular, but seldom perfectly so, being often apparently oval or slightly irregular. Two differently colored parts are noticeable—a central patch, whiter than the rest, and into which most of the bloodvessels dip; and a surrounding part of pink or grayish-pink. In many eyes, especially in old persons, we distinguish a third part, a narrow boundary line of lighter color, which represents the border of the sclerotic, *scleral ring*,[1] Fig. 34. The bloodvessels consist of several large trunks and a varying number of small twigs; the large trunks emerge from the central white part of the disc, and often bifurcate once or twice on its area; the small twigs may emerge separately from various parts of the disc, or form branches of the large trunks.

Variations.—The color of the disc appears paler or darker according to the color of the surrounding choroid, the brightness of the light used, and the patient's age and state of health. A curved line of dark pigment often bounds a part of the circumference of the disc, Fig. 36, and has no pathological meaning. The central white patch varies greatly in size, position, and distinctness; it may be so small as hardly to be perceptible, or very large; may shade off gradually or be abruptly defined; may be central or eccentric; when large it generally shows a grayish stippling or mottling, Fig. 36. This central white patch represents a hollow, the *physiological cup or pit*, compare Figs. 36 and 37, left by the nerve fibres as they radiate out from the centres of the disc toward the retina, like the tentacles of an open sea-anemone; and through it the chief bloodvessels pass on their way between the nerve and the retina. This depression is generally shaped like a funnel or a dimple, with gradually sloping sides, Fig. 37; but sometimes the sides are steep, or even overhanging; in other eyes it is wide, shallowed, and enlarged toward the outer side of the discs. The physiological pit is whiter than the rest of the disc, because the grayish-pink nerve fibres are absent at this part, and we can, therefore, see down to the opaque, white, fibrous tissue, which, under the name of *lamina cribrosa*, forms the floor of the whole disc, Fig. 37. The stippled appearance often noticed in the pit

---

[1] I fail to see the force of the objection to this term raised by Jaeger and Loring, Loring's Text-book, i. p. 57, since the inner sheath of the nerve and the fibres of the sclera are blended into one at this part.

is caused by the holes in this lamina, through which the
bundles of nerve-fibres pass on their way to the retina ; the
holes appear darker because filled by non-medullated nerve-
fibres, which reflect but little light.

The other parts of the fundus.—The groundwork is
of a bright fiery red—the choroid, *not the retina ;* in many
eyes this color is nearly uniform, but in persons of very
light or very dark complexion we see a pattern of closely-
set, tortuous, red bands (vessels of the choroid), separated
by spaces either of darker or of lighter color, Fig. 34.
For details see Chapter XII.

FIG. 34.

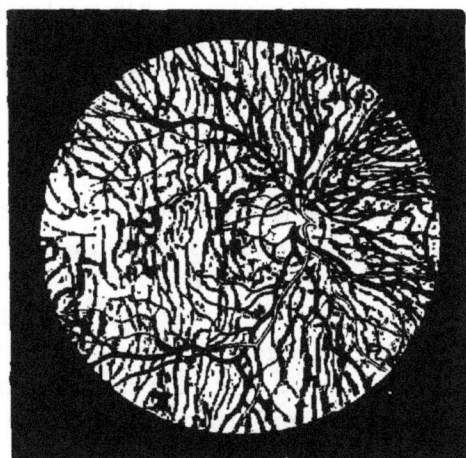

Ophthalmoscopic appearances of healthy fundus in a person of very
fair complexion. Scleral ring well marked. Left eye, inverted image.
(Wecker and Jaeger.)

Upon this red ground the vessels of the retina divide and
subdivide dichotomously. It will be noticed that the chief
trunks pass almost vertically upward and downward, and
that no large branches go to the part *apparently* inward

4

from the disc (to the left in the figure); that the visible
retinal vessels are comparatively few and are widely spread;
that they become progressively smaller as they recede from
the optic disc; and that they never anastomose with each
other. Special attention must be given to the part—apparently to the inner, nasal, side of the optic disc, really to its
outer temporal side—which is the region of most accurate
vision, the yellow spot, y. s., *macula lutea*, or, shortly,
"macula." In this region, which comes into view when
the patient looks straight at the ophthalmoscope, the choroidal red is duller and darker than elsewhere. It is
skirted by large retinal vessels which give off numerous
twigs towards its centre, though none of them can be seen
quite to reach that point. Compare Fig. 78, Chapter XIII.
In many eyes nothing but these indefinite characters mark
the y. s.; but in some, especially in dark eyes and young
patients, a minute bright dot occupies its centre, and is
encircled by an ill-bounded dark area, round which again
a peculiar shifting, white halo is seen. The minute dot is
the *fovea centralis*, the thinnest part of the retina. The
neighborhood of the disc and y. s. forms the *central region*
of the fundus. The *peripheral parts* are explored by telling the patient to look successively up, down, and to each
side, without moving his head. To see the extreme periphery the observer must move his head as well as the
patient his eye. Toward the periphery the choroidal
trunk-vessels are often plainly visible even when none were
distinguishable at the more central parts.

The vessels of the retina are easily distinguished from
those of the choroid by their course and mode of branching;
by the small size of all except the main trunks; by their
sharper outline and clearer tint; but especially by the
presence of a light streak along the centre of each, Fig.
34, which gives them an appearance of roundness, very
different from the flat, band-like look of the choroidal ves-

sels. They are divisible into two sets—a darker, larger, somewhat tortuous set—the veins; and a lighter, brighter red, smaller, and usually straighter set—the arteries; the diameter of corresponding branches being about as 3 to 2. The arteries and veins run pretty accurately in pairs. Pressure on the eyeball, through the upper lid, causes visible pulsation of the arteries on the disc.

The indirect method of examination is most generally useful, because it gives a larger field of view under a low magnifying power, about five diameters, and thus allows us to appreciate the general character and distribution of any morbid changes better than if we begin with the direct method, in which the field of view is smaller and the magnifying power much greater. It has also the great advantage of being equally applicable in all states of refraction; whereas, if the patient be myopic, his fundus cannot be examined by the direct method without the aid of a suitable concave lens, found experimentally, placed behind the mirror, p. 81. The inversion of the image seen by the indirect method is such that what appears to be the upper is lower, and what appears to be R. is L.

In the *Direct Method* the examination is made by the mirror alone, or with the addition of a lens in the clip or disc behind it, but without the intervention of the objective lens.

By this method the parts, unless the eye be myopic, are seen in their true position, Fig. 35, the upper part of the image corresponding to the upper part of the fundus, the right to the right, etc.; it is, therefore, often called the method of the "erect" or "upright" image, though, as will be seen below, these terms are not strictly convertible with "direct examination." It is used: (1) to detect opacities in the vitreous humor and detachments of the retina; (2) to ascertain the condition of the patient's refraction, *i. e.*, the relation of his retina to the focus of his

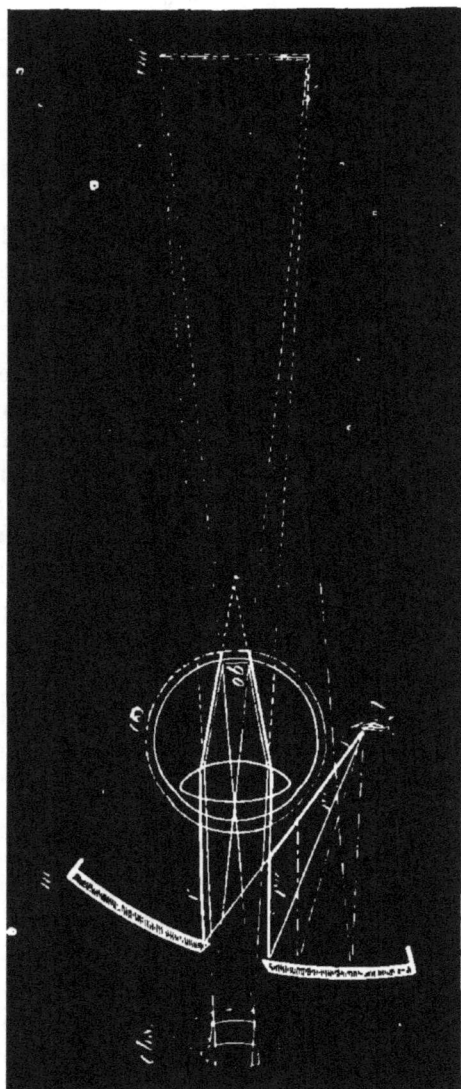

Examination of virtual erect image ("direct method"). Lettering as in Fig. 33. The rays r' r'' entering the eye divergent would be focussed behind the retina as at f, and hence illuminate the fundus diffusely. The returning pencils (thin lines) are parallel or divergent (according as the eye is E. or H.) on leaving the eye, and appear to proceed from a highly-magnified erect image id', behind the eye. It is seen that only those lamp-rays which strike close to the sight-hole are available; if the hole be too large, no rays will enter the pupil and the fundus will not be illuminated.

lens system; (3) for the minute examination of the fundus by the highly-magnified, virtual, erect image (Fig. 36); (4) for examining the cornea, iris, and lens with magnifying power.

(1) To examine the vitreous humor. The patient is to move his eye freely in different directions, whilst the light is reflected into it from a distance of a foot or more—for details see Diseases of Vitreous; detachments of the retina are seen in the same way. Opacities in the vitreous and folds of detached retina, being situated far within the focal length of the refractive media, are seen in the erect position under the conditions mentioned at p. 67, *c*, the observer being at a considerable distance from the eye. If the observer be close to the patient, Acc. must be used or a convex lens be placed behind the mirror, as in high degrees of H. See next page.

(2) To ascertain the refraction. If when using the mirror alone *at a distance of* 12″–18″, *or more*, from the patient's eye, we see some of the retinal vessels clearly and easily, the eye is either myopic or hypermetropic. If, when the observer's head is moved slightly from side to side, the vessels seem to move in the same direction, the image seen is a virtual one, and the eye is hypermetropic. The eye is myopic if the vessels seem to move in the contrary direction; the image in M. is, indeed, formed and seen in the same way as the inverted image seen by the "indirect" method of examination, compare Figs. 33 and 105, but except in the highest degrees of M. it is too large and too far from the patient to be useful for detailed examination. In low degrees of M. this image is formed so far in front of the patient's eye as to be visible only when the observer is distant perhaps 3′ or 4′; whilst in E. and in the lower degrees of H. the erect image will not be easily seen at a greater distance than 12″ or 18″, p. 67, *d*, and Fig. 14. If, therefore, in order to get a clear image by the

direct method, the observer has to go either very near to, or a long way from, the patient, no great error of refraction can be present.

The above tests only reveal qualitatively the presence of either M. or H., but by a modification of the method, the quantity of any error of refraction, e. g., H., can be determined with great accuracy. (*Determination of the refraction by the ophthalmoscope.*) In E., as already stated at p. 67, the erect image can be seen only if the observer be near to the patient, and also completely relax his accommodation; for, in experiment d there described, when the head was withdrawn from the lens the field of view and illumination rapidly diminished. The same occurs with the eye, but in a much greater degree, and hence in E. no useful view can be gained by the direct method without going very near to the eye.

In H., where the retina is within the focus of the lens system, the erect image is seen when close to the patient's eye only by an effort of accommodation in the observer, just as in the same experiment when the lens was within its focal length from the page, p. 67, c. And as in that experiment the print was also seen easily, even when the head was withdrawn, so in H. the erect image is seen at a distance, as well as close to the patient.

If now the observer, instead of increasing the convexity of his crystalline, place a convex lens of equivalent power behind his ophthalmoscope mirror, this lens will be a measure of the patient's H, i. e., it will be the lens which, when the patient's accommodation is in abeyance, will be needed to bring parallel rays to a focus on his retina. If a higher lens be used, the result will be the same as when in the experiment the convex lens was removed beyond its focal length from the print; the fundus will be more or less blurred.

Hence, to measure H.: (1) **Acc.** both in patient and

observer must be fully relaxed, usually by atropine in the
patient and by voluntary effort in the observer; (2) the
observer must go as close as possible to the patient; (3) he
must then place convex lenses behind his mirror, beginning
at the weakest and increasing the strength, till the highest
is reached which still permits the details of the o. d., or,
better, of the y. s., to be seen with perfect clearness.   By
practice the distance between the corneæ of patient and
observer may be reduced to about 1″.   The light must be
on the same side as the eye under examination.   The right
eye must examine the right, and *vice versâ*.

In the same way, though with less accuracy in the high
degrees, M. can be measured by means of concave lenses;
the lowest lens with which a clear erect image is obtained
being slightly more than the measure of the M.

It is sometimes useful to know how much lengthening or
shortening of the eye corresponds to a given neutralizing lens.
The following numbers, slightly altered from Knapp, are sufficiently near the truth.   The distance between the eye of the
observer and that of the patient is supposed to be not more
than 1 inch.

H. of	1	D. represents shortening of		0.3	mm.
"	2	"	"	0.5	"
"	3	"	"	1	"
"	5	"	"	1.5	"
"	6	"	"	2	"
"	9	"	"	3	"
"	12	"	"	4	"
"	18	"	"	6	"
M. of	1	D. represents lengthening of		0.3	"
"	2	"	"	0.5	"
"	3	"	"	0.9	"
"	5	"	"	1.3	"
"	6	"	"	1.75	"
"	9	"	"	2.6	"
"	12	"	"	3.5	"
"	18	"	"	5	"

Astigmatism (As.) may also be measured by this method, the refraction being estimated successively in the two chief meridians by means of appropriate retinal vessels. See Astigmatism. Any line, *e.g.*, a horizontally running vessel, is seen by means of rays which pass through the meridian of the cornea at a right angle to its course; hence, if a *vertical* vessel be clearly seen through a + 2 D. lens there is H. 2 D. in the *horizontal* meridian, etc.

This application of the direct method needs much practice. The lenses, of which there are twenty or more, are placed in a thin metal disc, which can be revolved behind the mirror so as to bring each lens in succession opposite the sight-hole. There are many forms of these "refraction ophthalmoscopes," varying in the details of their construction. See Appendix.

(3) The erect image is very valuable, on account of the high magnifying power, about 20 diameters in the E. eye,

FIG. 36.

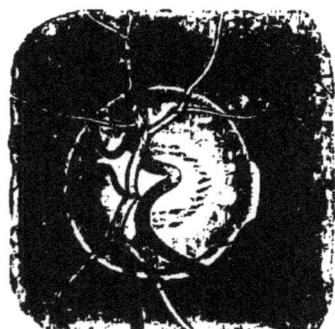

Ophthalmoscopic appearance of healthy disc, as seen in the erect image. Dark vessels, veins. Physiological pit stippled. × 15 diameters. (After Jaeger.)

for the examination of the finer details of the fundus. The disc looks less sharply defined, because more magnified, than when seen by the indirect method; both the disc and the retina often show a faint radiating striation, the nerve-fibres; the *lamina cribrosa* is often more brilliantly white; and the pigment epithelium of the choroid can be recognized as a fine uniform dark stippling.

If the refraction be E. or H., no lens is needed behind the mirror; if M., a concave lens must be placed in the clip behind the mirror, of sufficient strength to give a good, clear, erect image. The observer must come as near as possible to the patient.

FIG. 37.

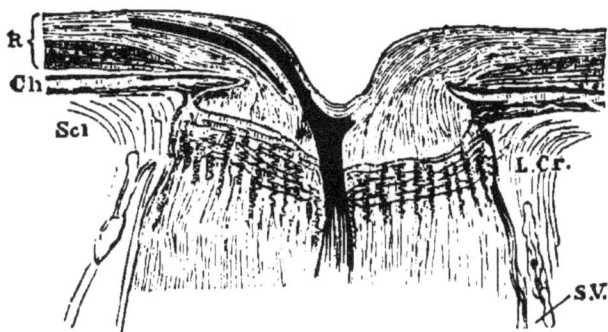

Vertical section of healthy optic disc, etc. × about 15. *R.* Retina, outer layers shaded vertically, nerve-fibre layer shaded longitudinally. *Ch.* Choroid. *Scl.* Sclerotic. *L. Cr.* Lamina cribrosa. *S. V.* Subvaginal space between inner and outer sheath of optic nerve. The central vein and one of the divisions of the central artery are seen in the nerve and disc.

By reference to Fig. 35 it will be seen that only those rays are useful which strike near the centre of the mirror, none others entering the patient's pupil; hence, if the aperture in the mirror be too large, the fundus will not be well lighted. It should not be larger than 3 mm., nor smaller than 2 mm.

(4) Minute changes in the cornea, iris, and lens can often be better studied by direct ophthalmoscopic examina-

4*

tion with a high $+$ lens behind the mirror than focal illumination (p. 64).   All opacities seen in this way, however,
look black against the red background, whilst by focal
light they are seen in their true colors.

RETINOSCOPY (KERATOSCOPY, PUPILLOSCOPY, OR THE SHADOW TEST).

By this method the refraction is determined by noticing
the direction of movement of the light thrown on to the
retina by the mirror when the latter is rotated.   The degree of error of refraction is measured by the lens, which,
placed close to the patient's eye in a case of ametropia,
renders the movement and other characters of the illumination the same as in emmetropia.

The test is most accurate when used at a great distance
from the patient. in practice a distance of about 1 m.—
100–120 cm., or 3′–4′—is chosen.   The observer, seated in
front of his patient, throws the light from an ophthalmoscope mirror into the patient's pupil.   He will then see the
area of the pupil illuminated, and on slightly rotating the
mirror will notice a movement in this lighted area, which
movement will have a direction either the same as, or
opposite to, that in which the mirror is turned, " with" or
" against " the mirror.   The lighted area is bordered by a
dark *shadow*, and it is to the edge of this shadow that the
attention must be directed.   The edge is parallel to the
axis on which the mirror is turned, but moves in, and
shows the refraction of, the meridian at right angles to
it, *e. g.*, the shadow whose edge passes vertically across the
pupil moves across the horizontal meridian, the refraction
of which it indicates, and *vice versâ*.   Retinoscopy may be
practised with a concave or a plane mirror.   With the former the shadow moves " against " the mirror in E. H. and
low M. ; and " with " the mirror in M. of more than 1 D.

FIG. 38.

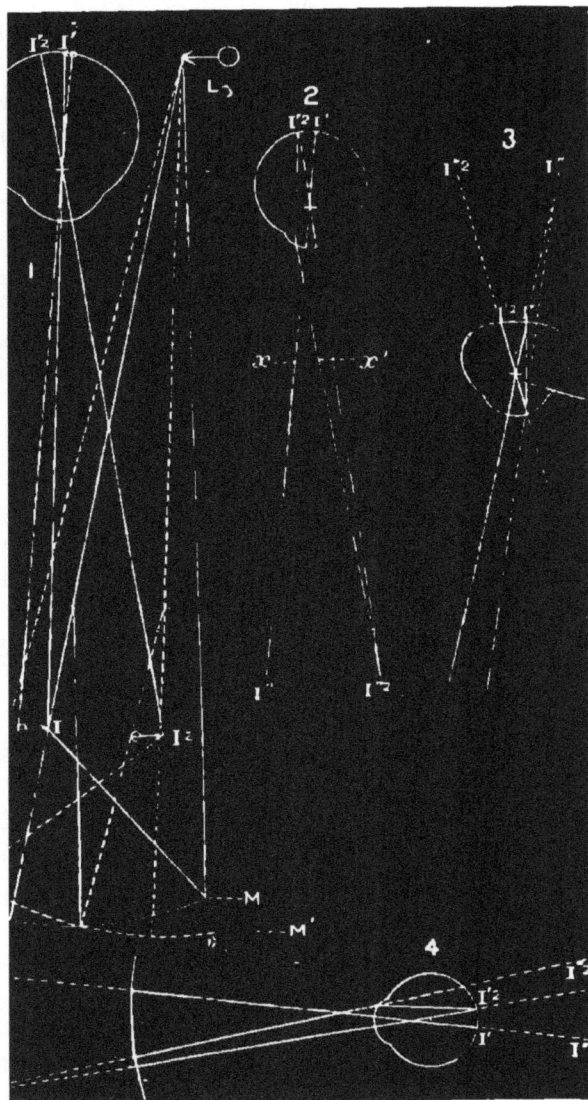

Retinoscopy (with square mirror).

With the latter these movements are exactly reversed. The light should be thrown as nearly as possible in the direction of the visual axis and the lamp be placed immediately over the patient's head rather than to one side.

(1) With a concave mirror (of about 22 cm. focus), Fig. 38. In Fig. 38, 1, the mirror, M, forms an inverted image, I, of the light, L, at its principal focus, and I becomes the source of light for the eye, E. A second image of I, again inverted, is formed at I′ on the retina of E If the far point of E be at I, this retinal image, I′, will be clear and distinct, but in every other case it will be more or less out of focus and indistinct. On rotating M to M′, I will move to I² and I′ to I′², and these movements (of I and I′) will occur no matter what the refraction of E may be.

The observer placed behind him, M, sees an image of I′ formed in the same way as the image of the fundus seen by the direct method, p. 67, and therefore either inverted and real, or erect and virtual, according as the refraction of the eye is M. or H., p. 77. If the observer's eye be accurately adapted for this image of I′, he will indeed see not only the light and shadow, but the retinal vessels; he neglects these, however, in attending to the movements of the shadow.

In the following description, L, I, and I² are disregarded, I′ or I′² being considered as the source of light.

If E *be myopic*, Fig. 38, 2, the image of I′ is real and inverted and formed at I″, the far point of E, compare Fig. 105. On rotating the mirror, as in Fig. 38, 1, I′ will move to I′², and I″ will move to I″², *i. e., the image* seen by the observer *moves in the same direction as* (or " *with*") *the mirror.*

If E *be hypermetropic*, Fig. 38, 3, *or emmetropic*, rays reflected from its retina leave the eye divergent or parallel and are not brought to a focus after emerging; the observer therefore sees a virtual image erect at I″, the virtual focus of $1'$, compare Fig. 13, and see its movements actually as they occur, $i.\ e.$, in the same direction as the movements of the real image $1'$ or $1'^2$, and therefore "against" the movements of the mirror.   Hence in H. and Em. *the shadow* moves "*against*" the mirror.

The above statement for myopia is true only if the observer be beyond the far point of the observed eye.   (See Myopia.)   In M. of 1 D. the rays returning from the patient's eye are focussed at a distance of 1 m., and if the observer intercept these rays before they meet, Fig. 38, 4, he will refer them toward $1''$ and $1''^2$ and obtain an erect virtual but unfocussed image of $1'$, the movements of which will be the same as those in H. or E., Fig. 38, 3, $i.\ e.$, "*against*" the mirror.   Hence, at a distance of about 1 m., movement "against" the mirror may indicate M., of about 1 D., or E. or H.   The lowest M. which can give the characteristic movement at this distance is slightly more than 1 D., say 1.25 D.

(2) With a plane mirror, Fig. 39.   Here the source of light for the observed eye is an erect and virtual image of the flame formed at the same distance behind the mirror as the lamp is in front of it.   In Fig. 39, 1, this image is at l, the virtual focus of L.   A second and inverted image of l is formed on the retina of E at 1.   The movements of these images, on rotation of the mirror, are the reverse of those of the image 1 (and its retinal image $1'$) Fig. 38, 1, obtained when the concave mirror is used.   When the mirror M is rotated to M', l will move in the opposite direction to l', but its retinal image 1 will move to $1'$; $i,\ e.$, in the same direction as, or "*with*" the mirror.   These movements of l and 1 occur in every eye, whatever its refraction.   In E. and H., however, the movement of the retinal image is seen as it occurs, and therefore "*with*" the mirror; but in M, Fig. 39, 2, the observer sees an inverted image of 1 formed at the far point of E, and its

EXAMINATION BY ARTIFICIAL LIGHT.

movements are exactly the reverse of those of the retinal image. Therefore, when, on rotating M to M', I moves to I² the image I' seen by the observer moves to I", *i. e.,* "*against*" the mirror. If the plane mirror be used at a distance of rather more than 1 m., 3'–4', from the patient, a movement of the shadow "*with*" the mirror will occur in M. of 1 D. or less, for the reasons given previously, Fig. 38, 4 ; but if the observer be about 2 m. (say 7') away, the characteristic movement "*against*" the mirror will be ob. tained, unless the M. be less than 0.5 D., since the far point of an eye with M. 0.5 D., and, therefore, the image seen, is at 2 m. As a plane mirror gives at a long distance a better illumination than a concave one, it can, if necessary, be used at a greater distance from the patient, and by this means low degrees of ametropia be very accurately meas- ured. Generally, however, the distance given, 3'–4', will be found most convenient.

In employing retinoscopy the patient is armed with a trial frame, into which lenses are successively put until one is reached which just reverses the movement of the shadow. This lens indicates nearly, but not quite, the refraction of the eye under observation. In H. we must subtract (about) 1 D. from the lowest + lens which reverses the shadow, because we know that this movement would not occur until a myopia of at least 1 D. had been produced. In M., for the same reason, 1 D. must be added to the lowest — lens which reverses the shadow.

Astigmatism is easily detected, and its amount measured by observing, on rotating the mirror, first from side to side, then from above downward, whether the shadow has the same movement and characters in each direction ; or by noting that when the shadow in one meridian is "cor- rected" by a lens, the meridian at right angles to it still shows decided ametropia. The lens is then found which corrects the latter meridian, and the As. equals the difference between the two lenses.

Apart from the direction in which the image (and shadow) moves, something may be learned from variations in (1) its brightness; (2) its rate of movement; (3) the form, straight or crescentic, of its border. The image is brightest, its movement quickest and most extensive, in very low M. and in Em. The higher the ametropia, whether M. or H., the duller the illumination, the slower and less extensive its movement, and the more crescentic and ill-defined its shadow border. The *brightness* of the image depends on how clearly 1, Fig. 38, 1, is focussed on the retina; the more accurately 1' is an image of 1, the brighter and larger will 1'', Fig. 38, 2 or 3, be; and as the flame is rectangular, the borders of the image will be nearly straight. These conditions occur when the eye is exactly adapted for the distance of 1, *i. e.*, in M. of 1 D. or less. If the M. be higher than 1 D., 1 will be out of focus, and, therefore, be spread over a larger retinal area, and being formed by the same number of rays as before, it will be less bright. The image 1'', Fig. 38, 2, will be correspondingly diffused and dull, and being formed nearer to the patient's eye, as, for example, at x, it will move only from x to x' in the same time as 1'' takes in moving to 1''², and hence its movement is slower and less extensive. The same is true in H., Fig. 38, 3, because the higher the H., the more diffused is 1' and the nearer is 1'' to the patient's eye. In both cases, high M. and high H., the border of the shadow is crescentic, because the diffused image forms a nearly round area on the retina.

Retinoscopy is a valuable means of objectively determining the quantity of any error of refraction, and as it is more easily learned, and, on the whole, more accurate in its results, than estimation by the direct method, p. 79, it has, in the hands of many of our students and assistants, almost displaced the latter method during the last four or five years as a preliminary to testing the patient with trial lenses. For the quick discovery of very slight astigmatism, and of the direction of the chief meridians in astigmatism of all degrees, retinoscopy probably excels all other methods.

Retinoscopy, however, carries with it none of the collateral advantages afforded by a thorough training in the more difficult "direct method;" for in retinoscopy we see nothing and think nothing of the condition of the fundus of the eye. Accurate retinoscopy is not quicker than measurement by the direct method; indeed, with a good instrument, the latter method certainly has the advantage in rapidity. I think there is reason to fear that the free use of retinoscopy by students, before they have mastered the more difficult "direct method," may tend to lower the present high quality of English ophthalmoscopic work. I cannot help thinking, therefore, that the importance of retinoscopy has been somewhat overrated, and that though in some difficult cases it will remain our best objective test, we shall do well generally to use it as an auxiliary rather than as a substitute for other methods.

PART II.

CLINICAL DIVISION.

CHAPTER IV.

DISEASES OF THE EYELIDS.

THE border of the lid, which contains the Meibomian glands, the follicles of the eyelashes, and certain modified sweat-glands and sebaceous glands, is often the seat of troublesome disease. Being half skin and half mucous membrane, it is moist and more susceptible than the skin itself to irritation by external causes; being a free border, its circulation is terminal, and therefore especially liable to stagnation. Its numerous and deeply-reaching glandular structures, therefore, furnish an apt seat for chronic inflammatory changes.

Blepharitis (ophthalmia tarsi, tinea tarsi, sycosis tarsi) includes all cases in which the border of the eyelid is the seat of subacute or chronic inflammation. There are several types. The skin is not much altered, but chronic thickening of the conjunctiva near the border of the lid is generally observed. The disease may affect both lids or only one, and the whole length or only a part.

In the commonest and worst form the glands and eyelash-follicles are the principal seats of the disease. The symptoms are, firm thickening and dusky congestion of the border region, with exudation of sticky secretion from its edge, glueing the lashes together into little pencils.

Very mild cases present merely overgrowth of lashes and excess of Meibomian secretion. But generally the disease progresses; little excoriations, and ulcers covered by scab, form along the free border, and often minute pustules appear; the thickening and vascularity increase; the lashes are loosened, and free bleeding occurs if they are pulled out After months or years of varying activity some or all of the hair-follicles become altered in size and direction, or quite obliterated; and the lashes stunted, misplaced, or entirely lost. As the thickening gradually disappears, little lines, or thin seams, of scar form just within the edge of the lid, and often cause slight eversion. The resulting exposure of the marginal conjunctiva, added to the scantiness of the cilia, causes the disagreeably raw and bald appearance termed *lippitudo;* and epiphora, from eversion, tumefaction, or narrowing of the puncta, often results. Often, however, the disease leads to nothing worse than the permanent loss of a certain number of the lashes.

In another type the changes are quite superficial—marginal eczema; the patient is liable, perhaps through life, to soreness and redness of the borders of the lids, and little crusts, scales, or pustules form at the roots of the lashes, the growth of the lashes not being much interfered with. In such people the eyes look weak or tender; the condition is made worse by exposure to heat, dust, and wind, and by long spells of work. See Chronic Lachrymal Conjunctivitis, Chapter VI.

Ophthalmia tarsi generally begins in childhood, and an attack of measles is a common exciting cause. It seldom becomes severe or persistent except from neglect of cleanliness in a child with sluggish circulation; the patients are generally anæmic, often scrofulous, and the condition is then often the result of a previous more acute ophthalmia. In adults severe sycosis of the eyelids may accompany sycosis of the beard, but, as a rule, no tendency to such disease of the skin is observed.

TREATMENT.—When the inflammatory symptoms are severe nothing has such a marked effect as pulling out all the lashes. Cases of a few weeks' standing may be cured and recurrence in older cases very much relieved by one or two such epilations, together with local remedies. Local applications are always needed (1) for the removal of the scabs, (2) to subdue the inflammatory symptoms. A warm alkaline and tar lotion, with which the lids are to be carefully soaked for a quarter of an hour night and morning, followed by a weak mercurial ointment applied along the edges of the lids after each bathing, is an efficient plan if the mother will take the pains. In bad cases painting, or pencilling, the border of the lid with nitrate of silver, either in strong solution, or the diluted stick, or the use of weak copper drops, is very useful in addition to the ointment. In old cases with much epiphora the canaliculus is to be slit up. The patients generally need a long course of iron. (F. 1, 2, 3, 6; 15, 16; 24, 25, 26.)

A stye is the result of suppurative inflammation of the connective tissue, or of one of the glands, in the margin of the lid. Owing to the close texture of the tarsus and the vascularity of the parts, the pain and swelling are often severe, and even alarming to the patient. The matter generally points around an eyelash; but if seated in a Meibomian gland, it may point either to the border of the lid or to the conjunctiva, rarely to the skin.

Styes almost always show some derangement of health especially of the stomach or reproductive organs. Overuse of the eyes, especially if ametropic, is the exciting cause in some cases; exposure to cold wind in others. Styes are very apt to recur, singly or in crops, for several weeks or months.

TREATMENT.—A stye may sometimes be cut short if seen quite early, by the vigorous use of an antiphlogistic lotion ; but an incision followed by hot fomentations or a poultice is usually more efficacious ; the puncture must be made parallel to the free border and extend rather deeply ; a Beer's knife or broad needle, Figs. 160 and 145, may be used. The health always needs attending to, and a purgative iron mixture often suits better than anything else.

Some persons are subject to very small postules or styes, much more superficial than the above, and less closely associated with derangement of health.

A Meibomian gland is often the scene of chronic overgrowth, a little tumor in the substance of the lid being the result—**Meibomian cysts, chalazion.** In a few weeks or months the growth becomes as large as a pea, forming a firm, hemispherical, painless swelling, over which the skin is freely movable. A dusky spot where the tarsal tissues are thinned marks the conjunctival aspect, and when spontaneous rupture has occurred a flattened mass of granulation is found there. The deeper part of the gland is the common seat of disease; if, as sometimes happens, the part near the edge of the lid is affected, the tumor usually remains very small. Occasionally the growth pushes forward and adhesion to the skin occurs ; even then it is easily distinguished from a sebaceous cyst by the firmness of its deep attachment. During its course the cyst may inflame and even suppurate, and in the latter case it forms one variety of "stye." The same tumor may inflame several times, and finally suppurate and shrink. Like styes, these tumors are apt to continue forming one after another. They are much commoner in young adults than earlier or later in life, but they are now and then seen in infants. Patients as often apply for the disfigurement as for any discomfort which these little growths occasion.

TREATMENT.—The cyst is to be removed from the *lower surface* of the lid ; but if it point forward the incision may be in the skin. The tumor generally consists of a soft, pinkish, gelatinous mass, or of a gruelly or puriform fluid, without a cyst wall. Sometimes the contents are very firm and adherent. See Operations.

Small yellow dots are sometimes seen on the inner surface of the lids, due to little cheesy collections in the Meibomian glands, and causing irritation by their hardness. They should be picked out with the point of a knife.

Warty formations are not very common on the border of the lid, and are of little consequence, except in elderly people, in whom they should be looked upon with suspicion as possible starting-points of rodent cancer. A small fleshy, yellowish-red, flattened growth is sometimes met with just upon the tarsal border, and apparently seated at the mouth of a Meibomian gland. It causes some irritation, and should be pared off. *Small pellucid cysts* are also not uncommon on the lid border. Cutaneous horns are occasionally seen on the skin of the eyelids.

Molluscum contagiosum is partly an ophthalmic disease, because so often seated on the eyelids. One or more little rounded prominences, showing a small dimpled orifice at the top, plugged by dry sebaceous matter, are seen in the skin, varying from the size of a mustard-seed to a cherry, but usually not larger than a sweet pea ; at first they are hemispherical, but afterwards become constricted at the base. The skin is tightly stretched, thinned, and adherent. The larger specimens sometimes inflame, and their true nature may then, without due care, be mistaken. Each molluscum must be removed, the white, lobulated, gland-like mass which forms the growth being squeezed out through the incision made by a knife or scissors.

Xanthelasma palpebrarum appears as one or more yellow patches like pieces of washleather in the skin, varying from mere dots to the size of a kidney bean, quite soft in texture, and very little raised. The disease is commonest near the inner canthus, and, unless symmetrical, is usually on the left side. It occurs chiefly in elderly persons who have previously been subject to become very dark around the eyes when out of health. The patches are due to infiltration of the deeper parts of the skin by groups of cells loaded with yellow fat. The frequency of xanthelasma in the eyelids is perhaps related to the normal presence of certain peculiar granular cells, some of which contain pigment, in the skin of these parts.

The pediculus pubis (crab-louse) in very rare cases will reach the eyelashes and flourish there. The lice cling close to the border of the lid, and look like little dirty scabs; the eggs are darker, and may also be mistaken for bits of dirt. The absence of inflammation and the rather peculiar appearances will lead, in doubtful cases, to the use of a magnifying glass, by which the question will be at once settled.

Ulcers on the eyelids may be malignant, or lupous, or syphilitic; and in the last case the sore may be either a chancre or a tertiary ulcer.

Rodent cancer, rodent ulcer, flat epithelial cancer, is by far the commonest form of carcinoma affecting the eyelids; although cases of eyelid cancer occasionally present both the clinical and pathological characters of ordinary epithelioma. The peculiarities of rodent cancer are that it is very slow, that ulceration almost keeps pace with the new growth, and that it does not cause infection of lymphatics. It seldom begins before, generally not until considerably after, middle life, and in its course often extends over many years. Beginning as a "pimple" or "wart," it slowly spreads, but years may pass before the ulcer is as large as a sixpence. When first seen we generally find a shallow ulcer, covered by a thin scab, most often involving the skin at the inner end of the lower lid. Its edge is raised, sinuous, nodular, and very hard, but neither inflamed nor tender. Slowly extending both in area and depth, it attacks all tissues alike, finally destroying the eyeball and opening into the nose. In a few very chronic cases the disease remains quite superficial, and cicatrization may occur at some parts of the ulcerated surface. Now and then a considerable nodule of growth forms in the skin before ulceration begins.

The diagnosis is generally easy. A long-standing ulcer of the eyelids in an adult is nearly certain to be rodent cancer. *Tertiary syphilitic ulcers* are much less chronic, more inflamed and punched out, and devoid of the very peculiar, hard edge of rodent ulcer; moreover, they are very rare. *Lupus* seldom occurs so late in life as rodent cancer, presents more inflammation and much less hardness, and is often accompanied by lupus elsewhere on the cutaneous or mucous surfaces. Lupus is seldom difficult to distinguish on the eyelids from tertiary syphilis, the latter being more acute, more dusky, and showing more loss of substance, with none of the little, ill-defined, soft tubercles seen in lupus.

When a *chancre* occurs on the eyelid [1] the induration and swelling are usually very marked, the surface abraded and moist, but not much ulcerated; the glands in front of the ear and behind the jaw become enlarged. The same glands enlarge, either with or without suppuration, in lupus and in many inflammatory conditions of the lid.

Several cases are on record in which a hard chancre formed on the palpebral conjunctiva so far from the border of the lid as to be quite concealed. I have seen two such, and Mr. James Adams and Mr. Wherry have each recorded one. In all of these cases the swelling bore considerable

---

[1] An interesting monograph on this subject was read by Dr. De Beck at the American Ophth. Soc., July, 1886.

resemblance to a large Meibomian cyst. In all there were enlarged glands and well-marked constitutional symptoms.

TREATMENT OF RODENT CANCER.—Early removal is of great importance, and probably the more so in proportion to the youth of the patient. Chloride of zinc paste or the actual cautery is necessary in addition to the knife in bad cases; scraping may also be employed. The disease is very apt to return locally. Even in very advanced cases, where complete removal is impossible, the patient may be made much more comfortable, and life probably prolonged, by vigorous and repeated treatment.

Congenital ptosis is not a very rare affection. It may be double or unilateral, is present from birth, and its causation is unknown. I believe it is never complete. It sometimes seems to diminish in the first few years of life, but probably never disappears. Although the lid droops, the skin is often scanty, the lid being tight and deficient in the natural folds. Operations have been devised for producing deep cicatricial bands, by means of subcutaneous sutures passed from the brow to the tarsus (Bowman, Pagenstecher, Wecker).[1] These rather tedious procedures avoid the risk of further shortening of the lid which attends the simpler operation of removing an elliptical fold of skin. I have obtained considerable improvement from Pagenstecher's operation. (See also Ocular Paralysis, Chapter XXI.)

Epicanthus is a rare condition, in which a fold of skin stretches across from the inner end of the brow to the side of the nose, hiding the inner canthus. If it does not disappear as the child's nose develops, an operation—removal of a piece of skin from the bridge of the nose, sometimes combined with canthoplasty—is indicated.

---

[1] Panas has devised a new operation more recently. Arch. d'Ophtalmologie, T. 6, p. 1, 1886.

CHAPTER V.

THESE may be divided into the affections of the secreting parts—the lachrymal gland and its ducts; and those of the drainage apparatus—the puncta, canaliculi, lachrymal sac, and nasal duct. In the great majority of cases the fault lies entirely in the drainage system.

The flow of tears over the edge of the lid, "watery eye," is called *epiphora* or *stillicidium lacrimarum*. No useful purpose is served by keeping the two names, and only the former will be here used. *Lachrymation* indicates the increased flow which often accompanies inflammation of the eyeball.

The drainage system may be at fault in any part from the puncta to the lower end of the nasal duct.

The slightest change in the position of the lower punctum causes epiphora. In health the punctum is directed backward against the eye; if it look upward or forward, the tears do not all reach it, and some will then flow over a lower part of the lid. Thus in paralysis of the facial nerve the patient sometimes comes to us for epiphora before he notices the other symptoms; the watering is caused partly by loss of the compressing and sucking action of the punctum that is effected in winking, by those fibres of the orbicularis which lie in relation with the lachrymal sac, partly by a slight falling of the lid away from the eye and a consequent displacement of the punctum. The various chronic diseases of the border of the lids, ophthalmia tarsi, and also

[1] For Diseases of Lachrymal Gland, see Diseases of Orbit, Chap. XIX.

granular disease of the conjunctiva, granular lids, are common sources of (1) tumefaction, with narrowing, of the puncta and canaliculi ; (2) cicatricial stricture of the same parts ; and in both cases the puncta are displaced as well as constricted. Narrowing, even to complete obliteration, of the puncta is sometimes seen as the result of former inflammation, of which all traces have long since passed away. Wounds by which the canaliculi are cut across cause their obliteration, and epiphora is the result.

In all the above cases epiphora is accompanied by a visible change in the size or position of the punctum, none of the signs of inflammation in the lachrymal sac or stricture in the nasal duct being present ; and simple division of the canaliculus will cure, or much relieve, the watering. (See Operations.) This is, however, seldom necessary in the epiphora of facial paralysis.

The canaliculus is occasionally plugged by the growth in it of a mycelial fungus, which, mingled with pus-cells and mucus, forms a yellowish, or greenish, putty-like concretion. These masses sometimes calcify, and are then called dacryoliths.[1]

Epiphora not explained by the above causes is usually due to obstruction in the nasal duct, and accompanied by distention and disease of the lachrymal sac from the same cause. *Primary* disease of the lachrymal *sac* is rare.

Obstruction of the nasal duct is usually caused by chronic thickening of the mucous and submucous tissues lining the canal. Dense, hard thickening causes a stricture, often very tight and unyielding ; but obstruction is often present, though the canal be of full size or perhaps even dilated,[2] excess of mucus being apparently the chief

[1] The same term is applied to concretions, still more rare, in the ducts of the lachrymal gland.

[2] There can be little doubt that the healthy nasal duct varies much in size in different persons (Noyes).

cause. Disease of the duct occurs at all ages, and is much commoner in females than in males.[1] In some cases the change evidently forms a part of a chronic disease of the naso-pharyngeal mucous membrane, but in many no cause can be assigned. Sometimes stricture is the result of periostitis or of necrosis, and of these conditions syphilis, either acquired or inherited, scarlet fever, and smallpox are the commonest causes. Injuries to and growths in the nose, or invading it, account for a few cases.

A stricture may be seated at any part of the duct; but the upper end, where there is often a natural narrowing, is the commonest spot.

Obstruction of the nasal duct, by preventing the escape of tears, leads to *distention of the lachrymal sac*, to chronic thickening of its lining membrane, and increased secretion of mucus. The mucus may be clear or turbid. At length a point is reached at which the distention can be seen as a little swelling under the skin at the inner canthus, *mucocele* or *chronic dacryo-cystitis.* This swelling can generally be dispersed by pressure with the finger, the mucus and tears either regurgitating through the canaliculi or being forced through the duct into the nose. In cases of old standing the sac is often much thickened, and may contain polypi, and the swelling cannot then be entirely dispersed by pressure.

A mucocele is always very apt to inflame and suppurate, the result being a *lachrymal abscess.* Most cases of lachrymal abscess, indeed, have been preceded by mucocele. Its formation gives rise to great pain, and to tense, brawny, dusky swelling, which, extending for a considerable distance around the sac, is sometimes mistaken for erysipelas. The matter always points a little below the tendo-palpebrarum; the pus often burrows in front of the sac, forming

[1] In a group of 113 consecutive cases I find 89 females and 24 males.

little pouches in the cellular tissue, and if allowed to open spontaneously, a fistula, very troublesome to cure, is likely to follow. If seen early, before there is decided pointing, it is best to open the abscess by slitting the lower canaliculus freely into the sac, and passing a knife down the nasal duct; anæsthesia is usually necessary. If interference be delayed, the skin over the sac soon becomes thinned, and the abscess is then best opened through the skin, by a free puncture inclined downward and a little outward; no anæsthetic is necessary, and the resulting scar is insignificant. When the thickening has subsided, under the use of warm lead lotion dressing, the stricture of the duct is to be treated; but the mucocele will form again, and another abscess may occur at any time, unless a free passage can be restored down the nasal duct.

Obstinate chronic conjunctivitis is often set up by unrelieved lachrymal obstruction (Chap. VI.). It has long been known that severe suppurative inflammation was very likely to occur after any operation performed on the cornea when there was pus in the lachrymal sac. (See Cataract.) These evidences of local irritation and infection are now believed often to depend upon septic organisms which, owing to the obstruction, collect in the lachrymal sac.

TREATMENT OF MUCOCELE AND LACHRYMAL STRICTURE.—The object aimed at is the permanent dilatation of the stricture; but, whether this can be gained or not, a free opening from the canaliculus into the sac should be maintained, so that the secretions may be often and easily squeezed out.

Dilatation by probing (Chap. XXII.) is the ordinary and best treatment for all strictures, whether there be mucocele or not, the rule being to use the largest probe that will pass readily. The probing is repeated every few days or less often, according to the duration of its effect, and often needs to be continued for weeks or months. The

patient may sometimes learn to use the probe himself.
When the stricture is tough and tight, it is best at once to
divide it by thrusting a strong-backed, narrow knife down
the duct, and afterward to use probes. In cases where the
stricture is quite soft, and the obstruction due rather to
general thickening of the mucous membrane and over-
secretion of mucus than to dense fibrous thickening, frequent washing out of the duct with water or weak astringents by means of a lachrymal syringe is quite as beneficial
as, and less painful than, probing. The diligent use of
astringent lotions to the conjunctiva is also useful, particularly in soft strictures, some of the lotion reaching the sac
and duct. In cases of long standing, where other treatment has failed and the sac is much thickened, its complete
obliteration by the actual cautery gives great relief; extirpation of the lachrymal gland is also occasionally practised.
For refractory children and for patients who cannot be
seen often, a style of silver or lead, passed in exactly the
same way as a probe, but worn constantly for many weeks,
is very useful; but it may slip into the sac out of reach
unless furnished with a bend or head so large as to be
somewhat unsightly. As a rule, probing should not be
begun until the inflammatory thickening and tenderness
following a lachrymal abscess have subsided. If the probe
be used too often, or with much violence, or if false passages be made, the case may easily be made worse instead
of better. It must be confessed, indeed, that in many
lachrymal cases, whether the stricture be soft or firm,
treatment, however skilful, gives only partial relief to the
epiphora.

Suppuration of the lachrymal sac, on one or both sides,
sometimes takes place in newborn infants without apparent cause; if there be much redness, the abscess should
be opened, but the suppuration is sometimes chronic, and

will cease under the use of astringent lotions. The cases of epiphora with contracted punctum, which are sometimes met with in older children, may perhaps be the consequences of this infantile suppuration.

Cases in which the sac or duct is obliterated by injury can seldom be relieved.

CHAPTER VI.

IT is convenient to distinguish those which, from the outset, are general and affect the whole membrane, ocular and palpebral alike, and of which the various forms of contagious ophthalmia are examples, from others which primarily affect either the ocular or the palpebral part alone. *The term "ophthalmia" includes all inflammations of the conjunctiva, and should not be applied to other diseases.*

GENERAL DISEASES.

The conjunctiva, like the urethra, is subject to purulent inflammation, and, like the respiratory mucous membrane, is liable to the muco-purulent and to the membranous or diphtheritic forms of disease. All cases in which there is yellow discharge are in greater or less degree contagious. The congestion which forms a part of conjunctivitis is much influenced by age, the younger the patient the less is the congestion in proportion to the discharge—a fact to be borne in mind in examining patients at both ends of the scale.

Purulent ophthalmia (O. neonatorum, Gonorrhœal O., Blenorrhœa of the conjunctiva) is generally due to contagion from the same disease, or from an acute or chronic discharge from the urethra or vagina, which may or may not be gonorrhœal. It is commonest in newborn infants whose eyes have been inoculated from the mother during birth; next in adults with gonorrhœa; it is also seen sometimes in young girls who have non-venereal discharges from the genitals. Muco-purulent ophthalmia, when quickly

5*

passed on from one to another, under conditions of health favorable to suppuration, *e. g.*, weakness after acute exanthems, may be intensified into the purulent form. The presence of a special form of micrococcus in the pus-cells of gonorrhœa and of purulent ophthalmia, described by Neisser in 1879, has been confirmed by Sattler, Widmark, and many others. The coccus is said (1) to be absent in some of the milder forms of infantile ophthalmia ; (2) when cultivated, to be capable of producing purulent ophthalmia by inoculation ; (3) to be usually present in the vaginal discharge of women whose babies have purulent ophthalmia. Gonorrhœa was experimentally produced by inoculation with pus from purulent ophthalmia long before the days of bacterial pathology. Like gonorrhœa, purulent ophthalmia may occur more than once. It varies greatly in severity, but is, on the whole, much worse in adults than in infants, perhaps because there is much more adenoid tissue in the conjunctiva of adults than of babies (Widmark). The quality of the infecting discharge, no doubt, has much influence, severe forms being generally caused by inoculation from a recent or severe case ; but chronic discharge may also give rise to a severe attack. The health of the recipient and the previous condition of the eyelids exert an important influence, and if the lids be granular, various slight causes sometimes bring on severe purulent ophthalmia.

The disease sets in from twelve to about forty-eight hours after inoculation ; in infants the third day after birth is almost invariably given as the date when discharge was first noticed. Itchiness and slight redness of conjunctiva soon pass on to intense congestion of conjunctiva, with chemosis, tense inflammatory swelling of the lids, great pain, and discharge. The discharge at first is serous, or like turbid whey, but soon becomes more profuse, creamy (purulent), and yellow, or even slightly greenish. Dark,

abrupt ecchymoses are often present. The lids, always
swollen, hot, and red, in bad cases become very tense and
dusky. The upper lid hangs down over the lower, and is
often so stiff that it cannot be completely everted. The
conjunctiva is succulent and easily bleeds.

The disease if untreated declines spontaneously, and the
discharge almost ceases in about six weeks, the palpebral
conjunctiva being left thick, relaxed, and more or less
granular. Cicatricial changes, identical with, but less
severe than, those resulting from chronic granular lids, and
analogous to what occurs in stricture of the urethra, sometimes follow; considerable permanent thickening of the
ocular conjunctiva may also occur.

There is a risk to the cornea in this disease, partly from
strangulation of the vessels, partly from the local influence
of the discharge. If within the first two or three days the
cornea becomes hazy and dull, like that of a dead fish,
there is great risk that total or extensive sloughing will
occur. In many of the milder cases ulcers form a little
below the centre, and rapidly cause perforation. In other
cases clear deep ulcers form close to the edge of the cornea.
There is less risk of ulceration of the cornea in the purulent
ophthalmia of infants than in that of adults, but a form of
corneal affection appears in infants which seems to be peculiar to them. This variety is generally seen when the discharge is getting scanty, or perhaps when too much nitrate
of silver has been used; it sometimes occurs when the attack
is of a diphtheritic type. The cornea becomes quickly and
almost entirely opaque throughout, with the exception of a
narrow zone at its edge; the surface is dull, and the epithelium irregular, but there is little, if any, loss of substance. In many cases the opacity clears up to a great
extent, even entirely, and eserine seems to help the recovery; it remains longest and densest at the centre. Either
one or both eyes may be attacked; in adults one eye often

escapes; in infants, where the inoculation occurs during birth, both eyes almost always suffer.

TREATMENT.—If only one eye be affected, and the patient be old enough to obey orders, the sound eye must be covered up with the shield introduced by Dr. Buller : Take two pieces of india-rubber plaster, one $4\frac{1}{2}''$, the other $4''$ square, cut a round window in the middle of each, and stick them together, with a small watch-glass inserted into the window. The plaster is fixed by its free border, and by other strips, to the nose, forehead, and cheek, and the patient looks through the glass; the lower outer angle is left open for ventilation; particular attention is to be paid to the fastening on the nose. All concerned are to be warned as to the risk of contagion and the means of conveying it. The essential curative measures are : (1) Frequent removal of the discharge by the free use of weak antiseptic or astringent lotions (F. 3, 19, 20, 23, 28, 29). Every hour, day and night, the lids are gently opened, and the discharge removed with soft bits of moistened rag or cotton-wool; or a syringe or irrigation apparatus, such as the hollow speculum or retractor described by Mr. Edgar Browne and Mr Collins, may be used.[1] In adults, where the swelling is often extreme and very brawny, the cleansing must be done very gently lest the congestion and irritability be increased. (2) Iodoform, at first extensively tried, has, I believe, not given satisfaction in this disease. Many surgeons greatly prefer weak nitrate of silver (F. 3) to all other remedies. (3) Strong solutions of nitrate of silver or the mitigated solid nitrate (F. 1 and 2) are of great service in shortening the attack and lessening the risks, and, whatever other treatment be adopted, they should be used in all severe cases, unless specially contraindicated. A ten- or twenty-grain solution is brushed

[1] British Medical Journal, 1885, vol. i.

freely over the conjunctiva of the lids, everted as well as possible and freed from discharge. If the mitigated stick is used, more care is needed ; and to prevent too great an effect it is to be washed off with water, after waiting about fifteen seconds. These strong applications must be made by the surgeon. The pain caused by them is lessened, and the benefit increased, by free bathing with cold or iced water afterward. The application is not to be repeated until the discharge, which will be markedly lessened for some hours, has begun to increase again ; once a day is enough in many cases. (4) Between the cleansings either warm or cold applications ; warmth is often preferred by the patient. (5) In the early stage, in adults, several leeches to the temple will give relief, or, if the swelling be very tense, we may divide the outer canthus with scissors or knife, and thus both bleed and relax the parts at the same time. Removal of the ring of conjunctiva which overlaps the cornea is valuable when the chemosis is severe. The late Mr. Critchett, in a very bad case, divided the upper lid vertically across, and kept its two halves turned upward by sutures fastened to the forehead, at once relieving the tension of the lids and rendering the conjunctiva accessible. (6) The lids should be often anointed with a simple ointment.

The following additional precautions are important: Strong nitrate of silver applications are unsafe in the earliest stage, before free discharge has set in, and also in cases where, even later in the disease, there is much hard, brawny swelling of the ocular conjunctiva and comparatively little discharge ; cases, in fact, approaching the condition known as diphtheritic ophthalmia. In these either very cold or very hot applications, leeches, cleanliness, and weak lotions should be chiefly relied upon. Ice and leeches are seldom advisable for infants. It is of extreme importance to begin treatment very early, for the cornea is often irreparably damaged within two or three days. The patients, if adults, are often in feeble health, and need supporting treatment. Ulceration of the cornea does not contra-indicate the use of strong nitrate of silver if the discharge is abundant. Treatment must be continued so long as there is any discharge, for a relapse of purulent discharge often takes place if remedies are discontinued too soon. Over-use of nitrate of silver sometimes seems to cause the diffuse opacity of the cornea referred to at p. 107 ; I have seen it clear quickly and entirely when eserine was used. I once saw hemorrhage continuing for some time, without apparent cause, from the conjunctiva of the lid, in a child recovering from purulent ophthalmia. Serious conjunctival hemorrhage has been noted by Pomeroy and Schmidt-Rimpler.

The systematic *prevention of ophthalmia neonatorum* by the cleansing and disinfection of the eyes of every infant immediately after birth, sometimes preceded by disinfection of the maternal passages, has been introduced by Credé during the last three or four years, and largely carried out in many lying-in hospitals, especially on the Continent. Credé applies a few drops of a 2 per cent solution of nitrate of silver (about 8 gr. to $\mathfrak{z}$j) to the conjunctival sac once. Various other agents or weaker solutions of silver have been used. The general result of such measures has been to reduce the number of cases in an astonishing degree ; and as it is calculated that about a third of all the blind in Europe have become so by the ravages of this disease, considerable importance is to be attached to the general adoption of Credé's principle by medical men and midwives.[1]

Muco-purulent ophthalmia.—The commonest and best characterized of the acute ophthalmiæ is the so-called

[1] Particulars and statistics may be found in " Edinburgh Medical Journal," April, 1883 (Dr. A. R. Simpson), and in more recent papers.

catarrhal ophthalmia. The name is a bad one, for neither does the disease form part of a general catarrh of the respiratory tract, nor does it show the tendency to relapse so characteristic of catarrh, nor does it seem to be caused by cold. The disease attains its height very quickly, almost always attacks both eyes, and gets well spontaneously in about a fortnight. There is great congestion, much gritty pain, which often prevents sleep, spasm of the lids, free muco-purulent discharge, and, in many cases, ecchymotic patches in the conjunctiva. The lids are somewhat swollen and red, but never tense, and the cornea seldom suffers.

This disease seems to be much oftener communicated from person to person than purulent ophthalmia, for which it is sometimes mistaken. It varies much in severity, even in different members of the same household, who catch it almost at the same time, but attacks all ages indiscriminately. It is, I believe, commonest in warm weather, or perhaps at the change from cold to warm. It is rare to find that the patient has suffered from the disease before. Any mild antiseptic lotion will cut it short, nitrate of silver (F. 3) being the best.

Troublesome *ophthalmia, with muco-purulent discharge,* is common in children *after exanthemata,* especially measles. It runs a less definite course than the preceding disease, shows but little tendency to spontaneous cure, and is very often complicated with phlyctenular ulcers of the cornea, blepharitis, and eruptions on the face; the patients are frequently strumous. The discharge is seldom so abundant as in the disease just considered. The treatment is often troublesome, and many changes have to be tried; weak nitrate of silver lotions (F. 3), with the use of the yellow ointment (F. 12 to 14), or boracic acid ointment, both to the skin and conjunctiva, or calomel dusted into the eye, are the best local means; atropine alone often increases the irritation. Careful attention to health is necessary. The patients should not be confined to the house, but with a large shade over both eyes should take plenty of exercise in fine weather. *The eyes should not be bandaged in any form of ophthalmia, and poultices are very seldom suitable.*

Some forms of acute conjunctivitis, with little or no discharge, are seen both in children and adults, which do not conform to the above types, and are of comparatively slight importance. Many such appear to depend on changes of weather or exposure to cold, and are complicated with phlyctenulæ. A few are distinctly rheumatic. The conjunctiva is involved more or less in herpes zoster of the ophthalmic division of the fifth nerve, in erysipelas of the face, in the early stage of measles, and slightly in eczema of the face. Slight degrees of chronic conjunctivitis are set up by various local irritants, dust, smoke, cold wind, etc., and by the strain attending the use of the eyes without glasses in cases of hypermetropia. Mention must be made of the cases sometimes seen in children, where an ophthalmia appears to form part of an impetiginous or herpetic eruption on the face, with which it is simultaneous. These again differ from the commoner cases in which the lids, cheek, and lining membrane of the nose are irritated into an eruption by tears and discharge from a pre-existing conjunctivitis.

Muco-purulent ophthalmia of any kind becomes a very important affair if it breaks out in schools or armies, etc., where granular disease of the eyelids is prevalent.

Membranous and diphtheritic ophthalmia. — In a few cases of ophthalmia, either purulent or muco-purulent, the discharge adheres to the conjunctiva in the form of a membrane, *membranous or croupous ophthalmia.* Still more rarely, in addition to membrane on the surface, the whole depth of the conjunctiva is stiffened by solid exudation, which much impairs the mobility both of the lids and eye-

balls, and, by compressing the vessels, prevents the formation of free discharge, and places the nutrition of the cornea
in great peril. It is to the latter cases that the term *diphtheritic* has been limited by most authors ; but we find
many connecting links between the two types, and between
each of them and the ordinary purulent and muco-purulent
cases.

It is of much consequence in practice, both for prognosis
and treatment, to recognize the presence of membranous
discharge and of solid infiltration in any case of ophthalmia ; for the liability to severe corneal damage is much
increased by either of these conditions, especially by the
latter. The membrane may cover the whole inside of the
lids, or it may occur in separate or in confluent patches ; it
often begins at the border of the lid, and is seldom found
on the ocular conjunctiva. It can be peeled off, the conjunctiva beneath bleeding freely unless infiltrated and solid ;
in the latter case the membrane is more adherent, the conjunctiva is of a palish color, and scarcely bleeds when
exposed, and there is little or no purulent discharge. In
most cases the solid products, whether membrane or deep
infiltration, pass after some days into a stage of liquefaction, with free purulent secretion. In rare cases the membrane forms and reforms for months. As regards cause:
(1) very rarely the process creeps up to the conjunctiva
from the nose in cases of primary diphtheria, or is caused
by inoculation of the conjunctiva with membrane; whilst
in a few the ophthalmia forms the first symptom of general
diphtheria, or of masked or anomalous scarlet fever. (2)
more commonly it is part of a diphtheritic type of inflammation following some acute illness ; (3) it may be caused
by the over-use of caustics in ordinary purulent ophthalmia;
(4) it may be due to contagion, either from a similar case
or from a purulent ophthalmia, or a gonorrhœa, the diphtheritic type depending on some peculiarity in the health

or tissues of the recipient.   Membranous and diphtheritic
ophthalmia are seen most often in children from two to
eight years old, less commonly in adults and infants.   It
is commoner in North Germany than in other parts of
Europe, but severe and even fatal cases are well known in
our own country.   In two cases I have seen the same condition attack the skin of the eyelids and cause sloughing
patches.

In *treatment* the cardinal point is not to use nitrate of
silver in any form when there are scanty discharge and
much solid infiltration of the conjunctiva.   The agents to
be relied on are : (1) either ice or hot fomentations ; ice, if
it can be used continuously and well; fomentations, to encourage liquid exudation and determination to the skin if
the cold treatment cannot be carried out, or fails to make
any impression on the case ; (2) leeches, if the patient's
state will bear them ; (3) great cleanliness.   The presence
of membrane is no bar to the use of caustics, provided
that the conjunctiva is succulent, red, and bleeds easily.
Mr. Tweedy strongly advises quinine lotion used very frequently (F. 27).

PARTIAL DISEASES.

Granular ophthalmia (trachoma) is a very important
malady, characterized by slowly progressive changes in the
conjunctiva of the eyelids, in consequence of which this
membrane becomes thickened, vascular, and roughened by
firm hemispherical elevations, instead of being pale, thin,
and smooth.   The change usually begins in the conjunctiva of the lower lid, extending to the submucous tissue of
both lids at a later period, and giving rise to the growth
of much organized new tissue in the deep parts of the
conjunctiva.   The tissue is afterward partly absorbed and
partly converted into dense, tendinous scar, which by very

close shrinking often gives rise to much trouble. It is
stated by Reid and others that trachoma follicles come to
the surface, open, discharge their contents, and leave minute
ulcers; but it cannot be said clinically that trachoma is an
ulcerative disease, and the prominences are not "granulations" in the pathological sense.[1] There have been, and
still are, extraordinary differences of opinion as to the
origin and nature of the "granulations" or "trachoma
bodies" in this disease. The latest researches favor the
view that they are derived either from natural lymphatic
follicles or from tubular glands. The question is very
difficult, whether from the histological or the clinical point
of view, though we may hope that it will be simplified if
Sattler's view that trachoma is due to a specific coccus be
confirmed, 1881 and 1882. Fig. 40 shows a section through
some recent trachoma bodies.

FIG. 40.

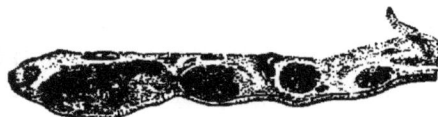

X 14

Microscopical section through four recent trachoma bodies ("sago-
grain granulations"), from the lower lid of a young Irish soldier whose
eyes became affected in the late Egyptian campaigns. The epithelial
cells became almost indistinguishable from those of the growth where
they cover the largest nodule. No reticulum can be made out between
the cells of which the growths are composed.

The disease is first shown by the presence, on the lower
lid, of a number of rounded, pale, semitransparent bodies
like little grains of boiled sago, or sometimes looking like
vesicles; the so-called "vesicular," or "sago-grain," or
"follicular" granulations, Fig. 41. Judging clinically,

_____
[1] I am aware that Rachlmann makes a contrary statement.

they are, to a certain degree, normal, and are seen, especially on the lower lids, in many young persons with slight ophthalmia, who never afterwards suffer from true granular lids. Such mild cases, in which no parts deeper than the normal lymphatic follicles and papillæ are affected, and in which recovery takes place without cicatricial

FIG. 41.

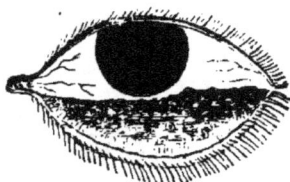

Granular lower lid. (After Eble.)

changes, are by Saemisch and some other authors placed, under the name of *conjunctivitis follicularis*, in a separate category from the granular disease; the two conditions being supposed due to radically different causes. But the frequent coincidence of transitional forms in the same case, the fact that both "follicular conjunctivitis" and well-marked granular disease admittedly occur under the same general conditions, and that in a given case the distinctions between "follicles" and "granulations" often cannot be made until it is known whether or no cicatricial changes will occur, certainly much lessen the clinical value of the asserted pathological difference.

Granular disease is very important because it greatly increases the susceptibility of the conjunctiva to take on acute inflammation and to produce contagious discharge; makes it less amenable to treatment, and very liable to relapses of ophthalmia for many years; and often gives rise to deformities of the lid and to serious damage of the cornea. In crowded poor-law schools we see many cases of granular lids in which there is no history of an acute attack having ever occurred, but in ordinary practice it is rare to see such.

Chronic granular disease is the result (1) of prolonged overcrowding, or rather of long residence in badly-ventilated and damp rooms; it used to be very abundant in the army and navy, and is still seen in great perfection in workhouse schools; (2) a generally low state of health, no doubt, increases the susceptibility to it; (3) it is, *cæteris paribus*, commonest and most quickly produced in children; (4) certain races are peculiarly liable to suffer, *e. g.*, the Irish, the Jews, and some other Eastern races, and some of the German and French races. The Irish and Jews carry it with them all over the world, and transmit the liability to their descendants wherever they live. Negroes in America are said to be almost exempt; (5) damp and low-lying climates are more productive of it than others; thus it is rare in Switzerland. Possibly what are now race tendencies may be the expression of climatal conditions acting on the same race through many generations. It is difficult clinically to decide whether the trachoma growths, apart from the discharge, are caused by contagion, or by the influence of non-vital causes, such as damp and impure air; many high authorities held for a long time that the chronic disease was contagious, and even communicable at a distance through the air, without the presence of any appreciable discharge. When accompanied by discharge, the disease is contagious: and it is generally held that the discharge from a case of trachoma is specific, *i. e.*, that it will give rise by contagion, not only to muco-purulent or purulent ophthalmia, but to the true granular disease.

Sattler in 1881–2 believed that he had discovered a specific microbe for trachoma; his results have been substantially confirmed by Michel and others, and it is held by Koch and other recent investigators that in mixed cases of catarrhal and granular disease two specific microbes exist.

Should this prove true, it will at once simplify and explain the varying characters of contagious ophthalmia complicated by granular lids.

Those who practise in the army, or who have charge of such institutions as pauper schools, will find that in practice the causes of the chronic granular condition are inextricably mixed up with all kinds of facilities for contagion, and that it will be necessary to fight against two enemies—the cause of spontaneous chronic granular disease, and the sources of contagious discharge. The former is to be combated by improved hygienic conditions, especially by free ventilation, dry air, abundant open-air exercise, and improvement of the general vigor. The sources of contagion are endless, especially since, as has been stated, granular patients are liable to relapses of muco-purulent discharge from almost any slight irritation. Frequent inspection of all the eyes, rigid separation of all who show any discharge or are known as especially subject to relapses, arrangements for washing such as will prevent the use of towels and water in common, extreme care against the introduction of contagious cases from without—such are the chief preventive measures. Extra precautions will be needed in time of war or famine, or when measles or scarlet fever is prevalent, or during marches through hot, sandy, or windy districts.

The *curative treatment*, when discharge is present, does not differ from that of the acute ophthalmiæ already given. The use of strong astringents (solid sulphate of copper) or caustics (nitrate of silver in strong solution, or in the mitigated solid pencil), however, is generally needed in order to make much impression on the granular state of the lids. The lids being thoroughly everted, are touched all over with one or other application, and this is repeated daily, or less often ; some experience being required before we can decide how often to touch the eyelids in each case.

By careful treatment on this principle most patients may
be kept comfortably free from active symptoms, many
relapses may be prevented, the duration of the disease
shortened, and the risks of secondary damage to the cornea
much lessened. Do what we will, however, granular disease when well established is most tedious, and fastens
many risks and disabilities on its subjects for years to
come.

For routine treatment on a large scale nothing is so
effectual as nitrate of silver, either a ten- or twenty-grain
solution or the mitigated solid point (F. 1 and 2). But
silver has the disadvantage of sometimes permanently
staining the conjunctiva after long use, and in very chronic
cases I think either sulphate of copper or the lapus divinus (F. 5) is to be preferred, especially as the patient may
sometimes be taught to evert his own lids and use it himself. The solid mitigated nitrate of silver needs washing
off with water at first, but in old cases it is often better not
to do so.

Results of granular disease.—Friction by the granulations of the upper lid, *a*, Fig. 42, especially in cases of long
standing where some scarring is present, *b*, often causes

Fig. 42.

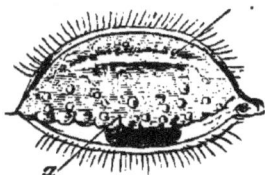

Granular upper lid.   *a.* Granulations.   *b.* Line of scar in typical
position, parallel with border of lid.

cloudiness of the cornea, partly from ulceration, but mainly
from the growth of a layer of new and very vascular tis-

sue, in the superficial layers of the cornea—*pannus*,[1] Fig.
43.   In later periods the conjunctiva and deeper tissues
are shortened and puckered by the scar following absorption of the "granulations," Fig. 42, *b*.   These changes,
when severe, often lead to inversion of the border of the lid,
entropion ; when slighter, some or all of the lashes may be
distorted so as to rub against the cornea, without actually
turning inward, *distichiasis,trichiasis;* and these conditions

FIG. 43.

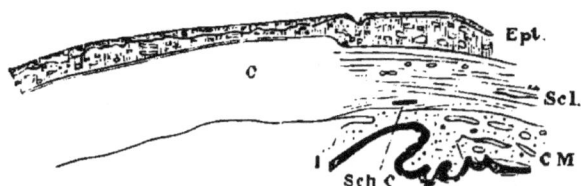

Section showing layer of new and vascular tissue (*pannus*) between
epithelium (*Ept.*) and cornea (*C*). *Scl.* Sclerotic. *C. M.* Ciliary muscle. *Sch. C.* Schlemm's canal. *I.* Iris. × about 10 diameters.

are often combined with pannus.   Pannus begins beneath
the upper lid, its vessels are superficial and continuous
with those of the conjunctiva, and are distributed in relation to the parts covered by the lid, not in reference to the
structure of the cornea, Fig. 44.   The proper corneal tissue suffers but little except where ulcers occur ; but when
the vascularity is extreme it may soften and bulge, even
without ulcerating.

[1] It is doubtful how far the development of pannus is due to friction,
or to extension of the trachoma over the sclerotic to the cornea.   Trachoma bodies may certainly be sometimes seen on the ocular conjunctiva.   Rachlmann states that the first sign of pannus consists in a collection of lymph-cells in the cornea beneath Bowman's membrane ;
subsequently a layer resembling adenoid tissue is found there containing
blood and lymphatic vessels.   That friction may alter the epithelium is
proved by certain cases in which the upper half of the cornea loses its
polish during a temporary papillary roughening of the upper lid.

Pannus disappears when the granular lid or the displacement of lashes is cured. Very severe and universal pannus is sometimes best treated by artificial inoculation with purulent ophthalmia, the inflammation being followed by obliteration of vessels and clearing of the cornea; but this

Fig. 44.

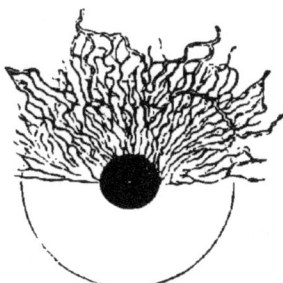

Pannus affecting upper half of cornea.

treatment needs great judgment and caution. More recently an infusion of the seeds known in commerce as "jequirity" (F. 40) has been introduced into Europe by de Wecker. It acts in much the same way as pus from purulent ophthalmia, but less severely; a very acute attack of diphtheritic or purulent ophthalmia with much swelling comes on a few hours after the infusion has been used, lasts a few days, and is followed by more or less shrinking of the trachoma bodies and of the vessels. It occasionally causes glandular swellings in the neck and considerable general disturbance. Repeated attacks may be induced with safety at intervals of a few weeks. Jequirity probably depends for its action upon a non-organized ferment such as is found in some other seeds. Sattler believed, from experiment, that a specific bacillus was the active agent, 1883, but his results have been negatived by Widmark, Klein, and several others; whilst an albuminous extract free from organisms, but possessing the peculiar properties of the infusion of the seed, has been separated by Warden and Waddell, Salomonsen, and others.[1] Much difference of opinion exists as to the clinical value of jequirity, owing to its having been often employed too strong and in unsuitable cases; it is not safe unless there are vessels on the cornea, and, safety apart, it is of little or no use if the conjunctiva be succulent and producing pus. It should be reserved for old, dry, granular lids with more or less pannus, and in such I have repeatedly had excellent results from it. Removal of a zone of conjunctiva and subconjunctival tissue, *syndectomy, peritomy*, from around the cornea is free from risk and sometimes very beneficial in old cases which, though severe, are not bad enough for inoculation. In old cases of granular disease, even where no complications have arisen, the upper lids often droop from relaxation of the loose conjunctiva above the tarsal cartilage, and the patient acquires a sleepy look.

For the cure of the displaced lashes and incurved eyelids we may: (1) repeatedly pull out the lashes with forceps; (2) extirpate all the lashes by cutting out a narrow strip of the marginal tissues of the lid; (3) attempt by operation to restore the lashes to their proper direction, Chap. XXII.; (4) employ electrolysis; for a few lashes I now use sewing needles, inserting several at a time into the hair follicles, and passing the current through all at once, by means of a broad eyelid forceps; such operations well selected and carefully performed give very good results; but as the inner surface of the lid continues to shorten, and this shortening tends to reproduce the original state of things, some of these procedures give only temporary relief.

Chronic conjunctivitis, chiefly of the lower lid, is a common disease, especially in elderly people. There is

[1] Mr. Martindale last year went to considerable trouble in trying to prepare such an active principle for me, but unfortunately the substance he separated was almost inert.

more or less soreness and smarting, redness and papillary roughness of the inner surface of the lid or of both lids, but very little discharge and no trachoma granulations. The caruncle is red and fleshy, as it is in all forms of palpebral conjunctivitis, and there is often soreness of the lids at the canthi. Lapis divinus is one of the best applications, and yellow ointment is sometimes useful (F. 5 and 12.)

Lachrymal conjunctivitis.—Troublesome chronic conjunctivitis, often complicated by small pustules at the roots of the lashes, or by chronic blepharitis, is a common result of lachrymal obstruction. Recently microörganisms of several kinds associated with pus-formation have been found in these little abscesses as well as in pus from the lachrymal sac (Widmark). Palpebral conjunctivitis of long standing with watering, gummy discharge, and more or less blepharitis, should, especially if confined to one eye, always lead to the suspicion of mucocele or chronic lachrymal abscess.

The rare disease described as Amyloid of the Conjunctiva seems scarcely to have been noticed in this country. Detailed accounts of its clinical and pathological characters may be found in Knapp's *Archives of Ophthalmology*, vols. x. and xi., and an excellent abstract of one of these papers appeared in the *Ophthalmic Review* for August, 1882.

Spring catarrh.—A peculiar and apparently specific chronic disease, affecting the conjunctiva of the globe and upper lid. In the former situation it takes the form of confluent broad patches of fleshy-looking thickening of a light brown-pink color, slightly overlapping the edge of the cornea for a considerable part of its circumference. In the latter situation it occurs as large, pale, flat-topped granulations, which are sometimes made to assume polygonal outlines by their pressure upon one another. They begin, like trachoma, at the inner and outer end of the lid : either variety may occur separately. The disease is worst in the warm part of the year, but it lasts in some cases many years, and gives but little trouble ; the growths on the upper lid do not produce pannus. The thickening is said to consist chiefly of epithelium, and not to affect the deep tissues.

Treatment by nitrate of silver is unnecessary ; occasional touching of the larger granulations by the galvano-cautery is the best treatment. Unlike trachoma, it occurs commonly in all classes of society, and is probably not contagious; hence its differential diagnosis in children at school is very important. Hitherto it has not been noticed much in this country, but probably it is not so rare as has been thought.

Conjunctivitis from drugs.—The local use of atropine sometimes gives rise to a peculiar inflammation of the conjunctiva and skin of the lid—*atropine irritation.* The conjunctiva of the lids becomes vascular, thickened, and even granular, and usually the skin is reddened, slightly excoriated, and somewhat shining. This effect of atropine is commonest in old people. Some persons are very susceptible, and cannot bear even a drop or two without suffering in some degree. Daturine and duboisin cause less irritation and may be used instead ; but it is better, if possible, not to use mydriatics at all for a few days. An ointment containing lead and zinc should be applied to the lids, and zinc or silver lotion to the conjunctiva ; sometimes glycerine suits better than ointment. In susceptible persons I have not found this peculiar inflammation prevented, either by the use of solutions made with antiseptics, or of solutions quite freshly made. Eserine sometimes causes identical symptoms. Congestion of the conjunctiva has been seen among those employed in aniline dye-works ; conjunctivitis was seen by Trousseau in 4 to 5 per cent. of patients treated for psoriasis by chrysophanic acid. If continued long enough, arsenic will in some persons produce redness and congestion of the conjunctiva. The action of jequirity is described on p. 121.

Primary shrinking of the conjunctiva (Pemphigus of Conjunctiva).—A very peculiar and rather rare disease, in which, with the phenomena of chronic inflammation, the whole conjunctiva slowly atrophies and contracts, owing to the formation in it of cicatricial tissue. During the earlier stages, the thickening of the tarsus and the congestion, with scarring of the palpheral conjunctiva, have sometimes led to the disease being mistaken for trachoma ; the two maladies are, however, quite distinct. Finally, the whole conjunctival sac disappears, and the free borders of the lids, fixed closely to the globe, are directly continuous with the cornea, which , irritated and dried by exposure and want of secretion, becomes opaque and covered with crusts—"xerosis." No treatment seems of any use.

In some of the cases there has been a history of general pemphigus, and reason to believe that the disease of the conjunctiva resulted from a modified form of pemphigus eruption.

CHAPTER VII.

DISEASES OF THE CORNEA.

A ULCERS AND NON-SPECIFIC INFLAMMATORY DISEASES.

INFLAMMATION of the cornea may be circumscribed or diffuse, and, though usually affecting the proper corneal tissue, may be limited to the epithelium on either of its surfaces. It may be a local process leading to formation of pus or to ulceration ; or the expression of a constitutional disease, such as inherited syphilis ; or it may form part, and perhaps only a minor part, of disease involving also the deeper parts of the eyeball—the iris (kerato-iritis) or sclerotic (sclero-keratitis), for example.

The different varieties of corneal ulceration and suppurative inflammation form a very large and important contingent of ophthalmic cases. The cornea, although a fibrous structure, is further removed from the bloodvessels than almost any other tissue, and its delicate surface is much exposed ; it is, therefore, extremely susceptible both to external irritants and to disturbances of nutrition from defective supply, or bad quality, of blood ; ulceration of the cornea always means deficient vitality. Lastly, its surface is so delicate, and its perfect transparency and regularity so important, that slight injuries and irritations are of more moment here than in any other part of the body.

When inflamed, the cornea always loses its transparency. If only the anterior epithelium be involved, the surface loses its polish, and looks like clear glass which has been breathed upon—"steamy," or finely pitted—a condition occurring in many states of disease. Thickening of the epithelium, and, still more, exudation into the corneal tissue, is shown by a white, grayish, or yellowish tint. If the corneal tissue be opalescent, while the surface is at the same time "steamy," the term "ground-glass" gives a good idea of the appearance, though, to make the simile correct, the glass ought to be milky throughout, as well as ground on the surface. Rapid suppurative inflammation is preceded by a stage of diffused opalescence; hence rapid opalescence is a sign of imminent danger in such diseases as purulent ophthalmia, severe burns, or paralysis of the fifth nerve. Fluorescence of the cornea has been seen as the result of the use of quinine lotions to the eye, and appears to be due to the deposit of crystals of quinine in the cornea.

Before describing the most important types of corneal ulcer, it is convenient to mention the principal *changes attendant on ulceration of the cornea* in general. An ulcer of the cornea is preceded by a stage of infiltration, and the inflamed spot is generally a little raised. After the centre of the spot has broken down into an ulcer, the extent, density, and color of the infiltration at its base and edges are important guides to its future course. The ulcer, when healed, leaves a hazy or opaque spot, *leucoma* if dense, *nebula* if faint, which is slight, and may disappear entirely if superficial, but will in part be permanent if the ulcer have been deep. These opacities are likely to clear, *cæteris paribus*, in proportion to the youth of the patient; time, also, is a very important element, nebulæ often continuing to clear slowly for years; local stimulation aids in the removal of the opacities, one of the best applications being the ointment of yellow oxide of mercury (F. 12, 13). Other modes of local stimulation have been recommended, such as tattooing, massage, electrolysis, and the use of various powders. Several successful attempts have been made to transplant circular portions of the clear cornea removed from the rabbit by a trephine, to replace portions of the human cornea rendered opaque by disease. To do this successfully it is necessary to leave behind Descemet's membrane in the diseased cornea (v. Hippel). Ulcers which have little or no infiltration often heal slowly, but leave a permanent facet or flattening; such facets destroy the regular curvature of the cornea, and thus often cause more damage to vision than a considerable degree of mere clouding. During repair bloodvessels often form and pass from the nearest part of the corneal edge to the ulcer, to disappear when healing is complete; phlyctenular ulcers, however, are vascular from the beginning. Corneal imperfections are, of course, most damaging to vision when placed over the pupil.

The chief *symptoms* of corneal ulceration are : (1) *photophobia*, with its consequence, spasm of the orbicularis, *blepharospasm;* (2) *congestion;* (3) *pain.* All three symptoms vary extremely in degree in different cases. As a broad rule with many exceptions, we may say that tolerance of light is worse in children than in adults, worse with superficial than with deep ulcers, and worse in persons who are strumous and irritable than in those with healthy tissues and good tone. Photophobia should always lead to a careful inspection of the cornea, and we shall then sometimes be surprised to find how slight a change gives rise to this symptom in its severest form. The degree of congestion varies with the seat and cause of the ulcer, and with the patient's age, being usually greatest in adults. The visible congestion is, as in iritis, due especially to distention of the subconjunctival twigs of the *ciliary zone*, Fig. 25, Ant. Cil., and Fig. 28, but there is often congestion of the conjunctival vessels as well. In some forms of marginal ulcer, only those vessels which feed the diseased part are congested. Great pain in and around the eye often attends the earlier stages of corneal abscess, and is common in many acute ulcers ; as a symptom, it, of course, always needs careful attention ; it is generally relieved by those local measures which are best for the disease itself.

Types of Corneal Ulceration.

(1) One of the simplest forms is the *small central ulcer* often seen in young children. A little grayish-white spot forms in the central part of the cornea, at first elevated and bluntly conical, afterward showing a minute shallow crater ; the congestion and photophobia vary, but are often slight. The ulcer is usually single, but it is apt to recur in the same or the other eye. The infiltration often extends into the corneal tissue, and the residual opacity remains for a long time, if not permanently. The patients are always badly nourished. In most cases the ulcer quickly heals, but now and then the infiltration passes into an abscess, or a spreading, suppurating ulcer.

(2) Less commonly we meet with a central ulcer, or a succession of ulcers, of a much more chronic character, and attended with little or no infiltration. After lasting for months the loss of tissue is only partly repaired, and a shallow depression or a flat facet is left with but little loss of transparency. Some of the best examples are seen in anæmic or strumous patients with granular lids of long standing.

(3) *Phlyctenular ophthalmia* and *phlyctenular ulcers* of cornea (phlyctenulæ, herpes corneæ, pustular ophthalmia, marginal keratitis, " strumous ophthalmia ").—The formation of little papules, or pustules, on or near the corneal margin is exceedingly common, either independently or as a complication of some existing ophthalmia. Although there are many varieties and degrees of phlyctenular inflammation in respect to the seat, extent, and course of the disease, the following features are common to all : They

show a strong tendency to recur during several years; they are seldom seen in very young children, and comparatively seldom after middle life; they occur so often in strumous subjects, that we are justified in suspecting scrofulous tendencies in all who suffer much from them; ophthalmia tarsi is often seen in the same patients; the first attack often follows closely after an acute exanthem, and especially after measles; the cases are much influenced by climate and weather, and their condition often varies extremely from day to day without making either progress or regress.

An elevated spot, like a papule, commonly about the size of a small mustard-seed, is seen either on the white of the eye near the cornea, or upon, or just within, the corneal border. It is preceded and accompanied by localized congestion. Its top sometimes becomes as yellow as that of an acne pustule, but more often when seen it has become abraded and aphthous-looking. Pustules at a little distance from the cornea, Fig. 45, although generally larger than those seated on the corneal border, occasion less photophobia and are more easily cured. Pustules at the corneal border, though often very small, cause troublesome, and even very severe, photophobia; they are troublesome in proportion rather to their number than their size, and if so numerous as to form a ring around the cornea, their cure is often very tedious.

A pustule is always liable, even when it has begun on the conjunctiva, to advance as a superficial ulcer on to the cornea, though it never extends in the opposite direction over the sclerotic. Such a *phlyctenular ulcer*, if it do not stop near the corneal border, will make, in an almost radial direction, for the centre, carrying with it a leash of vessels which lie upon the track of opacity left in the wake of the ulcer, Fig. 46. Finally, the ulceration stops, the vessels dwindle and disappear, but the path of opacity seldom clears up entirely. The term *recurrent vascular ulcer* is used when such ulcers are solitary ; but they are often multiple as well as recurrent, and then, in the end, we find the cornea covered by a thin, irregular network of superficial vessels on a patchy, uneven, hazy surface, the socalled *"phlyctenular pannus."*

FIG. 45.

FIG 46.

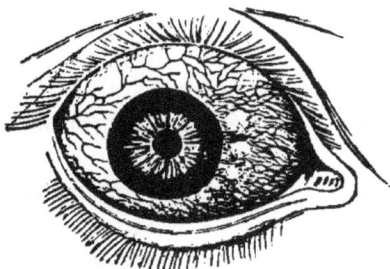

Phlyctenular ophthalmia, conjunctival form. (Dalrymple.)

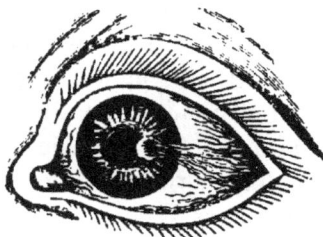

Phlyctenular ulcer. (Travers.)

A common variety of phlyctenular inflammation, aptly called *marginal conjunctivitis*, perhaps allied to the *"spring catarrh"* of Continental authors, occurs in the form of a slight, granular-looking, often vascular, swelling, beginning crescentially above or below, but often extending all around the edge of the cornea. If the process continue, the cornea is invaded by a densely vascular, superficially ulcerated, and yet thickened zone. It is to be distinguished from a deeper variety of marginal keratitis alluded to at p. 140.

In another variety a single pustule just within the border of the cornea ulcerates deeply, becomes surrounded by swollen, softened, suppurating tissue, and may perforate : such cases are seen in weakly women and strumous children. In very rare cases, what appears to be an ordinary conjunctival pustule, persists, grows deeply, and may even perforate the sclerotic in the form of an ulcer; or it may infiltrate the sclerotic and ciliary body beneath, forming a soft, semi-suppurating tumor, whence the inflammation is likely to spread to the vitreous and destroy the eye. Stopping short of these extreme results, such a case forms one type of episcleritis. Chapter IX.

Occasionally a large, sometimes solitary blister forms under the anterior corneal epithelium; it rises quickly, is attended by severe neuralgic pain, which is often relieved when the vesicle bursts, about a day after the onset. The condition is liable to relapse in the same cornea, and seems often, though not always, to have its origin in a superficial injury. See Abrasion.

The corneal changes produced by the friction of granular lids have been considered under that subject. The pannus of granular lids usually differs from the "phlyctenular pannus" just mentioned in being more uniform and worse beneath the upper lid, Fig. 44; any doubt is dispelled by everting the lid. But it must be borne in mind that ulceration of the cornea often occurs as a complication of trachomatous pannus.

(4) In old persons a crescentic ulcer sometimes forms in the situation of, or actually upon, an arcus senilis. Though these cases generally do well, they should be watched, for at first they may be indistinguishable from more serious forms about to be described.

(5) *Infective corneal ulcers.*—Several varieties of dangerous corneal ulcer may be grouped together as probably depending upon local infection, and there seems to be no doubt that destructive inflammation of the cornea may occur *in utero.* Differing widely in rapidity and depth, they agree in being often the result of slight injuries by chips of metal, beards of corn, etc., in tending to spread at one border, whilst healing at another, in the absence of "vessels of repair," such as are usually formed during the

healing of other ulcers, and in being often complicated with hypopyon. Fig. 48.

The most important variety is the acute serpiginous ulcer, which begins as a gray spot showing slight ulceration, and having a sharply-cut border, *one part of which is more*

FIG. 47.

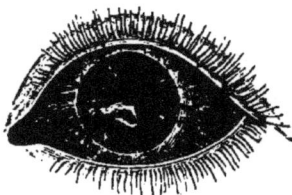

Acute serpiginous ulcer of cornea with crescentic border of infiltration. (From a sketch by Dr. Herbert Habershon.)

densely opaque than the rest, Fig. 47 ; this infiltrated, advancing edge is the distinguishing mark of the ulcer.   If the ulcer have lasted for some little time, a portion of its edge, usually that nearest the corneal border, will be more or less filled up ; in such a state the most conspicuous part of the ulcer is crescentic. Fig. 47.   Unless quickly checked, the process often spreads widely, eats deeply, becomes complicated with iritis and hypopyon, and leads to perforation of the cornea.

Probably many cases of corneal abscess and acute suppurating ulcer of less distinct type than the above are, like it, due to infection.

Abscess may occur at any age, but, like serpiginous ulcer, is commonest in those who are old, underfed, or damaged by drink ; but the little gray central ulcers of children may go on to abscess.   Abscess usually forms at the centre of the corneal area as a small, round, raised spot, with great pain and congestion; rapidly enlarging, it usually bursts forward, leaving a round ulcer covered with lymphy pus, but it may perforate the hinder surface of the cornea; hypopyon often occurs. The purulent infiltration may spread rapidly and destroy almost the whole cornea.

Hypopyon signifies a collection of pus or puro-lymph at the lowest part of the anterior chamber ; its upper boundary is usually, but not always, level. Fig. 48. It may occur with any ulcer, whether deep or not, which is accompanied

FIG. 48.

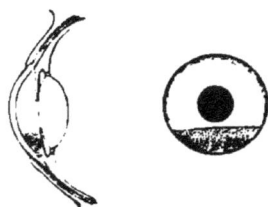

Hypopyon, seen from the front, and in section, to show that the pus is behind the cornea.

FIG. 49.

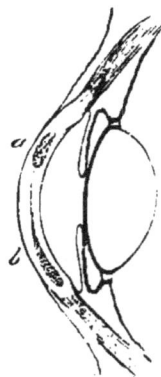

a. Abscess. b. Onyx.

by purulent infiltration of the surrounding cornea ; or with corneal abscess. The pus may be derived either from an abscess breaking through the posterior surface of the cornea, or from suppuration of the epithelium covering Descemet's membrane, or from the surface of the iris. Simple iritis now and then gives rise to hypopyon. The diameter of the anterior chamber being rather greater than the apparent diameter of the clear cornea, a very small hypopyon may be hidden behind the overlapping edge of the sclerotic. In some cases of severe corneal suppuration (*a*, Fig. 49) the pus sinks down between the lamellæ of the cornea (*b*). To this condition the term *onyx* is applied and should be limited, though it is sometimes used in other senses. The term, however, may very well be discarded. Onyx and hypopyon often co-exist, and then the distinction between them can hardly be made without tapping the anterior chamber. Hypopyon, if liquid, will, but onyx will not, change its position if the patient lies down ; as, however, the pus of hypopyon is often gelatinous or fibrinous, this test loses much of its value. The distinction can sometimes be made by means of oblique illumination, if the cornea in front of an hypopyon remain clear.

Chronic and subacute serpiginous ulcers are seen from time to time spreading for weeks or even months. They sometimes have the form above described, Fig. 47, but occasionally the ulceration takes the form of a stem with irregular broad buds or branches not unlike a liverwort, the disease being superficial from beginning to end, and showing no tendency to the formation of pus, but spoiling the surface of the cornea—*dendritic creeping ulcer.*

Treatment of ulcers of the cornea.

The principles of local treatment for the various types of corneal ulceration are : (1) To favor healing by keeping the surface at rest. (2) To relieve pain, photophobia, and severe congestion. (3) To promote absorption of pus, whether in the corneal layers or in the anterior chamber. (4) To check the spread of local infection by scraping, actual cautery, and antiseptics. (5) By incision to evacuate pus between the corneal layers (abscess), or in the anterior chamber (hypopyon), when abundant or increasing. (6) To stimulate the surface of ulcers which have begun to heal, or of indolent ones which are stationary. (7) Counter-irritation by a seton in certain chronic cases. (8) When the corneal ulceration is caused by granular lids, or associated with any form of acute ophthalmia, the treatment of the conjunctiva is usually more important than that of the cornea.

Often we have no difficulty in deciding upon the treatment; but in some cases, especially the severer ones, much judgment is needed, and it is sometimes impossible to predict with certainty what measures will be best.

Ulcers of the cornea are so often a sign of bad health that every care should be bestowed upon the patient's general state.

Treating the matter clinically, we shall find that local stimulation (6) is best for a large number of the cases as they first come under notice, including phlyctenular cases, chronic superficial ulcers of various kinds, and even many recent ulcers if not threatening to suppurate. As a general rule, this plan alone is not suitable when there is much photophobia; but exceptions occur, especially in old-standing cases. The most convenient remedy is the ointment of amorphous yellow oxide of mercury (F. 12 and 13), of which a piece about as large as a hemp-seed is to be put inside the eyelids once or twice a day. If smarting continue for more than half an hour, the ointment should be washed out with warm water; and if the irritability increase after a few days' use of the ointment, the preparation must be weakened or discontinued. The same ointment, combined with atropine, gives excellent results in cases of superficial ulcer with much photophobia (F. 14). Calomel flicked into the eye daily or less often is also an admirable remedy. Nitrate of silver in the form of solid mitigated stick (F. 1) is useful if carefully applied to large conjunctival pustules, and occasionally to indolent corneal ulcers; its use, however, needs some skill, and is seldom really necessary: solutions of from 5 to 10 grains to the ounce may be cautiously used by the surgeon instead of the yellow ointment, and are particularly valuable in old vascular ulcers and in ulcers with conjunctivitis. When in doubt it is best to depend for a few days on atropine alone, used once or twice a day.

Division of the outer canthus by scissors is sometimes employed for children with severe photophobia, but is only of temporary use; free douching of the head and face, by putting the child's head under a tap of cold water, is sometimes successful. In all cases of corneal disease attended with intolerance of light, the patient is to wear a large shade over *both* eyes, or, better, a pair of "goggles;" a little patch over one eye does not relieve photophobia. Many a child is kept within doors, to the injury of its health, who, with suitable protection, can go out daily without the least detriment to its eyes.

In chronic and relapsing cases, with photophobia and irritability, where other methods have had a fair trial, a seton gives the best results, whether the eye be much congested or not. The silk must be very thick ; the punctures should be at least an inch apart, and be so placed that the scars may be hidden by the hair on the temple or behind the ear. The seton is to be moved daily, and if acting badly may be dressed with savin ointment ; it should be worn at least six weeks. Severe inflammation, and even abscess, sometimes sets in a few days after the insertion of the thread, and in very rare cases secondary bleeding has occurred from a branch of the temporal artery. To avoid wounding this artery the skin is to be held well away from the head.

Very severe, recent phlyctenular cases are occasionally difficult to influence, and remain practically "blind" with spasm of the lids for weeks. There is seldom any risk, provided that the cornea be examined at intervals of a few days, and in the end such cases do well. Calomel dusted on the cornea sometimes helps more than any other local measure, and change of air, especially to the seaside, frequently effects a more rapid cure than any local treatment.

Cases for which the stimulating treatment is suitable seldom need the eye to be bandaged, though, as mentioned, they often need a shade or goggles.

The remaining methods are applicable to the severer forms of ulceration—the serpiginous ulcer, deep suppurating ulcers, abscess, and generally all ulcers with hypopyon, and all acute ulcers in elderly persons. In many cases of severe type, at an early stage, the pain may be relieved and the ulceration stopped by *very hot* fomentations (of water, poppy-head, or belladonna) to the eyelids for twenty minutes every two hours, the eye being tied up in the intervals with a large pad of cotton-wool and bandage, and atropine used two or three times a day; the patient must rest, have good food, often with alcohol, and take quinine, or bark and ammonia. If, nevertheless, the ulceration spread, or an hypopyon form or increase, incision of the cornea and the use of topical remedies are called for. Of such remedies the best seems to be the actual cautery, preceded by scraping with a sharp spoon, and followed by iodoform or boracic acid. The actual cautery may be either the fine galvano-cautery, or a very small Paquelin; the edge of the ulcer is to be well burnt before the heat is applied to the floor, and I like to burn a little beyond the opaque edge.

Iodoform, which is probably the most useful corneal antiseptic, may be used in powder or strong ointment (20 or 30 gr. to ʒj; F. 19), freely three times a day or more; it gives no pain. Boracic acid may be used in the same way; perchloride of mercury, of the strength of 1 in 1000, has also been used in cases of dendritic creeping ulcer.

Hypopyon, if large, Fig. 48, or increasing, must be let out, and, on the whole, for most cases, Saemisch's plan of cutting through the cornea quite across the ulcer is the best for this purpose, because if there be pent-up pus in the cornea this section will allow its removal at the same time;

the section should be made with a Graefe's cataract knife, Fig. 154, entered with its back toward the lens at one border of the ulcer, carried across the anterior chamber, and brought out at the other side of the ulcer. It is sometimes an advantage to keep up leakage by reopening the wound with a probe for a few days. Corneal section also often instantly relieves the severe pain of these cases, and it has been strongly advocated for this purpose by Mr. Teale and others. The section may sometimes be made with equally good effect in the lower part of the cornea away from the ulcer. If the ulcer have already perforated and the eye be worth saving, iridectomy should be done, either by drawing the prolapsed iris freely through the perforation and cutting it off, or by making an incision in a sound part of the cornea. I believe that careful scraping and burning will do much to reduce the severity of infective corneal ulcers.

Some of these ulcers are accompanied by a good deal of muco-purulent conjunctivitis, for which a ten-grain solution of nitrate of silver, painted inside the lower lid with a brush about once a day, may generally be used ; its effect must be watched, and its employment discontinued if it increase irritability.

Use of atropine and eserine in severe ulcers of the cornea. Formerly either atropine or belladonna lotion was used for nearly every case of severe corneal ulcer. Atropine often relieves pain, prevents or lessens iritis, and probably lessens engorgement of the vessels of the iris and ciliary region ; it may generally be used, sparingly, as an auxiliary in suppurating and serpiginous cases. But atropine tends to increase any existing conjunctival inflammation, and by narrowing the area and contracting the vessels of the iris, it probably retards, rather than hastens, the absorption of pus in the anterior chamber. During the last few years eserine has come into use for certain cases which would formerly have been treated chiefly by atropine. The deep, funnel-shaped, suppurating ulcer which sometimes develops from a marginal pustule (p. 131) is the most suitable for treatment by eserine, whether complicated with hypopyon or not. Although in a bad case of this sort, hot fomentations and the compress are necessary, I have seen a certain number of less severe ones recover quickly under eserine alone, used about six times a day (F. 35). Eserine probably acts partly by enlarging the surface of the iris and dilating the ciliary arteries, and thus favoring absorption ; possibly, also, it acts locally on the ulcerated surface. There is no clinical proof that eserine lowers tension unless this were previously increased, as it seldom is in corneal ulcers. Eserine causes congestion of the deep vessels of the ciliary region, and after a time increases the photophobia and irritability of the eye : these symptoms usually coincide with disappearance of the corneal infiltration and the commencement of vascularization of the ulcer, and when this stage is reached the eserine should be discontinued

The alternate use of heat and cold for short periods is recommended in some obstinate cases of corneal ulceration, the object being to improve nutrition by causing frequent changes in the quantity and rate of the blood-supply.

Rapidly destructive ulceration of the cornea is common in children dying of meningitis, and is probably due to the exposure and drying associated with the patients' semi-comatose state, but its occasional limitation to one eye suggests the thought that it may be in part directly due to trophic influence. Dr. Barlow tells me that very similar ulceration may occur in the severe exhaustion following infantile diarrhœa. Ulceration from exposure may also occur in severe cases of exophthalmic goitre. In all the above cases the ulceration usually takes place between the centre and the lower edge, the part of the cornea which is last covered when the lids are closed and first exposed when they are opened.

General dense opacity of the cornea occasionally comes on with extreme quickness in infants who are recovering from purulent ophthalmia. If it lead to destructive ulceration, the term *kerato-malacia* is not inappropriate; the opacity sometimes, however, clears up in a remarkable and very unexpected manner. I have seen two such recoveries under the use of eserine.

Conical cornea.—In this condition the central part of the cornea very slowly bulges forward, forming a bluntly conical curve. The focal length of the affected part of the cornea is thereby shortened, and the eye becomes myopic. The curvature, however, is not uniform, and hence irregular astigmatism complicates the myopia. Chapter XX.

The disease, which is rare, occurs chiefly in young adults, especially women, and is often associated with chronic dyspepsia; its onset is sometimes dated from a severe, exhausting illness; it appears to be due to defective nutrition of that part of the cornea which is furthest from the bloodvessels. In advanced cases the protrusion of the cornea is very evident, whether viewed from the front or from the side, but slight degrees are less easily distinguished from ordinary myopic astigmatism. In high degrees the apex of the cone, which is situated rather below the centre of the cornea, often becomes nebulous. The disease may progress to a high degree, or stop before great damage has been done. Concave glasses alone are of little use; but they are sometimes useful in combination with a screen perforated by a narrow slit or small central hole, which allows the light to pass only through the centre, or through some one meridian of the cornea. In advanced cases an operation must be performed which, by substituting a contracting cicatrix for the corneal tissue at or near the apex of the cone, shall lead to a diminution of the curvature. Chapter XXII.

B. Diffuse Keratitis.

Syphilitic, interstitial, parenchymatous, or "strumous" keratitis.

In this disease the cornea in its whole thickness undergoes a chronic inflammation, which shows no tendency either to the formation of pus or to ulceration. After several months the inflammatory products are either wholly or in great part absorbed, and the transparency of the cornea restored in proportion.

The changes in the cornea are usually preceded for a few days by some ciliary congestion and watering. Then a faint cloudiness is seen in one or more large patches, and the surface, if carefully looked at, is found to be "steamy" (p. 126). These nebulous areas may lie in any part of the

Fig. 50.

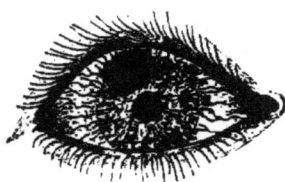

Interstitial keratitis.

cornea. In from two to about four weeks the whole cornea has usually passed into a condition of white haziness with steamy surface, of which the term "ground-glass" gives the best idea. Even now, however, careful inspection, especially by focal light, will show that the opacity is by

no means uniform, that it shows many whiter spots, or
larger denser clouds, scattered among the general mist; in
very severe cases the whole cornea is quite opaque and the
iris hidden ; but, as a rule, the iris and pupil can be seen,
though very imperfectly. Fig. 50. In many cases iritis
occurs and posterior synechiæ are formed. Bloodvessels
derived from branches of the ciliary vessels, Fig. 25, are
often formed in the layers of the cornea, Fig. 51; they are
small but set thickly, and in patches; as they are covered
by a certain thickness of hazy cornea, their bright scarlet
is toned down to a dull reddish-pink color ("salmon
patch" of Hutchinson). The separate vessels are visible
only if magnified, when we see that the trunks, passing
from the border, divide at acute angles into very numerous
twigs, lying close to each other, and taking a nearly straight
course toward the centre. Fig. 52. These salmon patches
when small are often crescentic, but if large tend to assume

FIG. 51.

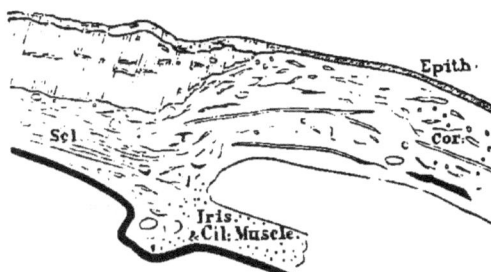

Thickening of cornea and formation of vessels in its layers in
syphilitic keratitis. Subconjunctival tissue thickened. × about 10
diameters. Compare with Fig. 36.

a sector-shape. In another type the vascularity begins as
a narrow fringe of looped vessels which are continuous
with the loop-plexus of the corneal margin, Fig. 53, *com-*
pare Fig. 25, *l*, and gradually extend from above and below

toward the centre. The vessels in these cases are somewhat more superficial, and the corneal tissue in which they
lie is always swollen by infiltration. This type, which forms
a variety of "*marginal keratitis,*" *compare* p. 131, usually

FIG. 52.

FIG. 53.

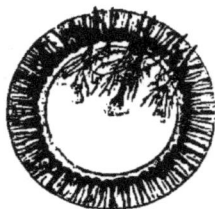

Vessels in interstitial
keratitis.

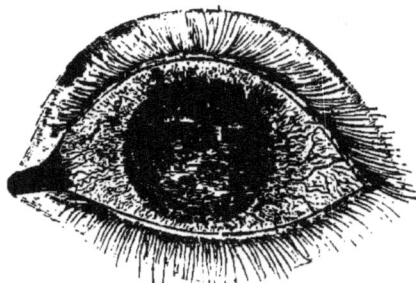

Marginal vascular keratitis.

occurs in syphilitic subjects, but I believe that some of the
patients are at the same time strumous. A similar condition, sometimes leading to secondary glaucoma, occurs now
and then in elderly people. In extreme cases of either
type of vascular keratitis the vessels cover the whole
cornea, except a small central island.

The degree of congestion and the subjective symptoms
in syphilitic keratitis vary very much; as a general rule,
there is but moderate photophobia and pain, but when the
ciliary congestion is great these symptoms are sometimes
very severe and protracted.

The attack can be shortened and its severity lessened by
treatment; but the disease is always slow, and from six to
twelve months may be taken as a fair average for its duration from beginning to end. Very bad cases, with excessively dense opacity, sometimes continue to improve for
several years, and may recover an unexpected degree of

sight. Perfect recovery of transparency is less common,
even in moderate cases, than is sometimes supposed, but the
slight degree of haziness which so often remains does not
much affect the sight. The epithelium usually becomes
smooth before the cornea becomes transparent; but in
severe cases irregularities of surface may remain, and render
the diagnosis difficult. Very minute vessels (as in Fig. 52)
seen by direct ophthalmoscopic examination with a high
+ lens (p. 81), nearly straight, and branching at acute
angles with short abrupt rectangular bends here and there,
are often left, and when found are good evidence of previous interstitial keratitis.

Syphilitic keratitis is almost always symmetrical, though
an interval of a few weeks commonly separates its onset in
the two eyes : rarely the interval is several months, a year,
or even more. It generally occurs between about the ages
of six and fifteen ; sometimes as early as two and a half or
three years ; in rare instances it may set in after forty ;
many of the very late cases are severe and complicated.
If it occur very early the attack is generally mild. Relapses of greater or less severity are common. Not only
does iritis occur with tolerable frequency, but we occasionally meet with deep-seated inflammation, in the ciliary
region, giving rise either to secondary glaucoma, or to
stretching and elongation of the globe in the ciliary zone,
or to softening and shrinking of the eyeball.[1] Dots of
opacity may sometimes be seen on the back of the cornea
at its lower part, before the cornea itself is much altered :
sometimes, too, the interstitial exudation is much more
dense at the lower part of the cornea than elsewhere.

---

[1] When the cornea has cleared, ophthalmoscopic signs of past choroiditis (Chap. XII.) are often found at the fundus. The choroiditis often
dates much further back than the keratitis, but there is little doubt
that it may relapse, or occur as an accompaniment of the corneal disease. (Chap. XXIII.)

Syphilitic keratitis in strumous children often shows more irritability, photophobia, and conjunctival congestion, than in others; but it is very seldom that ulceration occurs, and although in the worst cases the cornea becomes softened and yellowish, and for a time seems likely to give way, actual perforation is one of the rarest events. Pannus from granular disease may coexist with syphilitic keratitis.

TREATMENT.—A long but mild course of mercury is certainly of use. It is customary to give iodide of potassium also, and it probably has some influence. If the patients be very anæmic, and they often are so, iron, or the syrup of its iodide, is more advisable than iodide of potassium as an adjunct to the mercury. Locally it is well to use atropine by routine until the disease has reached its height, on the ground that iritis may be present. Setons in my experience are seldom of use; but in cases attended by severe and prolonged photophobia and ciliary congestion iridectomy is occasionally followed by rapid improvement; this operation, however, is seldom needed or justifiable unless there be decided glaucomatous symptoms. When all inflammatory symptoms have subsided, the local use of yellow ointment of calomel (F. 11 and 12) appears to aid the absorption of the residual opacity.

The form of keratitis above described is caused by *inherited* syphilis. In rare cases it has been seen as the result of secondary *acquired* syphilis. Other cases of diffuse keratitis occur in which syphilis has no share, but they are seldom symmetrical, nor do they occur early in life. That diffuse, chronic keratitis, affecting both eyes of children and adolescents, is, when well characterized, almost invariably the result of hereditary syphilis, is proved by abundant evidence. A large proportion of its subjects show some of the other signs of hereditary syphilis in the teeth, skin, ears (deafness), physiognomy, mouth, or bones. When the patients themselves show no such signs, a history of infantile syphilis in the patient or in some brothers and sisters, or of acquired syphilis in one or other parent, may often be obtained.[1] That this keratitis stands in no causal relation to struma, is clear, because the ordinary signs of struma are not found oftener in its victims than in other children, because persons who are decidedly strumous do not suffer from this keratitis more often than others, and because the forms of eye disease which are universally recognized as "strumous" (ophthalmia tarsi, phlyctenular disease, and relapsing ulcers of cornea) very seldom accompany this diffuse keratitis. Illustrations of the teeth in inherited syphilis are given in Fig. 164, Chap. XXIII.

Other Forms of Keratitis.

Inflammation of the cornea forms a more or less conspicuous feature in several diseases where the primary, or the principal, seat of mischief lies in another part of the eye. It is important for purposes of diagnosis to compare these *secondary or complicating forms of keratitis* with the primary diseases of the cornea already described.

In iritis the lower half of the cornea often becomes steamy, and more or less hazy. In some cases a number of small, separate, opaque dots are seen on the posterior elastic lamina (Descemet's membrane), often so minute as to need magnifying. These dots are sharply defined, large ones looking very like minute drops of cold gravy-fat, the smallest like grains of gray sand; in cases of long standing they may be either very white or highly pigmented. They are generally arranged in a triangle, with its apex toward the centre and its base at the lower margin of the cornea,

---

[1] I have found other personal evidence of inherited syphilis in 54 per cent. of my cases of interstitial keratitis. and evidence from the family history in 14 per cent. more ; total 68 per cent. ; and in most of the remaining 32 per cent. there have been strong reasons to suspect it.

the smallest dots being near the centre, Fig. 54 ; but in
some cases, sympathetic ophthalmitis, especially, the dots
are scattered over the whole cornea.   They are, of course,

FIG. 54.

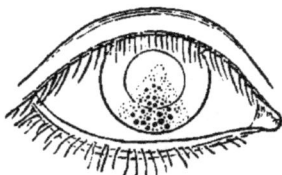

Keratitis punctata.   (From a sketch by Dr. Herringham.)

difficult to detect in proportion as the corneal tissue itself
is hazy.

The term *keratitis punctata* is used to express this accumulation of dots on the back of the cornea, and by some
authors is allowed to include also allied cases in which
small spots with hazy outlines are seen in the cornea proper.
Keratitis punctata is, almost without exception, secondary
to some disease of the cornea, iris, or choroid and vitreous.
But a few cases are seen, chiefly in young adults, where
the corneal dots form the principal, if not the sole, visible
change ; the number of such cases diminishes, however, in
proportion to the care with which other lesions are sought.

It is now and then difficult to say, in a mixed case,
whether the iritis or keratitis have been the initial change;
but when this doubt arises the cornea has generally been
the starting-point; and with care we are seldom at a loss
to decide whether the case be one of syphilitic keratitis
with iritis, or sclerotitis with corneal mischief and iritis,
or of primary iritis with secondary haze of cornea.   See
Chaps. VIII. and IX.

Slight loss of transparency of the cornea occurs in most
cases of *glaucoma*.   The earliest change is a fine, uniform

steaminess of the epithelium. In very severe, acute cases, the cornea becomes hazy throughout, though not in a high degree. The same haze occurs in chronic cases of long standing with great increase of tension, but the epithelial "steaminess" often then gives place to a coarser "pitting" with little depressions and elevations (vesicles), especially on the part which is uncovered by the lids.

In buphthalmos (hydrophthalmos) the corneal changes are often very conspicuous, although not essential. In this rare and very peculiar malady there is general and slowly progressive enlargement of cornea, anterior part of sclerotic, and iris, together with extreme deepening of the anterior chamber and slight increase of tension. The cornea often becomes hazy and semi-opaque. The disease, which may, perhaps, be looked upon as a congenital or infantile form of glaucoma, is either present at birth or comes on in early infancy, and usually causes blindness. Operative treatment generally fails, but eserine is said to be useful. See Glaucoma.

A rare but peculiar form of corneal disease, generally seen in elderly persons, is the *transverse calcareous film*, forming an oval patch of light-gray opacity, which runs almost horizontally across the cornea. It lies beneath the epithelium, and consists of minute crystalline granules chiefly calcareous.

Arcus senilis is caused by fatty degeneration of the corneal tissue just within its margin, Fig. 55. It first appears beneath the upper lid, next beneath the lower, thus forming two narrow, white or yellowish crescents, the horns of which finally meet at the sides of the cornea ; it always begins, and remains most intense, on a line slightly within the sclero-corneal junction, and the degeneration is most marked in the superficial layers of the cornea beneath the anterior elastic lamina ; in other words, the change is greatest at the part most influenced by the marginal blood-

vessels.   Arcus, though seldom seen except in senile persons, is not found to interfere with the union of a wound
carried through it, though the tissue of the arcus is often
very tough and hard.

FIG. 55.

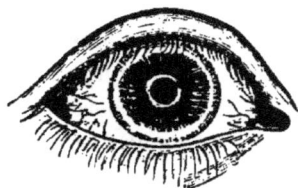

Arcus senilis.   (From a sketch by Dr. Herringham.)

Less regular forms of arcus are seen as the result of prolonged or relapsing inflammations near the corneal border,
whether ulcerative or not.   It is generally easy to distinguish such an arcus, because the opacity is denser and more
patchy, and its outlines are less regular than in the primary
form; when arcus is seen unusually early in life it is generally of this inflammatory kind, for simple arcus is rare
below forty.

Opacity of a very characteristic kind is likely to follow
the use of a lotion containing *lead* when the surface of the
cornea is abraded.   An insoluble, densely opaque, very
white film of lead salts is precipitated on, and adheres
very firmly to, the ulcerated surface; the spot is sharply
defined, and looks like white paint.   If precipitated on a
deep and much inflamed ulcer, the layer of tissue to which
the film adheres is often thrown off, but when there is only
a superficial abrasion or ulcer, the lead adheres very firmly,
and can only be scraped off imperfectly.   But even in the
latter cases the film is probably, after a time, thrown off or
worn off, if we may judge by the fact that nearly all the
lead opacities which come under notice are comparatively

new. The practical lesson is never to use a lead lotion for the eye when there is any suspicion that the corneal surface is broken.

The prolonged use of *nitrate of silver*, whether in a weak or strong form, is sometimes followed by a dull, brownish-green, permanent discoloration of the conjunctiva, and even the cornea may become slightly stained.

CHAPTER VIII.

IRITIS.

INFLAMMATION of the iris may be caused by certain specific blood diseases, especially syphilis; or may be the expression of a tendency to relapses of inflammation in certain tissues under the influence largely of climate and weather—*rheumatic iritis;* it often occurs in the course of ulcers, and of wounds and other injuries of the cornea; also with diffuse keratitis and sclerotitis. Iritis also forms a very important part of the remarkable and serious disease known as sympathetic ophthalmitis.

Acute iritis, whatever its cause, is shown by a change in the color of the iris, indistinctness or "muddiness" of its texture, diminution of its mobility and the formation of adhesions (*posterior synechiæ*) between its posterior (uveal) surface and the capsule of the lens; there is, besides, in most cases, a dulness of the whole iris and pupil, caused by muddiness of the aqueous humor, and partly, also, by slight corneal changes. The eyeball is congested and sight usually dimmed. There may or may not be pain, photophobia, and lachrymation.

The congestion is often almost confined to a zone about one-twelfth or one-eighth of an inch wide, which surrounds the cornea, its color pink (not raw red), the vessels small, radiating, nearly straight, and lying beneath the conjunctiva, *ciliary or circumcorneal congestion,* Fig. 28. These are the episcleral branches of the anterior ciliary arteries,

Fig. 25. Quite the same congestion is seen in many other conditions, e. g., corneal ulceration; whilst on the other hand, in some cases of iritis, the superficial (conjunctival) vessels are engorged also, especially in their anterior divisions, which are chiefly offshoots of the ciliary system. We therefore never diagnose iritis from the character of the congestion alone; but the disease being proved by the other symptoms, the kind and degree of congestion help us to judge of its severity.

The altered color of the iris is due to its congestion, and the effusion of lymph and serum into its substance; a blue or gray iris becomes greenish, a brown one is but little changed. The inflammatory swelling of the iris also accounts both for the blurring (muddiness) of its beautifully reticulated structure, and for the sluggishness of movement noticed in the early period. Lymph is soon thrown out at one or more spots on its posterior surface, and still further hampers its movements by adhering to the lens capsule; and most cases do not come under notice till such synechiæ have formed. The quantity of solid exudation, whether on the hinder surface or into the structure of the iris, varies much; it is usually greatest in syphilitic iritis, when distinct nodules of pink or yellowish color are sometimes seen projecting from the front surface, generally close to the pupil. In rare cases pus thrown off by the iris into the aqueous subsides and forms hypopyon; a corresponding deposit of blood constitutes hyphæmia. Firm adhesions to the lens capsule may be present without much evidence of exudation into the structure of the iris. Exudative changes are usually most abundant at the inner ring of the iris, where its capillary vessels are far the most numerous. Fig. 56.

Apparent discoloration of the iris is, however, often due entirely to suspension of blood-corpuscles, or inflammatory products in the aqueous humor; sometimes this altered fluid coagulates into a slightly turbid gelatinous mass,

7*

which almost fills the chamber ("spongy exudation"). The aqueous sometimes becomes yellow without losing transparency.

FIG. 56.

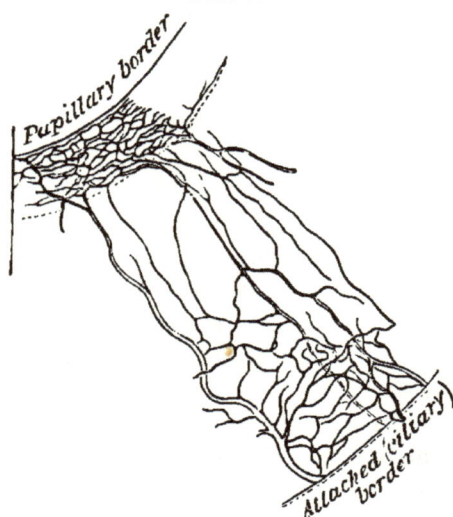

Vessels of human iris artificially injected; capillaries most numerous at pupillary border, and next at ciliary border.

The tension of the eyeball, usually unaltered in acute iritis, may be a little increased; rarely it is considerably diminished, and in such cases there are generally other peculiarities.

The condition of the pupil alone is diagnostic in all except very mild or incipient cases of iritis. It is sluggish or motionless, and not quite round; it is also rather smaller than its fellow (supposing the iritis to be one-sided), because the surface of the iris is increased (and the pupil, therefore, encroached on) whenever its vessels are distended. Atropine causes it to dilate between the synechiæ; the synechiæ being fixed, appear as angular projections when the iris on each side of them has retracted. If there be only one adhesion it will merely notch the pupil at one spot; if the adhesions be numerous the pupil will be crenated or irregular, Fig. 57. If the whole pupillary ring, or still more, if the entire posterior surface of the iris be adherent, scarcely any dilatation will be effected; the former condition is called annular or circular synechia, and its result is "*exclusion*" *of the pupil;* the latter is known as *total posterior*

FIG. 57.

FIG. 58.

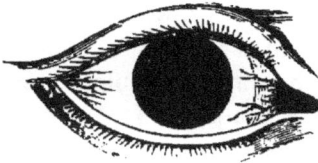

Iritic adhesions (posterior synechiæ) causing irregularity of pupil. (Wecker and Jaeger.)

Spots of pigment and lymph at seat of former iritic adhesions.

synechia. If the synechiæ be new and the lymph soft the repeated use of atropine will break them down and the pupil become round; but even then some of the uveal pigment, which is easily separable from the posterior surface of the iris, often remains behind, glued to the lens capsule by a little lymph, Fig. 58. The presence of one or more such spots of brown pigment on the capsule is always conclusive proof of present or of past iritis. The pupillary area itself in severe iritis is often filled by grayish or yellowish lymph, which spreads over it from the iris; if such exudation become organized a dense white membrane or a delicate film (often, however, presenting one or more little clear holes), is formed over the pupil ("*occlusion*" *of the pupil*). The iris may be inflamed without any lymph being effused from its hinder surface, and then the pupil, though sluggish, acting imperfectly to atropine, and never dilating widely, will present no posterior synechiæ nor any adhesion of pigment spots to the lens, but it will always be discolored (serous iritis); iritis of this kind often occurs with ulceration of the cornea, and as a complication of deeper inflammations.

Pain referred to the eyeball and to the parts supplied by the first, and sometimes by the second division of the fifth nerve, is common with iritis, especially in the early period. It is, however, a very variable symptom, and gives no clue to the amount of structural change, being sometimes quite insignificant when much lymph is thrown out. The pain is seldom constant, but comes on at intervals, is often worst at night, and is described as shooting, throbbing, or aching. It is commonly referred to the temple or forehead, as well as to the eyeball; sometimes also to the side of the nose and to the upper teeth. Photophobia and watering are generally proportionate to the pain.

The duration of acute iritis varies from a few days when mild, to many weeks when severe. The defect of sight is proportionate to the haziness of the cornea, aqueous, and pupillary space, but in some cases is increased by changes in the vitreous. Iritis sometimes sets in very gradually, causing no marked congestion or pain, but slowly giving rise to the formation of tough adhesions, and often to the growth of a thin membrane over the pupillary area; in some of these cases the iris becomes thickened and tough, and its large vessels undergo much dilatation, whilst in others keratitis punctata occurs. See Cyclitis, Chap. IX., Diseases of Cornea, p. 147; and Sympathetic Ophthalmitis, Chap. IX.

Permanent results of iritis.—Reference has been made to the adhesions, which are often permanent, and to the spots of uveal pigment on the lens capsule, which are always so; either condition tells a tale of past iritis, and is thus a valuable aid to diagnosis. A blue iris which has undergone severe inflammation may remain greenish.

Patches of atrophy may follow severe plastic exudations into the iris, and are recognized by their whitish color and thinness. Large patches of new pigment occasionally form, extending from the pupillary border on the anterior surface.

When the pupil is "excluded" or "occluded," the remainder of the iris being free, fluid collects in the posterior aqueous chamber, and by bulging the iris forward, and diminishing the depth of the anterior chamber, except at its centre, gives the pupil a funnel-like appearance; if the bulging be partial, or be divided by bands of tough membrane, the iris looks cystic. *Secondary glaucoma* is likely to follow, and the tension of the globe should, therefore, be carefully noted whenever bulging is present; in not a

FIG. 59.

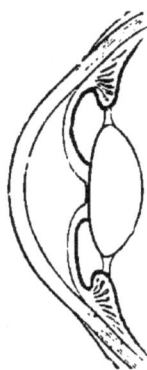

Diagram to show the result, upon the iris, of exclusion of the pupil (p. 155). (From a specimen.)

few of these cases, however, we find the eye soft and beginning to shrink, the sequel, perhaps, of a glaucomatous state. "Total posterior synechia" always shows a severe, though often a chronic, iritis; it is often accompanied by deep-seated disease, and followed by opacity of the lens, secondary cataract, and in some cases ultimately the lens becomes absorbed. Relapses of iritis are believed to be induced by the presence of synechiæ, even where there is no protrusion of the iris by fluid; but their influence in this direction has, I believe, been much overrated.

It must, however, be observed that there is still much difference of opinion on the point last referred to. The iritis of syphilis is still held by some to be liable to recur, and to be by no means limited to the secondary stage; and we still often hear it stated that iritic adhesions, by preventing free movement of the iris, operate as sources of irritation, and thus predispose to relapse. I have seldom succeeded in getting a history of recent syphilis in cases of recurring iritis, whilst in a number of cases of old iritis with the history that the attack occurred during secondary syphilis years before, I have scarcely found one with well-marked history of relapses. On the other hand, I have several times seen severe relapses in rheumatic cases after iridectomy had been performed as a preventive. All the evidence seems to me to favor the view that recurrences of iritis depend, as a rule, upon the constitutional cause of the disease.

The following are the most important points as to the causes of iritis, and the chief clinical differences between the several forms.

CONSTITUTIONAL CAUSES. *Syphilis.*—The iritis is acute; it shows a great tendency to effusion of lymph and formation of vascular nodules (plastic iritis), and the nodules, when very large, may even suppurate; it is symmetrical in a large proportion, probably at least two-thirds, of the cases. But asymmetry and absence of lymph-nodules are common. It occurs only in secondary syphilis, either acquired or inherited, and seldom relapses. Its significance is thus entirely different from that of the iritis which often complicates syphilitic keratitis.

Rheumatism is the cause of most cases of relapsing unsymmetrical iritis; there is but little tendency to effusion of lymph, and nodules are never formed, but there is occa-

sionally fluid hypopyon; the congestion and pain are often
more severe than in syphilitic iritis. An attack is usually
unsymmetrical, though both eyes commonly suffer by turns.
It relapses at intervals of months or years. Even repeated
attacks sometimes result in but little damage to sight.
Gout is apparently a cause of some cases of both acute and
insidious chronic iritis. It is perhaps doubtful whether
the gout or the chronic rheumatism from which the same
patients sometimes suffer is the cause of the iritis. In its tendency to relapse, and to affect only one eye at a time, gouty
resembles rheumatic iritis. The children of gouty parents
are occasionally liable to a very insidious and destructive
form of chronic iritis, with disease of the vitreous, keratitis
punctata, and glaucoma. Chaps. IX. and XXIII.

Chronic iritis (*plastic irido-choroiditis*).—In a few
cases symmetrical iritis, of a chronic, progressive, and destructive character, is complicated with choroiditis, disease
of vitreous, and secondary cataract. These cases, for which
it is at present impossible to assign any cause, either general or local, are chiefly seen in adults below middle life.

Sympathetic iritis.—See Sympathetic Ophthalmitis.

LOCAL CAUSES. *Injuries.*—Perforating wounds of the
eyeball, particularly if irregular, contused, and complicated
with wound of the lens, are often followed by iritis, and
more often if the patient be old than young. If the corneal wound suppurate, or become much infiltrated, the
iritis is likely to be suppurative, and the inflammation to
spread to the ciliary processes and cause destructive panophthalmitis. Iritis may follow a wound of the lens-capsule without wound of the iris, and with only a mere
puncture of the cornea. Examples of traumatic iritis from
these several causes are seen after the various operations
for cataract. The iritis, or more correctly irido-capsulitis,
following extraction of senile cataract is often prolonged,
attended by chemosis, much congestion, and the formation

of tough membrane behind the iris. Iritis may also follow superficial wounds and abrasions of the cornea, or direct blows on the eye; but it is of great importance, whenever the question of injury comes in, to ascertain whether or not there has been a perforating wound. Iritis often accompanies ulcers and other inflammations of the cornea, especially when deep, or complicated with hypopyon, or occurring in elderly persons. Iritis may accompany deep-seated disease of the eye.

TREATMENT.—(1) In every case where iritis is present atropine is to be used often and continuously, in order to break down adhesions already formed, and to allow any lymph subsequently effused to be deposited outside the ordinary area of the pupil. A strong solution, four grains of sulphate of atropine to one ounce of distilled water, is to be dropped into the conjunctival sac every hour in the early period. Even if the synechiæ are, when first seen, already so tough that the atropine has no effect on them, it may prevent the formation of new ones on the same circle. Atropine also greatly relieves pain in iritis, and lessens the congestion, and through these means it no doubt helps materially to arrest exudation. Mild acute iritis may sometimes be cured by atropine alone.

(2) If there be severe pain with much congestion, three or four leeches should be applied to the temple, to the malar eminence, or to the side of the nose. They may be repeated daily, in the same or smaller numbers, with advantage, for several days, if necessary; or, after one leeching, repeated blistering may be substituted. Some surgeons use opiates instead of, or in addition to, leeches. Leeches occasionally increase the pain. Severe pain in iritis can nearly always be quickly relieved by artificial heat, either fomentations or dry heat, as hot as can be borne, to the eyelids. To apply dry heat, take a piece of cotton-wool the size of two fists, hold it to the fire or against a tin pot

full of *boiling* water, till quite hot, and apply it to the lids; have another piece ready, and change as soon as the first gets cool; continue this for twenty minutes or more, and repeat it several times a day.[1] Paracentesis of the anterior chamber should be resorted to in severe iritis if the aqueous humor remain very turbid after a few days of other treatment; it may be repeated every day or two unless there is marked improvement.

(3) Rest of the eye is very important. Many an attack is lengthened out, and many a relapse after partial cure is brought on, by the patient continuing at, or returning too soon to, work. It is not in most cases necessary to remain in a perfectly dark room; to wear a shade in the room with the blinds down is generally enough, provided that no attempt be made to use the eyes. Work should not be resumed till at least a week after all congestion has gone off.

(4) Cold draughts of air on the eye and all causes of " catching cold " are to be very carefully avoided by keeping the eye warmly tied up with a large pad of cotton wool.

(5) The cause of the disease is to be treated, and into this careful inquiry should always be made. If the iritis be syphilitic, treatment for secondary syphilis is proper, mercury being given just short of salivation for several months, even though all the active eye symptoms quickly pass off. The rheumatic and gouty varieties are less definitely under the influence of internal remedies: iodide of potassium, alkalies, colchicum, salicylate of soda, and turpentine, each have their advocates; when the pain is severe tincture of aconite is sometimes markedly useful; mercury is seldom needed, but in protracted and severe cases it may be given with advantage. It is sometimes advisable to

---

[1] I owe my knowledge of the value of dry heat to Mr. Liebreich.

combine quinine or iron with the mercury in syphilis, or to give them in addition to other remedies in rheumatic cases.

(6) As a rule no stimulants are to be allowed, and the bowels should be kept well open.

(7) Iridectomy is needed for cases of severe iritis, even when there is no increase of tension, if judicious local and internal treatment have been carefully tried for some weeks without marked relief to the symptoms. It is chiefly in cases of constitutional origin, either syphilitic or rheumatic, and in the iritis accompanying ulcers of the cornea, that iridectomy is useful ; it is not admissible in sympathetic iritis, nor in iritis after cataract extraction. Iridectomy has been largely employed to prevent relapses of iritis, but the operation has much less effect in this way than has often been supposed ; it should not, therefore, be employed until the other means of cure have been fairly tried. It must be borne in mind, that unless iridectomy is necessary, it is injurious, by producing an enlarged and irregular pupil through which, for optical reasons, the patient will often not see so well as through the natural pupil, even though this be partially obstructed. In regard to all methods of local treatment we must bear in mind that acute iritis occurs in all degrees of severity, and that the mildest cases often need only atropine and rest.

Traumatic iritis, in the earliest stage, is best combated by atropine, continuous cold obtained by laying upon the closed eyelids pieces of lint wetted in iced water and changed every few minutes, and by leeches. *Cold is not to be used in any other form of iritis*, and is useless even for traumatic cases after the first day or so ; later, warmth is more appropriate.

Congenital irideremia (absence of iris) is occasionally seen, and is often associated with other defects of the eye, especially opacities in the lens.

Coloboma of the iris (congenital developmental cleft in the iris) gives the effect of a very regularly made iridectomy. It is always downwards or slightly down-in, and is often, but not always, symmetrical. It occurs in different degrees, and sometimes a mere line or seam in the iris indicates the slightest form of the defect. It often occurs without coloboma of the choroid.

Pupillary and capsulo-pupillary membranes.—In early fœtal life, the capsule of the lens is vascular, supplied with blood by the hyaloid artery; when the iris grows in from the anterior part of the choroid, and comes into contact with the capsule, its vessels anastomose with those of the capsule, and the membrane so formed fills the pupil. Normally this membrane disappears entirely with the vessels of the lens capsule; sometimes the part attached to the capsule only disappears, leaving behind the anterior part of the structure, which is known as the pupillary membrane. In this, bands of tissue, resembling that of the iris, run from one part of the anterior surface of the iris to another, springing from near the pupillary edge. Sometimes the whole thickness of the membrane remains, in which case bands of tissue pass from the anterior surface of the iris to the capsule; this forms the capsulo-pupillary membrane. Some of the latter cases have probably been described as the remains of intra-uterine iritis.

CHAPTER IX.

THIS chapter is intended to include cases in which the ciliary body itself, or the corresponding part of the sclerotic, or the episcleral tissue, is the sole seat, or at least the headquarters, of disease. From the abundance of vessels and nerves in the ciliary body, and the importance of its nutritive relations to the surrounding parts, we find that many of the morbid processes of the ciliary region show a strong tendency to spread, according to their precise position and depth, to the cornea, iris, or vitreous, and, by influencing the nutrition of the lens, to cause secondary cataract. Although alike on pathological and clinical grounds it is necessary to subdivide the class into groups, we may observe that the various diseases of this part show a general agreement in some of their more important characters; thus all of them are protracted and liable to relapse, and in all there is a marked tendency to patchiness, the morbid process being most intense in certain spots of the ciliary zone, or even occurring in quite discrete areas. It is convenient to make three principal clinical groups, the differences between which are accounted for to a great extent by the depth of the tissue chiefly implicated. The most superficial may be taken first.

(1) **Episcleritis** (more correctly *Scleritis*) is the name given to one or more large patches of congestion in the ciliary region, with some elevation of the conjunctiva from thickening of the subjacent tissues. The congestion generally affects the conjunctival as well as the deeper vessels,

and the yellowish color of the exudation tones the bright blood-red down to a more or less rusty tinge, which is especially striking at the central, thickest part of the patch. The thickening seldom causes more than a low, widely-spread mound of swelling.

Episcleritis is a rather rare disease. It occurs chiefly on the exposed parts of the ciliary region, and especially near the outer canthus; but the patches may occur at any part of the circle, and exceptionally the inflammation is diffused over a much wider area than the ciliary zone, extending far back, out of view. The iris is often a little discolored and the pupil sluggish, but actual iritis is the exception. There is often much aching pain. The disease is subacute, reaching its acme in not less than two or three weeks, and requiring a much longer time before absorption is complete. Fresh patches are apt to spring up while old ones are declining, and so the disease may last for months; indeed, relapses at intervals, and in fresh spots, are the rule. It usually affects only one eye at a time, but both often suffer sooner or later. After the active changes have disappeared, a patch of the underlying sclerotic, of rather small size, is generally seen to be dusky, as if stained; it is doubtful whether such patches represent thinning of the sclerotic from atrophy, or only staining; it is but seldom that they show any tendency to bulge as if thinned. In rare cases the exudation is much more abundant, and a large swelling is formed, which may even contain pus; such cases pass by gradations into conjunctival phlyctenulæ, and are generally seen in children.

Episcleritis is seldom seen except in adults, and is commoner in men than women. Inquiry often shows that the sufferer is, either from occupation or temperament, particularly liable to be affected by exposure to cold or by changes of temperature. Some of the patients are rheumatic, some gouty. Similar patches, but of brownish, rather translucent appearance, are occasionally caused by tertiary syphilis, acquired or inherited (*gummatous scleritis*).

In the treatment, protection by a warm bandage, rest, the yellow ointment (F. 12), the use of repeated blisters, and local stimulation of the swelling, are generally the most efficacious. Atropine is very useful in allaying pain. Internal remedies seldom seem to exert much influence, except in syphilitic cases. Salicylate of soda has been highly spoken of by some. Systematic kneading of the eye through the closed lids ("massage"), and scraping away the exudation with a sharp spoon, after turning back the conjunctiva, have also been recommended, and are worth trial.

(2) **Sclero-keratitis and sclero-iritis** ("scrofulous sclero-titis," "anterior choroiditis"). A more deeply-seated, very persistent, or relapsing, subacute inflammation, character-ized by congestion of a violet tint (deep scleral congestion, p. 55), abruptly limited to the ciliary zone, and affecting some parts of the zone more than others (tendency to patchiness). Early in the case there is a slight degree of bulging of the affected part, due partly to thickening; whilst patches of cloudy opacity, which may or may not ulcerate, appear in the cornea close to, and often continuous with, its margin; iritis generally occurs later; pain and photophobia are often severe. After a varying interval, always weeks, more often months, the symptoms recede; at the focus of greatest congestion, or it may be around the entire zone, the sclerotic is left of a dusky color, some-times interspersed with little yellowish patches, and per-manent haziness of the most affected parts of the cornea remains. The disease is almost certain to relapse sooner or later; or a succession of fresh inflammatory foci follow each other without any intervals of real recovery, the whole process extending over months or years. After each attack more haze of cornea and fresh iritic adhesions are

left.   The sclerotic, in bad cases of some years' standing, is much stained, and may become bulged (ciliary or anterior staphyloma), and the cornea becomes more opaque and altered in curve; the eye is then useless, though seldom liable to further active symptoms.

The characteristic appearance of an eye which has been moderately affected is the dusky color of the sclerotic and the irregular, patchy opacities in the cornea (Fig. 60), which

FIG. 60.

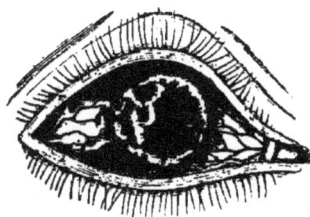

Relapsing sclero-keratitis.   (From nature.)

are often continuous with the sclerotic.   The disease does not occur in children, nor does it begin late in life; most of the patients are young or middle-aged adults, and, unlike the former variety, most are women.   It is not associated with any special diathesis or dyscrasia, but generally goes along with a feeble circulation and liability to "catch cold;" in some cases there is a definite family history of scrofula or of phthisis.   Predisposed persons are more likely to suffer in cold weather, or after change to a colder or damper climate, or after any cause of exhaustion, such as suckling.

TREATMENT is at best but palliative.   Local stimulation by yellow ointment or calomel is very useful in some cases, particularly in those which verge toward the phlyctenular type.   In the early stages, especially when the congestion is very violent and altogether subconjunctival, atropine often gives relief, and it is, of course, useful for the iritis. Repeated blistering is also to be tried, though not all cases are benefited by it. I have not seen much benefit from setons. Warm, dry applications to the lids are, as a rule, better than cold. Mercury, in small and long-continued doses, is certainly valuable when the patient is not anæmic and feeble, but it is to be combined with cod-liver oil and iron. Protection from cold and bright light by "goggles" is a very important measure, both during the attacks and in the intervals between them. There is no rule as to symmetry; both eyes often suffer sooner or later, but sometimes one escapes whilst the other is attacked repeatedly. Transition forms occur between this disease and episcleritis.

(3) **Cyclitis with disease of vitreous and keratitis punctata** (chronic serous irido-choroiditis, "serous iritis"). A small but important series of cases, in which there is congestion, as in mild iritis, and dulness of sight, but usually no pain or photophobia. Flocculi are found in the anterior part of the vitreous or numerous small dots of deposit are seen on the posterior surface of the cornea, keratitis punctata, Fig. 54; the anterior chamber is often too deep, and insidious iritis often follows. Patches of recent choroiditis (Chap. XII.) are sometimes to be seen at the fundus. In bad cases buff-colored masses of deposit form in the lower part of the angle between iris and cornea; or distinct nodules may be present on the iris near its periphery, but not, as in syphilitic iritis, at the pupillary border. Persistence, variability, and liability to relapse are almost as marked here as in other members of the cyclitic group. The tension is often slightly augmented at the beginning, but usually becomes normal again. Sometimes, however, the eye passes into a permanent state of chronic glaucoma,[1]

---

[1] Perhaps from blocking of the ligamentum pectinatum with cells.

without the intervention of plastic iritis (see Glaucoma) ; but usually the final condition in bad cases depends on the extent of the iritic adhesions, for when the synechiæ are numerous and tough, and the iris is much altered in structure, or the pupil blocked by exudation, secondary glaucoma is likely to arise from imprisonment of fluid behind the iris, Fig. 59. When seen quite early the diagnosis will probably be "serous iritis" or "ciliary congestion," unless the eye be carefully examined; for the pupil is generally free in all parts, or shows, at most, one or two adhesions after atropine has been used. In a few cases the punctate deposits on the back of the cornea constitute almost the only objective change (simple keratitis punctata), but these are rare. The refraction sometimes becomes temporarily myopic in serous iritis.

The cases occur in adolescents or young adults, and the disease is often sooner or later symmetrical. Many mild cases recover perfectly, and in most others the final result is satisfactory. In respect to cause, there is strong reason to believe that many of these cases are the result of gout in a previous generation, the patient himself never having had the disease. The disease seems often to be excited in predisposed persons by prolonged overwork or anxiety, combined with underfeeding, or defective assimilation ; the patients often describe themselves as delicate; some are phthisical. On the other hand, in some of the worst cases, leading to secondary cataract, and ultimately to shrinking of the eyes, the patient appears to be, from first to last, in good health, and free from any ascertainable morbid diathesis.

In the treatment, prolonged rest of the eyes is important. Atropine is usually necessary, but if there be increase of tension its effect must be carefully watched, and in cases where there are no iritic adhesions eserine may have to be substituted. If the increase of tension keeps up, and

8

seems to be damaging the sight, iridectomy is necessary. Small doses of iodide of potassium and mercury appear to be useful in the earlier stages, given with proper precautions, and accompanied by iron and cod-liver oil. Change of climate would probably often be very beneficial. In the worst cases, where the changes are like those resulting from sympathetic ophthalmitis, no treatment seems to have any effect.

Cases of acute inflammation are occasionally seen in which most of the symptoms resemble those of acute iritis, but with the iris so little affected that it is evidently not the headquarters of the morbid action. The tension may be much reduced, whilst repeated and rapid variations, both in sight and objective symptoms, occur. To some of these the term *idiopathic phthisis bulbi* has been applied. Again, some cases of syphilitic inflammation, which are classed as syphilitic "iritis," might more correctly be called "cyclitis." In some cases of heredito-syphilitic keratitis there is much cyclitic complication, and these are always difficult to treat.

Plastic inflammation of the ciliary body, following injury, *traumatic iritis* or *irido-cyclitis*, is the usual starting-point of the changes which set up sympathetic inflammation of the fellow-eye; the tension is often lowered, and the symptoms subacute The onset of *purulent traumatic cyclitis panophthalmitis* is signalized by congestion, pain, chemosis, and swelling of the lids, and the appearance of opacity at the wound. The inflammation quickly spreads to the iris, ciliary body, and vitreous, and then to the capsule of Tenon and the muscles, so that the eye becomes glued to the surrounding parts and fixed. If the lens be transparent a yellow or greenish reflection is, after a few days, sometimes seen behind it, indicating the presence of pus in the vitreous humor; but usually the cornea and aqueous are too turbid, even should the lens be clear, to

allow deep inspection.   Suppurative panophthalmitis occasionally sets in acutely and without apparent cause in eyes
which have long been blind from corneal disease or from
glaucoma.   It may also occur in pyæmia (Chap. XXIII).
See also Pseudo-glioma.

SYMPATHETIC IRRITATION AND SYMPATHETIC OPHTHALMITIS.

Certain morbid changes in one eye may set up either
functional disturbance or destructive inflammation in its
fellow.   The term *sympathetic irritation* is given to the
former, and *sympathetic ophthalmitis*, or *ophthalmia*, to the
latter.   Though these conditions may be combined, they
more often occur separately, and it is very important to
distinguish between them.

Although at present the exact nature of the changes
which precede sympathetic inflammation is unknown, and
their path has not been fully traced out, we are sure (1)
that the changes start from the region most richly supplied
with vessels and nerves, viz.: the ciliary body and iris; (2)
that the first changes recognized by the surgeon in the
sympathizing eye are generally in the same structures; (3)
that the *exciting eye* has nearly always been wounded, and
in its anterior part, and that plastic inflammation of its
uveal tract is always present; (4) that inflammatory
changes have in some cases been found in the ciliary
nerves, and in the coverings of the optic nerve, of the
exciting eye.

Within the last few years the hypothesis of transmission
along the ciliary nerves, which had many adherents, has
been almost given up in favor of the theory of infection.
Deutschmann has shown (1882-84) that the introduction
of certain septic organisms into the interior of the eyeball,
in rabbits, is followed by acute inflammatory changes in the
other eye, and Gifford (1886), and others more recently,

have obtained results which tend to confirm the infection theory. Most of Deutschmann's subjects died in a few days, and though in many of them the ocular changes were those of inflammation traceable along the optic nerve-sheaths of the "exciting" eye, by way of the chiasma, and down the optic nerve to the optic disc of the "sympathiser," still in one or two the morbid process had spread to the vitreous and uveal coat. Berlin[1] had previously suggested that the second eye was infected by a special organism which could flourish only in the eye-tissues, and which was carried by the blood from the first eye ; and Hutchinson[2] afterwards independently propounded a nearly identical view. Though there are difficulties to be explained and gaps to be filled in our knowledge before the infection theory in any form can be accepted, yet at the present time it claims more and stronger adherents than any other ; and the difficulties are, perhaps, not greater than for any other theory.

In almost every case sympathetic inflammation is set up by a perforating wound, either accidental or operative, in the ciliary region of the other eye, i. e., within a zone, nearly a quarter of an inch wide, surrounding the cornea. The risk attending a wound in this " dangerous zone" is increased if it be lacerated, or heal slowly, or if the iris or ciliary body be engaged between the lips of the sclerotic, or if the eye contain a foreign body ; under all conditions, indeed, which make the occurrence of plastic or purulent irido-cyclitis probable. Sympathetic inflammation may also be set up by a foreign body lodged in the eye, whether the wound be in the ciliary region or not; by an eye containing a tumor, perhaps even if the eye have not been perforated by operation or ulceration ; by a purely corneal wound, or a perforating ulcer, if complicated by adhesion of the iris, with dragging on the ciliary body.

[1] Berlin, 1880.   [2] Hutchinson, 1885.

Symptoms in the exciting eye.—The exciting eye, when it is causing sympathetic *irritation*, generally shows ciliary congestion and photophobia, and often suffers neuralgic pain. In an eye which is causing sympathetic *inflammation*, obvious iritis, often with lowered tension, is usually present; but the iritis is often painless and without noticeable congestion, and thus may easily be overlooked; it is especially important to remember that the exciting eye, though its sight is always damaged, need not be blind, and that under certain circumstances it may in the end be the better eye of the two.

Symptoms in the sympathizing eye. *a. Sympathetic irritation.*—The eye is, in common speech, " weak " or " irritable." It is intolerant of light and easily flushes and waters if exposed to bright light, or if much used; the accommodation is weakened or irritable, so that continued vision for near objects is painful, or even impossible; and the ciliary muscle seems liable to give way for a short time, the patient complaining that near objects now and then suddenly become misty for a while. Neuralgic pains, referred to the eye and side of the head, are also common. Temporary darkening of sight, indicating suspension of retinal function, and subjective sensations of colored spots, clouds, etc., occur in certain cases. Such attacks may occur again and again in varying severity, lasting for days or weeks, and finally ceasing without ever passing on to structural change. Sympathetic irritation is always and, as a rule, promptly, cured by removal of the exciting eye; but occasionally the symptoms persist for some time afterwards. A condition which cannot be distinguished from hysterical blindness is sometimes seen in the " sympathizing " eye, but the term sympathetic irritation does not then seem suitable.[1]

[1] Mr. Gunn tells me that he has noticed that marked oscillation of the iris often occurs when sympathetic *irritation* is about to give place to *inflammation*.

b. Sympathetic inflammation (Ophthalmitis).—The disease may arise out of an attack of "irritation," but more commonly it sets in without any such warning   It may be acute and severe, or so insidious as to escape the notice of the patient until well advanced.   It is in nearly all cases a prolonged and a recurring disease; when once started it is self-maintaining, and its course usually extends over many months, or even a year or two.   In mild cases a good recovery eventually takes place, but in a large majority the eye becomes blind.   The disease usually takes the form of a plastic irido-cyclitis or irido-choroiditis with exudation from the entire posterior surface of the iris, leading to total posterior synechia.   Its chief early peculiarities are great liability to dotted deposits on the back of the cornea, clouding of the vitreous by floating opacities, and often neuro-retinitis; there is a dusky ciliary congestion with marked engorgement of the large vessels which perforate the sclerotic in the ciliary region.   In acute and severe cases the congestion is intense, there is severe pain, photophobia, and tenderness on pressure, and the iris, besides being thick, is changed in color to a peculiar buff or yellowish brown, and shows numerous enlarged bloodvessels.   Attacks of intense neuralgia of the fifth nerve characterize some cases. In cases of all degrees the tension is often increased, the eye becoming decidedly glaucomatous for a longer or shorter time.   Many dotted opacities appear in the lens, which afterwards becomes completely cataractous and in some cases is finally quite absorbed.   In the worst cases the eye finally shrinks, but in many it remains glaucomatous with total posterior synechia, corneal haze, and more or less ciliary staphyloma.   In the mildest cases, the so-called "serous" form, the disease never goes beyond a chronic iritis with punctate keratitis and disease of the vitreous, with which neuro-retinitis often, perhaps always, coexists.

Sympathetic ophthalmitis generally begins between six

weeks and about three months after the injury to the exciting eye; very seldom sooner than three weeks, *i. e.*, not until time has elapsed for well-marked inflammatory changes to occur at the seat of injury. On the other hand, the disease may set in at any length of time, even many years, after the lesion of the exciting eye. It occurs at all ages. Distinct inflammatory changes are probably always present in the exciting eye; but, as already stated, these may be very slight and difficult of detection. When carefully observed, these changes are found to precede by some days, if not longer, the onset of structural disease in the sympathizing eye, the morbid process apparently taking some time to travel from one eye to the other.

TREATMENT.—By far the most important measure refers to prevention. When once sympathetic inflammation has begun we can do little to modify its course. The clear recognition of this fact leads us to advise the excision[1] of every eye which is at the same time useless and liable to cause sympathetic mischief, *i. e.*, of all eyes which are blind from injury or destructive corneal disease; and to give this advice most urgently when the blind eye is already tender or irritable, or is liable to become so, when it has been lost by wound, and when it is probable that it may contain a foreign body. Any lost eye in which there are signs of past iritis, even if there be no history of injury, is best removed, especially if shrunken. But much judgment is needed if the damaged eye, though irritable and likely to cause mischief, still retains more or less sight. Every attention must then be paid to the exact position of the wound, the evidence as to its depth, the evidence of

---

[1] Feeling doubtful whether either abscission or op tico-ciliary neuro_ tomy confers as great safety from sympathetic disea se as does excision, I have not performed those operations. The more newly revived evisceration has not yet been performed often enough for trustworthy conclusions to be drawn on this point.

hemorrhage, and especially to the condition of the lens, and to the presence of the yellowish haziness behind the lens which indicates lymph or pus in the vitreous. The date of the injury and the condition of the wound, whether healed by immediate union, or with scarring, puckering, or flattening, are very important points. *Irritation* of the fellow-eye may set in a few days after the injury; but since *inflammation* very seldom begins sooner than two or three weeks, we may, if we see the case early, watch it for a little time. Complete and prolonged rest in a darkened room is a very important element in the prevention of sympathetic irritation and inflammation, and should always be insisted on when we are trying to save an injured eye. In rare cases sympathetic inflammation sets in *after* the removal of the exciting eye, even after an interval of several weeks, a contingency which emphasises the importance of excising every condemned eye at the earliest possible moment.

When sympathetic ophthalmitis has set in we can do comparatively little.

A. *The exciting eye*, if quite blind or so seriously damaged as to be for practical purposes certainly useless, is to be excised at once, though the evidence of benefit from this course is slender. But it is not to be removed if there is reason to hope for restoration of useful sight in it; if there is simply a moderate degree of subacute iritis, with or without traumatic cataract, and with sight proportionate to the state of the lens, the eye is to be carefully treated, since it may very probably in the end be the better of the two.

B. *The sympathizing eye.*—The important measures are: (1) atropine, used very often, as for acute iritis; (2) absolute rest and exclusion of light by residence in a dark room and with a black bandage over both eyes; (3) repeated leeching if the symptoms are severe, or counter-irritation by blisters or by a seton in chronic cases. (4) Mercury is believed by some to be beneficial. Quinine is sometimes

given.   (5) As a rule no operation is permissible whilst
the disease is still active, since iridectomy, performed whilst
there are active symptoms, is followed by closure of the
gap with fresh lymph.   Operations in severe cases which
have become quiet are seldom of use, the eye being generally then past recovery.

The *prognosis* is, as will be gathered, very grave ; even
in the mildest cases, when seen quite early, we must be very
cautious, for the disease often slowly progresses for many
months.

8*

CHAPTER X

A CLEAR distinction is to be made between contusion and concussion injuries, and wounds of the eyeball.

(1) **Contusion and concussion injuries.**—*Rupture of the eyeball* is commonly the result of severe direct blows. The rent is nearly always in the sclerotic, either a little behind or close to the corneal margin, with which it is concentric; the cornea itself is but seldom rent by a blow. The rupture is usually large, involves all the tunics, and is followed by immediate hemorrhage between the retinal and choroid and into the vitreous and anterior chambers; the lens and some of the vitreous often escape; sight is usually reduced to perception of light or of large objects. The conjunctiva, however, often escapes untorn, and in such a case if the lens pass through the rent in the sclerotic, it will be held down by the conjunctiva and form a prominent, rounded, translucent swelling over the rupture. The diagnosis of rupture is generally easy, even if the rent be more or less concealed. The eyeball often shrinks; but occasionally it recovers with useful vision. Immediate excision is generally best when the wound is "compound;" but if the conjunctiva be not torn, and occasionally even when it is, we should wait a few days until the disappearance of the blood from the anterior chamber allows the deeper parts to be seen. The treatment is the same as for wounds of the eye. When the lens is lying beneath the conjunctiva it should be removed when the scleral wound has healed, if we decide to save the eye.

It may be here mentioned that copious hemorrhage, accompanied by severe pain, sometimes occurs between the choroid and sclerotic as the result of sudden diminution of tension, either by an operation, such as extraction of cataract or iridectomy, or by a glancing wound of the cornea. Eyes in which this occurs are for most part already unsound and often glaucomatous.

Blows often cause *internal damage without rupture of the hard coats* of the eye. The iris may be torn from its ciliary attachment (*coredialysis*), so that two pupils are formed,

FIG. 61.

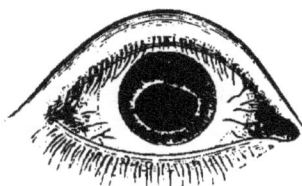

Separation of iris following a blow.

Fig. 61, or the lens may be loosened or displaced by partial rupture of its suspensory ligament, so that the iris, having lost its support, will shake about with every movement (*tremulous iris*). Such lesions are likely to be obscured for a time by bleeding into the anterior chamber and into the vitreous. The lens often becomes opaque afterward. Detachment of the retina is often found after severe blows, which have caused hemorrhage into the vitreous. Blows on the front of the eye may cause *rupture of the choroid* or hemorrhage from choroidal or retinal vessels. These changes are found at the central part of the fundus, and if the yellow spot is involved visual acuteness is much damaged. The rents in the choroid appear after the blood has cleared up, as lines or narrow bands of atrophy bordered by pigment, and often slightly curved toward the

disc, Fig. 74. Hemorrhages from the choroidal vessels
without rupture of the choroid usually leave some residual
pigment after absorption.   In an eye predisposed to detachment of retina, a blow will sometimes determine its occurrence. *Paralysis of the iris and ciliary muscle,* with partial
and often irregular dilatation of the pupil, are often the
sole results of a blow on the eye; the defect of sight can
be remedied by a convex lens.   Complete restitution is
moderately common; the ciliary muscle recovers before
the iris.   Partial dilatation or imperfection of the pupil
after a blow is sometimes dependent on a rupture of the
sphincter, one or more notches in the pupillary border of
the iris indicating the seat of the lesion or lesions.   For
Traumatic Iritis see p. 159.

Great defect of sight following a blow, and neither remedied by glasses nor accounted for by blood in the anterior
chamber, will generally mean copious hemorrhage into
the vitreous, with one or another of the changes just mentioned in the retina and choroid. The red blood may sometimes be seen by focal light, but often its presence can only
be inferred from the opaque state of the vitreous.   Probably in most of these cases the blood comes from the large
veins of the ciliary body, but sometimes from the vessels
of the choroid or retina.   There may be no external ecchymosis.   The tension of the globe is to be noted; it is not
often increased unless inflammation have set in, or the eye
were previously glaucomatous, and in some cases it is below
par. The prognosis should be very guarded whenever there
is reason to think, from the opaque state of the parts behind
the lens, that much bleeding has taken place, or that the
retina is detached, or when the iris is tremulous or partly
detached, or if any rupture of the choroid can be made
out.   Blood in the anterior chamber is often completely
absorbed in a day or two, or even sometimes in a few
hours; but in the vitreous humor absorption, though rapid,

is less complete, and permanent opacities are often left. The use of atropine, the frequent application, during the first twenty-four hours, of iced water, or of an evaporating lotion to the lids, and occasional leeching if there be inflammatory symptoms, will do all that is possible for the first week or two after a severe blow with internal hemorrhage. If the lens be loosened it may at any time act as an irritating foreign body, or set up a glaucomatous inflammation : Dislocation of Lens, p. 208. Now and then optic neuritis occurs in the injured eye as the immediate effect of the blow. Hemorrhage behind the choroid is believed to account for certain well-known cases in which, after a blow, there is defect of sight without a visible change, or with localized temporary haze of retina ("*commotio retinæ*"). Temporary myopia or astigmatism may also follow a blow on the eye ; they depend on altered curvature of the lens, and are sometimes entirely removed by paralyzing the ciliary muscle with atropine. See also Hysterical Amblyopia.

(2) **Wounds.**—A. Superficial *abrasions* of the cornea cause much pain, with watering, photophobia, and ciliary congestion. They are frequently due to a scratch by a finger-nail of a baby at the breast. The abraded surface is often very small and shows no opacity ; it is detected by watching the reflection of a window from the cornea, whilst the patient slowly moves the eye. Now and then the symptoms return after a long interval of cure. Many, if not all of the cases of relapsing bullæ of the cornea seem to have originated in a slight superficial injury.

Minute fragments of metal or stone flying from tools, etc., often partly imbed themselves in the cornea, *foreign body on the cornea*, and give rise to varying degrees of irritability and pain. The fragment soon becomes surrounded by a hazy zone of infiltration, but it remains easily visible unless it be very small or covered by mucus or epithelium.

When in doubt always examine the cornea by focal light with magnifying power.

The pupil is often smaller than its fellow, and the color of the iris altered, in cases of superficial injury to the cornea, indicating congestion of the iris. Actual iritis sometimes occurs, but not unless the corneal wound inflame.

TREATMENT.—(For removal of foreign bodies, see Operations.) After surface injuries a drop of castor oil may be applied, and the eye kept closed for the day with a pad of wadding and a bandage. Atropine is required if there be much irritation or threatened iritis. If hypopyon appear the case becomes one of hypopyon ulcer.

Foreign bodies often adhere to the inner surface of the upper lid; whenever a patient states that he has "something in his eye" and nothing can be found on the cornea, the upper lid must be everted and examined.

Large bodies sometimes pass far back into the upper or lower conjunctival sulcus and lie hidden for weeks or months, causing only local inflammation and some thickening of the conjunctiva. Search must be made, if needful, with a small scoop or probe whenever the suspicion arises. (See Orbit.)

B. *Burns, scalds, and injuries by caustics, etc.*—The conjunctiva and cornea are often damaged by splashes of molten lead, or by strong alkalies or acids, of which lime, either quick or freshly slaked, is the commonest. The eyeball is not often scalded, the lids closing quickly enough to prevent the entrance of steam or hot water. As in no such cases is the full effect apparent for some days, a cautious opinion should be given in the early stages.

The effects of such accidents are manifested by (1) inflammation of the cornea passing into suppurative keratitis with hypopyon, in bad cases; (2) scarring and shortening of the conjunctiva, and in bad cases adhesion of its palbebral and ocular surfaces, *symblepharon.*

The most superficial burns whiten and dry the surface

and in a few hours the epithelium is shed. This is shown
on the cornea by a sharply outlined, slightly depressed
area. The surface is clear if the damage be quite superficial and recent, but more or less opalescent, or even yellowish, if the case be a few days old, and the burn be deep
enough to have caused destruction or inflammation of the
true corneal tissue. When there is much opacity it does
not completely clear, and considerable flattening of the
cornea and neighboring sclerotic often occurs at the seat
of deep and extensive burns. The conjunctival whitening
is followed by mere desquamation and vascular reaction,
or by ulceration and scarring, according to the depth of
the damage.

TREATMENT.—In recent cases, seen before reaction has
begun, a drop of castor oil once or twice a day, a few
leeches to the temple, and the use of a cold evaporating
lotion, or of iced water, will sometimes prevent inflammation. If seen immediately after the accident, the conjunctival sac is to be carefully searched for fragments, or washed
with very weak acid or alkaline solution if a liquid caustic
of the opposite character have done the damage. If inflammatory reaction be already present, treatment by compress, hot fomentations, and the other means recommended
for suppurating ulcers, p. 138, is most suitable. There
is often much pain and chemosis. (See Operation for
Symblepharon.)

c. *Penetrating wounds and gunshot injuries.*—When a
patient says that his eye is wounded, the first step is to
examine the seat, extent, and character of the wound,
ascertain the interval since the injury, and test the sight
of the eye; the next to make out all we can about the
wounding body, and especially whether any fragment has
been left within the eyeball.

Very large foreign bodies, such as pieces of glass, sometimes lie long in the eye without causing much trouble,

the large wound having given exit to the contents of the
globe, and been followed by rapid shrinking without inflammation.

TREATMENT.—Penetrating wounds are least serious
when they implicate the cornea alone, or the sclerotic
behind the ciliary region, *i. e.*, ¼ inch or more behind the
cornea. Penetrating wounds of the cornea without injury
to the iris or lens, and without any prolapse of iris, are
rare; they generally do very well, and if the case be not
seen until one or two days after the injury, the wound will
often have healed firmly enough to retain the aqueous, and
it may be difficult to decide whether the whole thickness
of the cornea have been penetrated or not. Wounds of
the sclerotic seldom unite without the interposition of a
layer of lymph; when seen early they should, if gaping,
clean, and uncomplicated by evidence of internal injury,
be treated by the insertion of fine sutures, which should
be passed only through the conjunctiva, followed by the
use of ice.

But penetrating wounds are usually very serious to the
injured eye; the iris is frequently lacerated and included in
the track of the wound; the lens is punctured and becomes
swollen and opaque from absorption of the aqueous humor,
traumatic cataract, and liable in its swollen state to press
on the ciliary processes and cause grave symptoms; extensive bleeding perhaps takes place in the vitreous; within
the first few days purulent inflammation may destroy the
eye. The fellow-eye is, of course, often in danger of sympathetic inflammation. Every case has therefore to be
judged from two points of view, the damage to the injured
eye and the risk to the sound one; and the question
whether to sacrifice or attempt to save the former, is sometimes very difficult to decide.

(I.) In the two following cases the eye should be sacrificed
at once: (1) If the wound, lying wholly or partly in the

"dangerous region" be so large and so complicated with injury to deeper parts that no hope of useful sight remains. (2) If, even though the wound be small, it lie in the dangerous region, and have already set up severe iritis (pp. 159 and 170).

(II.) There is a large class of cases in which it is certain or very probable that the eye contains a foreign body, although the injury is not of itself fatal to sight and has not as yet led to inflammation or to shrinking of the eye.

The first question then is whether the foreign body can be seen, the second, whether or not it is steel or iron, and therefore possibly removable by a magnet. A foreign body, if lying on or embedded in the iris, the lens being intact, should be removed, usually with the portion of iris to which it is attached; if loose in the anterior chamber its removal may be difficult. If it can be seen embedded in the lens and the condition of the eye be otherwise favorable, a scoop extraction may be done in the hope of removing the fragment with the lens; or the lens may be allowed, or by a needle operation induced, to undergo partial absorption and shrinking so as to enclose the foreign body more firmly, and when subsequently extracted bring it away. If we are certain that the foreign body has passed into the vitreous, whether through the lens or not, and whether by gunshot or not, we can seldom save the eye. The foreign body can in such a case seldom be seen, but a track of opacity through the lens, with blood in the vitreous, or even the latter alone, with conclusive history that the wound was made by a fragment or a shot, and not by an instrument or large body, will generally decide us in favor of excision. These rules need some modification when the foreign body is of iron or steel, since it is possible in certain cases, by means of a strong electro-magnet, to remove such fragments, even when lying in the vitreous. This may be done either through the wound of entrance more or less

enlarged, or through a fresh wound made where the body
is seen or believed to lie. Many forms of magnet have
been employed, the most successful usually being those in
which a probe-ended instrument powerfully magnetized by
being attached to the core of an electro-magnetic coil, is
introduced into the eye in search of the body.   The terminal of the instrument used at Moorfields will, when the
circuit is complete, lift nine ounces. Though a certain
number of eyes have now been saved with useful sight by
means of the magnet, it must be remembered that the extraction of the foreign body does not insure the safety of
the eye; that the eye may inflame or shrink and remain
as potent a source of sympathetic disease as before, especially so if iritis or threatened panophthalmitis were present
at the time of operation.[1]   Foreign bodies occasionally become embedded at the fundus beyond the dangerous region
and cause no further trouble.   In gunshot cases the shot
often passes out through a counter-opening and remains
without doing harm in the orbit, though the eye is destroyed.   Occasionally the choroid and retina are damaged
by hemorrhage caused by a shot or bullet traversing the
orbit close to but without demonstrable lesion of the
sclerotic.

(III.) There remain cases of less severe character, in
which there is no foreign body in the eye : (1) the wound
is in the dangerous region and complicated with traumatic
cataract; (2) in the dangerous region without traumatic
cataract; (3) the injury is entirely corneal, and therefore
not in the dangerous zone, but the lens and iris are
wounded; (4) there is wound of cornea and iris only, the

[1] Mr. Snell, of Sheffield, who has probably had a larger experience
of this method than anyone else, has published (June, 1883) an excellent monograph, in which all the cases hitherto recorded are given, in
addition to his own. Hirschberg's monograph on the subject (1885)
brings the subject up to later date.

lens escaping. In group (2) there will often be much difficulty in deciding what to do, it being presumed that the
wounded eye shows no iritis or other signs of severe inflammation; some of the most difficult cases are those of wounds
by sharp instruments close to the corneal border, with considerable adhesion of the iris, or in which there is evidence
that the track lies between the lens and the ciliary processes, the lens not being wounded, and useful sight remaining. If the patient be seen within two or three weeks of
the injury, and the sound eye show no irritation, we may
safely watch the case for a few days. If decided sympathetic irritation be present and do not yield after a few
days' treatment, excision is advisable, even though the lens
of the wounded eye be uninjured. In regard to group (1),
excision is without doubt the safest course in all cases,
whether or not the eye be causing sympathetic symptoms,
or be itself especially irritable; for there is little prospect
of regaining useful vision in an eye with a ciliary wound
and traumatic cataract. In group (3) excision is necessary
if the wound be very large or irregular, and in some cases
with small wound but persistent symptoms. In group (4)
removal of the eye is very seldom justifiable, unless the
iris having healed into the wound chronic inflammatory
changes are present, or severe iritis and threatened panophthalmitis come on. The patient in all open cases must
be warned, and must be seen every few days for many
weeks.

When sympathetic ophthalmitis has set in before the
patient asks advice, the rule as to the excision of the exciting eye is different.

The treatment of wounded eyes which are not excised is
the same as for traumatic iritis and cataract, viz., atropine,
rest, and local depletion. If seen before inflammation
(iritis) has begun, ice is to be used. If the iris have prolapsed into the wound the protusion should be drawn

further out and a large piece of iris cut off so that the ends when replaced by the curette may retract and remain quite free from the wound, see Iridectomy; this may be done as much as a week after the injury.   Even when seen within an hour or two of the wound, the prolapse can seldom, in my experience, be either returned by manipulation or made to retract by eserine or atropine.

It is sometimes important to determine whether an excised eye contain a foreign body.   If nothing can be found in the blood or lymph, etc., by feeling with a probe, it is best to crush the soft parts, little by little, between finger and thumb, when the smallest particle will be felt.   If a shot have entered and left the eye, the counter-opening may, if recent, be found from the inside, although no irregularity be noticeable outside the eyeball.

CHAPTER XI.

CATARACT means opacity of the crystalline lens, and is due to changes in the structure and composition of the lens-fibres. The capsule is often thickened, but otherwise not much altered. The changes seldom occur throughout the whole lens at once, but begin first in a certain region, *e. g.*, the centre, *nucleus*, or the superficial layers, *cortex*, whilst in some forms of partial cataract the change never spreads beyond the part first affected.

Senile changes in the lens.—With advancing age the lens, which is from birth firmest at the centre, becomes harder, and acquires a very decided yellow color ; its refractive power usually decreases, its surface reflects more light, and its substance becomes somewhat fluorescent. The result of all these changes is, that at an advanced age the lens is more easily visible than in early life, the pupil becoming grayish instead of being quite black. This grayness of the pupil may easily be mistaken for cataract, but ophthalmoscopic examination shows that the lens is transparent, the fundus being seen without any appreciable haze. It has hitherto been supposed that the lens became smaller in old age, but the researches of Priestley Smith have lately shown that the lens continues to increase in all dimensions, so long as it remains transparent. As a rule, however, cataractous lens are undersized.

The consistence of a cataract depends chiefly on the patient's age. The wide physical differences between cataracts depend less on variations in the cause, position, or character of the opacity than on the degree of natural hardness which is proper to the lens at the time when the opacity sets in.   Below about thirty-five all cataracts are "soft."

Forms of General Cataract.

(1.) **Nuclear cataract.**—The opacity begins in, and remains more dense at, the nucleus of the lens, thinning off gradually in all directions toward the cortex, Fig. 64; the nucleus is not really opaque, but densely hazy.   As the patients are generally old, nuclear cataract is usually senile and hard, and also often amber-colored or light brownish, like "pea-soup" fog.

(2.) **Cortical cataract.**—The change begins in the superficial parts, and generally takes the form of sharply defined lines or streaks, or triangular patches, which point toward the axis of the lens, and whose shape is dependent on the arrangement of the lens fibres, Fig. 65.   They usually begin at the edge, *equator*, of the lens, where they are hidden by the iris, but when large enough they encroach on the pupil as whitish streaks or triangular patches.   They affect both the anterior and posterior layers of the lens, and the intervening parts may be quite clear.   Sooner or later the nucleus also becomes hazy, mixed cataract, and the whole lens eventually gets opaque.

Some cases of the large class known as "senile" or "hard" cataract are nuclear from beginning to end, *i. e.*, formed by gradual extension of diffused opacity from the centre to the surface; more commonly they are of the mixed variety.

A few cataracts beginning at the nucleus, and many beginning at the vortex, are not senile in the sense of accompanying old age, and are, therefore, not hard.   Some such are caused by diabetes, but in many it is impossible to say why the lens should have become diseased.[1] Mey-höfer, observing that opacities in the lens are disproportionately common in glassblowers, suggests that radiant heat may act as a direct cause of cataract. Many of them are known as "soft" cataracts when complete. They generally form quickly, in a few months. A few are congenital. Whether nuclear or cortical, they are whiter and more uniform looking than the slower cataracts of old age, and the cortex often has a sheen, like satin or mother-of-pearl, or looks flaky like spermaceti.

In some cortical cataracts we find only numerous very small dots or short streaks—"dotted cortical cataract." Occasionally a single large wedge-shaped opacity will form at some part of the cortex and remain stationary and solitary for many years. Sometimes in suspected cataract, though no opaque striæ are visible by focal illumination, one or more dark streaks, "striæ of refraction"—Bowman, are seen with the mirror, altering as its inclination is varied, and having much the same optical effect as cracks in glass; these "flaws" should always be looked on as the beginning of cataract.

PARTIAL CATARACT.

Three forms need special notice.

(1) **Lamellar (zonular) cataract** is a peculiar and well-marked form in which the superficial laminæ and the nucleus of the lens are clear, a layer or shell of opacity being present between them, Fig. 67. An examination of three or four specimens here and abroad shows a degenerated layer between the nucleus and cortex; in all the

---

[1] Lowered blood-supply from atheroma of the carotid has lately been suggested as a cause in some cases (Michel). Cataract does not seem to be often related to renal disease; but when renal albuminuria is present in a case of cataract, the prognosis for operation is decidedly less favorable than usual.

cases the nucleus has been found degenerated, but it is not
yet determined whether this is due to post-mortem change
or not (Lawford, Beselin).   It is probable that the opacity
is present at birth; it certainly never forms late in life.
The great majority of its subjects give a history of infantile
convulsions   The size of the opaque lamella or shell, and
therefore its depth from the surface of the lens, is subject
to much variation, and it may be much smaller than is
shown in the figure.   The opacity is often stationary for
years, perhaps for life, but cases are sometimes met with in
which we cannot doubt, from the history, that the opacity
has, without extending perceptibly, become more dense;
instances of lamellar opacity spreading to the whole lens
are, however, apparently very rare.

(2) **Pyramidal cataract.**—A small, sharply-defined spot
of chalky-white opacity is present in the middle of the
pupil, (at the *anterior pole* of the lens), looking as if it lay
upon the capsule.   When viewed sideways it seems to be
superficially embedded in the lens, and also sometimes
stands forward as a little nipple or pyramid, Fig. 62.   It

Fig. 62.

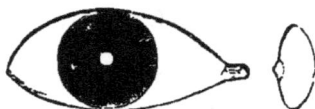

Pyramidal cataract seen from the front and in section.

consists of the degenerated products of a localized inflammation just beneath the lens-capsule, with the addition of
organized lymph derived from the iris and deposited on
the front of the capsule, the capsule itself being puckered
and folded, Fig. 63.   It is a stationary form, scarcely ever
becoming general.

Pyramidal cataract is the result of central perforating
ulceration of the cornea in early life, and of this ophthalmia
neonatorum is nearly always the cause; it is, therefore,

often associated with corneal nebula. The contact between the exposed part of the lens-capsule and the inflamed cornea, which occurs when the aqueous has escaped through the hole in the ulcer, appears to set up the localized sub-

FIG. 63.

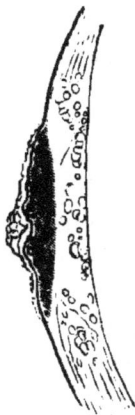

Magnified section through a pyramidal cataract, with the immediately subjacent layers. The fine parallel shading shows the thickness of the opacity, the double (black and white) outline is the capsule; above and below are the cortical lens-fibres, many being broken up into globules beneath the opacity. Lying upon the puckered capsule over the opacity is a little fibrous tissue, the result of iritis.

capsular inflammation. Iritis in very early life may also cause similar opacities at points of adhesion between the iris and lens.

The term *anterior polar cataract* is applied both to the form just described and to certain rare cases in which general cataract begins at this part of the lens.

(3) Cataract, which afterwards becomes general, may begin as a thin layer at the middle of the hinder surface of the lens, **posterior polar cataract**, Fig. 66. There are many varieties, but in general the pole itself shows the most change, the opacity radiating outward from it in more

or less regular spokes. The color appears grayish, yellowish, or even brown, because seen through the whole thickness of the lens. Sometimes the opacity is due to formations adherent to the back of the capsule, *i. e.*, in front of the vitreous; but this can seldom be proved during life. Cataract beginning at the posterior pole is often a sign of disease of the vitreous depending on choroidal mischief; it is common in the later stages of retinitis pigmentosa and severe choroiditis, and in high degrees of myopia with disease of the vitreous. The prognosis, therefore, should always be guarded in a case of cataract where the principal part of the opacity is in this position.

When a cataract forms without known connection with other disease of the eye, it is said to be *primary*. The term *secondary cataract* is used when it is the consequence of some local disease, such as severe irido-cyclitis, glaucoma, detachment of the retina, or the growth of a tumor in the eye. Primary cataract is symmetrical in most cases, but an interval, which may even extend to several years, usually separates its onset in the two eyes. Secondary cataract, of course, may or may not be symmetrical.

DIAGNOSIS OF CATARACT.—The subjective symptoms of cataract depend almost solely on the obstruction and distortion of the entering light by the opacities. Objectively, cataract is shown in advanced cases by the white or gray condition of the pupil at the plane of the iris; in earlier stages by whitish opacity in the lens when examined by focal light, and by corresponding dark portions, lines, spots, or patches in the red pupil when examined by the ophthalmoscope mirror.

Both subjective and objective symptoms differ with the position and quantity of the opacity. When the whole lens is opaque the pupil is uniformly whitish; the opacity lies almost on a level with the iris, no space intervening, and consequently, on examining by focal light, we find that the iris casts no shadow on the opacity; the brightest light from the mirror will not penetrate the lens in quantity enough to illuminate the choroid, and hence no red reflex will be obtained. Such a cataract is said to be mature or "ripe," and the affected eye will be, in ordinary terms, "blind." If both cataracts be equally advanced, the patient will be unable to see any objects; but he will distinguish quite easily between light and shade when the eye is alternately covered and uncovered in ordinary daylight, good *perception* of light, *p. l.*, and will tell correctly the *position* of a candle flame (good *projection*). The pupils should be active to light and not dilated, the tension normal.

In a case of incipient cataract the patient complains of gradual failure of sight, and we find the acuteness of vision impaired, probably more in one eye than in the other, and more for distant than for near objects. In the earliest stages of senile cataract some degree of myopia may be developed (Chap. XX.), or, owing to irregular refraction by the lens, the patient may see with each eye two or more images of any object close together, *polyopia uniocularis.* If he can still read moderate type, the glasses appropriate for his age and refraction, though giving some help, do not remove the defect. If, as is usual, he be presbyopic, he will be likely to choose over-strong spectacles, and to place objects too close to his eyes, so as to obtain larger retinal images, and thus compensate for want of clearness. In nuclear cataract, as the axial rays of light are most obstructed, sight is often better when the pupil is rather large, and such patients tell us that they see better in a dull light, or with the back to the window, or when shading the eyes with the hand. In the cortical and more diffused forms this symptom is less marked.

On examining by focal light (the pupil having been dilated) an *immature nuclear cataract* appears as a yellowish,

rather deeply-seated, haze, upon which a shadow is cast by
the iris on the side from which the light comes, 3, Fig. 64.
On now using the mirror this same opacity appears as a dull
blur in the area of the red pupil, darkest at the centre,

FIG. 64.

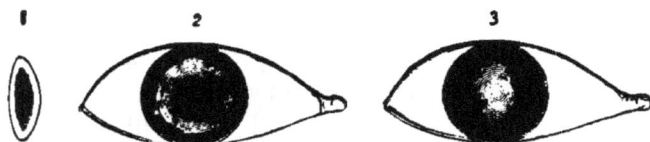

Nuclear cataract. 1. Section of lens; opacity densest at centre. 2.
Opacity as seen by transmitted light (ophthalmoscope mirror) with
dilated pupil. 3. Opacity as seen by reflected light (focal illumination). The pupil is supposed to be dilated by atropine.

and gradually thinning off on all sides, so that, at the
margin of the pupil, the full red choroidal reflex may still
be present; the details of the fundus, if still visible, are
obscured by the hazy lens, the haze being thickest when
we look through the centre of the pupil, 2, Fig. 64. If
the opacity be dense and large, a faint dull redness will
be visible, and that only at the border of the pupil.

Cortical opacities, if small and confined to the equator,
or edge, of the lens, do not interfere with sight; they are
easily detected with a dilated pupil by throwing light very
obliquely behind the iris. When large and encroaching

FIG. 65.

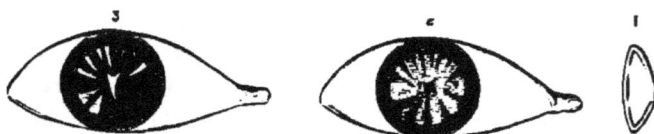

Cortical cataract. References as in preceding figure.

on the pupil they are visible in ordinary daylight. They
occur in the form of dots, streaks, or wedges; seen by focal
light they are white or grayish, and more or less sharply

defined according as they are in the anterior or posterior layers, 3, Fig. 65. With the mirror they appear black or grayish, and of rather smaller size, 2, Fig. 65; and if the intervening substance be clear, the details of the fundus can be seen sharply between the bars of opacity. Some forms of cataract begin with innumerable minute dots in the cortical layer.

Posterior polar opacities are seldom visible without careful focal illumination, when we find a patchy or stellate figure very deeply seated in the axis of the lens, 3, Fig. 66; if large it looks concave, like the bottom of a shallow cup. With the mirror it is seen as a dark star, 2, Fig. 66, or network, or irregular patch, but smaller than when seen by focal light.

The diagnosis of *lamellar cataract* is easy if its nature be understood, but by beginners it is often diagnosed as "nuclear." The patients are generally children or young adults; they complain of "near sight" rather than of

FIG. 66.

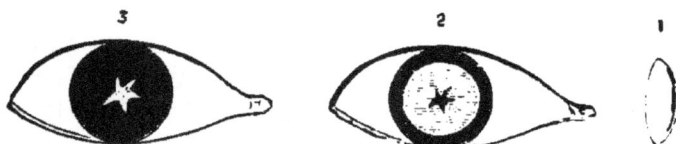

Posterior polar cataract.   References as before.

"cataract;" for the opacity is not usually very dense, and whether the refraction of their eyes be really myopic or not, they (like other cataractous patients) compensate for dull retinal images by holding the object nearer, and so increasing the size of the images. The acuteness of vision is always defective, and cannot be fully remedied by any glasses. They often see rather better when the pupils are dilated either by shading the eyes or by means of atropine; in the latter case convex glasses ($+4$, or $+4$ D.) are necessary for reading. The pupil presents a deeply-seated, slight grayness, 4, Fig. 67, and when dilated with atropine the outline of the shell of opacity is exposed within it. This opacity is sharply defined, circular and whitish by focal light, interspersed, in many cases, with white specks, which at its equator appear as little projections, 3, Fig. 67. By focal illumination we easily make out that the opacity consists of two distinct layers, that there is a layer

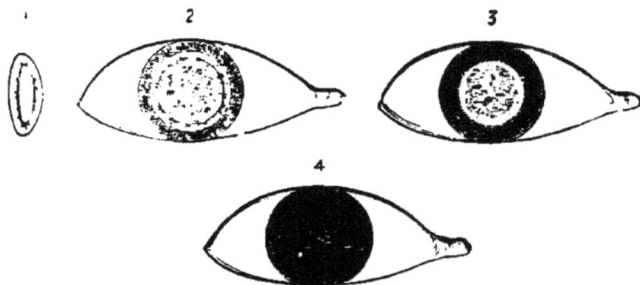

FIG. 67.

Lamellar cataract. Figs. 1, 2, 3, as before. Fig. 4 shows *slight* grayness of the undilated pupil, owing to the layers of opacity being deeply seated.

of clear lens substance, cortex, in front of the anterior layer, and that the margin, equator, of the lens is clear. By the mirror the opacity appears as a disc of nearly uniform grayish or dark color, sometimes with projections, or darker dots, and surrounded by a zone of bright-red reflection from the fundus corresponding to the clear margin of the lens, 2, Fig. 67. The opacity often appears rather denser at its boundary, a sort of ring being formed there, and in some cases quite large spicules or patches project from the part. Not only does the size of the opaque lamella, and, therefore, its depth from the surface of the lens, differ greatly in different cases, but its thickness or degree of opacity varies also. The disease is nearly always symmetrical in the two eyes. Occasionally there are two shells of opacity, one within the other, separated by a certain amount of clear lens substance.

The lens may be cataractous at birth, *congenital cataract.* This form, of which there are several varieties, is nearly always symmetrical, and generally involves the whole lens. Often the development of the eyeball is defective, and though there are no synechiæ, the iris may act badly to atropine. Cases are seen from time to time in which juvenile or perhaps congenital cataract appears in many members of a family, even in several generations.

PROGNOSIS OF CATARACT. *a. Course.*—Although opacities in the lens never clear up,[1] they advance with very varying rapidity in different cases. As a rough rule, the progress of a general cataract is rapid in proportion to the youth of the patient. Cataracts in old people commonly take from one to three years in reaching maturity—sometimes much longer; there are cases of nuclear senile cataract where the opacity never spreads to the cortex, and the cataract never becomes "complete," though it may become dry and "ripe" for operation. If the lens be allowed to remain very long after it is opaque, further degenerative changes generally occur; it may become harder and smaller, calcareous and fatty granules being formed in it; or the cortex may liquefy whilst the nucleus remains hard, *Morgagnian cataract.* A congenital cataract may undergo absorption and shrink to a thin, firm, membranous disc. Soft cataract in young adults, from whatever cause, is generally complete in a few months.

b. Sight.—The prognosis *after operation* is good when there is no other disease of the eye, and when the patient (although advanced in years) is in fair general health. It is not so good in diabetes, nor when the patient is in obviously bad health, the eyes being then less tolerant of operation. In the lamellar and other congenital varieties it must be guarded, for the eyes are often defective in other respects,

---

[1] Except sometimes in diabetes (Chap. XXIII.).

and sometimes very intolerant of operation; the intellect, too, is sometimes defective, rendering the patient less able to make proper use of his eyes. In traumatic cataract, of course, everything depends on the details of the injury, but, as a rule, the younger the patient the better the prospect of a quiet and uncomplicated absorption of the lens.

In every case of immature cataract the vitreous and fundus should be carefully examined by the ophthalmoscope, and the refraction ascertained. The presence of high myopia is unfavorable, and the same is true of opacities in the vitreous, indicating, as they usually do, that it is fluid. Any disease of the choroid or retina will, of course, be prejudicial in proportion to its position and extent. In every case, before deciding to operate, the state of the conjunctiva and lachrymal passages, the tension of the eye, and the size and mobility of the pupils to light, are to be carefully noted.

TREATMENT.—In the early stages of senile and nuclear cataract, sight is improved by keeping the pupil moderately dilated with a weak mydriatic solution, one-eighth of a grain of atropine to the ounce, used about three times a week. Dark glasses, by allowing some dilatation of the pupil, also assist. Stenopaic glasses are sometimes useful. With these exceptions, nothing except operative treatment is of any use. The management of lamellar cataract requires separate description.

Operations for the removal of cataract are of three kinds: (1) *Extraction of the lens entire* through a large wound in the cornea, or at the sclero-corneal junction, the lens-capsule remaining behind. By a few operators the lens is removed entire in its capsule. (2) For soft cataracts, *gradual absorption*, by the agency of the aqueous humor admitted through needle punctures in the capsule, just after accidental traumatic cataract-needle operations, *solution, discission.* The operation needs repetition two or three times, at intervals of a few weeks, and the whole process therefore occupies three or four months. (3) For soft cataracts, *removal by a suction syringe or curette*, introduced into the anterior chamber through a small wound near the margin of the cornea, the whole lens having, if thought necessary, been freely broken up by a discission operation a few days previously (Chap. XXII.).

Extraction is necessary for cataracts after about the age of forty. The lens from this age onwards is so firm that its absorption after discission occupies a much longer time than in childhood and youth; moreover, as already stated, the swelling of the lens, after wound of the capsule, is less easily borne as age advances, and hence solution operations become not only slower, but attended by more danger. Indeed, though suction and solution operations are applicable up to about the age of thirty-five, extraction is often practised in preference at a much earlier age. Suction is more difficult, and it is thought by some to be attended by more risk of irido-cyclitis than the "solution" operation; its advantage lies in its saving of time, almost the whole lens being removed at one sitting. Evacuation along the groove of a curette barely passed through the wound is a very safe proceeding.

If one present a complete cataract whilst the sight of the other is perfect, or at least serviceable, removal of the cataract will confer little immediate benefit to the patient. Indeed, if one eye be still fairly good, the patient will often be dissatisfied by finding his operated eye less useful than he expected, perhaps even not so useful as the other. In senile cataract, therefore, it is usually best not to operate so long as the lens of the other eye remains nearly clear; but so soon as it becomes sufficiently affected to interfere seriously with vision, extraction of the cataract from the first is advisable, provided that the patient have a fair prospect of life. The cataract in the first eye may be

over-ripe and less favorable for operation, if it be left until
the second eye be quite ready. The removal of a single
cataract in young persons is often expedient on account of
appearance. In all cases of single cataract it must be
explained that after the operation the two eyes will not
work together on account of the extreme difference of refraction. See Anisometropia.

Even when both cataracts are mature at the same time,
it is safer to remove only one at once, because the after-
treatment is more easily carried out upon one eye than
both, and because after the double operation any untoward
result in one eye adds to the difficulty of managing its
fellow; while a bad result after single extraction enables
us to take especial precautions, or to modify the operation
for the second eye. Even if the patient be so old or feeble
that the second eye may never come to operation, we shall
consult his interests better by endeavoring to give him one
good eye than by risking a bad result in attempting to restore both at the same time.

Cataract occurring after the age of forty can seldom be
safely extracted until it is complete or "ripe." The transparent portions of an immature cataract cannot be completely removed, partly because they are sticky, partly
because they cannot be seen; and, remaining behind in
the eye, they act as irritants and often set up iritis. Incomplete juvenile cataract, e. g., lamellar cataract, may be
safely ripened by tearing the capsule with a needle (see
Discission and Suction); but hard cataract cannot be so
treated because the lens is too hard to absorb the aqueous
well, and the senile eye is intolerant of injury to the lens.

Some years ago, Professor Förster, of Breslau, proposed a
plan for hastening the completion of very slow senile cataracts:
immediately after the iridectomy he bruises the lens by rubbing
the cornea firmly over the pupil with a cataract spoon or other
smooth instrument; the capsule is not ruptured, but the lens-

fibres are broken up or so changed that they often become opaque a few weeks or months after. Priestley Smith and others adopt the safer plan of bruising the lens directly by means of a small bulbous spatula passed through the corneal wound. These methods are very uncertain, sometimes having no effect, but the latter modification may be employed without risk in suitable cases. More recently McKeown and Wickerkiewicz have advocated the plan of washing out the capsule, after expulsion of the bulk of the lens, by means of a stream of water or weak antiseptic lotion ; either a syringe or syphon may be used. The authors hope that this proceeding, by facilitating the removal of clear cortical matter, will render the extraction of *immature* senile cataract safe and expedient. It must be borne in mind, however, that the lens substance is more sticky and adherent to the capsule when clear, and that, therefore, it may be most difficult of removal by this method, as by others, just when its removal is most important. The method is being largely tried by several operators.

The **principal causes of failure** after extraction of cataract are—

(1.) *Hemorrhage* between the choroid and sclerotic coming on, usually with severe pain, immediately after the operation. The blood fills the eyeball, and often oozes from the wound and soaks through the bandage.

(2.) *Suppuration*, beginning in the corneal wound, spreading to the iris and vitreous, and in many to the entire cornea, and ending in a total loss of the eye. It occasionally takes a less rapid course, and stops short of a fatal result. The alarm is given in from twelve hours to about three days after operation by the occurrence of pain, inflammatory œdema of the lids, particularly the free border of the upper lid, and the appearance of some mucopurulent discharge. On raising the lid the eye is found to be greatly congested, its conjunctiva œdematous, the edges of the wound yellowish, and the cornea steamy and hazy. In very rapid cases the pupil, especially near to the wound,

will already be occupied by lymph.   Suppuration is probably always caused by infection, though the source of the
mischief of course often remains hidden.   Chronic dacryo-
cystitis is a very dangerous concomitant of cataract operations, the pus escaping through the puncta and infecting
the wound.   Suppuration is more probable if the wound
lie in clear corneal tissue than if it be partly scleral, and
if the patient be in bad or feeble health.

The use of hot fomentations for an hour three or four
times a day, leeches, if there be much pain, and internally
a purge, followed by quinine and ammonia, and wine or
brandy if the patient be feeble, should be at once resorted
to.   As to other measures, opinions differ.   From what I
have seen of my own and others' cases I am, at present,
inclined to agree with Horner and those who direct most
attention to the vigorous antiseptic treatment of the wound
itself; I have found that the actual (galvano-) cautery
applied deeply along the whole length of the wound is more
successful than any other measures, assisted, however, by
hot fomentations, and the use of iodoform or of weak
lotions of chloride of zinc or bichloride of mercury, and by
leaving the eye open.[1]   But only in the cases of moderate
rapidity and intensity can we hope, even partly, to arrest
the disease, for the great majority of these cases go on to
suppurative panophthalmitis, or to severe plastic irido-
cyclitis with opacity of cornea and shrinking of the eyeball.

(3.) *Iritis* may set in between about the fourth and tenth
days.   Here also pain, œdema of the eyelids, and chemosis
are the earliest symptoms.   There is lachrymation, but
no muco-purulent discharge, and the cornea and wound
usually remain clear.   The iris is discolored (unless it
happen to be naturally greenish-brown), and the pupil dilates badly to atropine.   Whenever, in a case presenting

---

[1] Mr. C. T. Collins, our house surgeon at Moorfields, suggested to me
the last-named measure.

such symptoms, a good examination is rendered difficult on account of the photophobia, iritis should be suspected. If the early symptoms are severe, a few leeches to the temples are very useful. Atropine and warmth are the best local measures. If atropine irritate, daturine or duboisine should be tried (F. 32, 33).

This inflammation is plastic, ending in the formation of more or less dense membrane in the pupil. Such membrane by contracting and drawing the iris with it toward the operation scar often contracts and displaces the pupil. Fig. 161 shows this in an extreme degree. The membrane is formed partly by exudation from the iris and ciliary processes, *iritis, cyclitis*, partly by the lens-capsule and its proliferated endothelial cells, *capsulitis*. Mixed forms of chronic keratitis and iritis sometimes occur, the corneal haze spreading from the wound in the form of long lines or stripes. Iritis of obstinately plastic type is liable to occur after extraction of cataract in diabetes.

(4.) The iris may become incarcerated in or prolapse through the wound at the operation or a few days afterward by the reopening of a weakly united wound. When iridectomy has been done the prolapse appears as a little dark bulging at one or both ends of the wound, and often causes prolonged irritability, without actual iritis. The best treatment is to draw the protruding part further out, and to cut it off as freely as possible, as in accidental wounds.. The occurrence of prolapse is a reason for keeping the eye tied up longer. The capsule may also be incarcerated in or adherent to the wound after extraction, suction, or curette, simple linear extraction. *After-operations* are needed if the pupil be much obstructed by capsular opacities or by the results of iritis; but nothing should be done until active symptoms have subsided and the eye been quiet for some weeks.

Sight after the removal of cataract.—In accounting for the state of the sight we have to remember that the acuteness of sight naturally decreases in old age; that slight iritis, producing a little filmy opacity in the pupil, is common after extraction; and that some eyes with good sight remain irritable for long after the operation, and therefore cannot be much used. Thus, putting aside the graver complications, we find that even of the eyes which do best only a moderate proportion reach normal acuteness of vision. Cases are considered good when the patient can with his glasses read anything between Nos. 1 and 14 Jaeger and $\frac{6}{18}$ Snellen; but a much less satisfactory result than this is very useful. About 5 per cent. of the eyes operated upon are lost from various causes. The eye is rendered extremely hypermetropic by removal of the lens, and frequently there is a good deal of astigmatism due to flattening of that meridian of the cornea which is at a right angle with the operation wound. Strong convex glasses are necessary for clear vision; these should seldom be allowed until three months after the operation, and at first they should not be continuously worn. Two pairs are needed; one makes the eye emmetropic and gives clear distant vision ($+ 10$ or 11 D.); the other (about $+ 16$ D.) is for reading, sewing, etc., at about $10''$ (25 cm.), as during strong accommodation. When there is astigmatism it should usually be corrected. As all accommodation is lost, the patient has no *range* of distinct vision.

Lamellar cataract.—If the patient can see enough to get on fairly well at school, or in his occupation, it may be best not to operate; but when, as is the rule, the opacity is dense enough to interfere seriously with his prospects, something must be done. The choice lies between artificial pupil when the clear margin is wide and quite free from spicules, and solution or extraction when it is narrow, or when large spicules of opacity project into it from the opaque lamella, Fig. 67. It is difficult to say which method gives on the whole the better results, and we must judge each case on its own merits. If atropine, by dilating the pupil, improves the sight, an artificial pupil, made by removing the iris quite up to its ciliary border, will generally be beneficial; the clear border of the lens is thus exposed in the coloboma, and light passes through it more readily than through the hazy part. A very good rule is to operate on only one eye at a time, thus allowing the choice of a different operation on its fellow. My own experience is decidedly in favor of removing the lens in the majority of cases.

When a cataractous eye is absolutely blind (no p. l., see p. 49), some more deeply-seated disease must be present, and no operation should be undertaken; and when projection and p. l. are bad, great caution is needed.

Cataract following injury.—Severe blows on the eye may be followed by opacity of the lens, the capsule and often the suspensory ligament being no doubt torn in some part, *concussion cataract*. Lawford has shown that rupture of the posterior capsule may occur from a blow, while the anterior capsule remains intact (*Ophth. Rev.*, vi. 281). Such a cataract may remain incomplete and stationary for an indefinite period, but often it becomes complete. *Traumatic cataract* proper is the result of wound of the lens-capsule; the aqueous passing through the aperture is imbibed by the lens-fibres, which swell up, become opaque, and finally disintegrate and are absorbed. The opacity begins within a few hours of the wound; it progresses quickly in proportion as the wound is large and the patient young; but both the symptoms and consequences are often more severe in old persons. A free wound of the capsule, followed by rapid swelling of the whole lens, may give rise, especially after middle life, to severe glaucomatous symptoms and iritis. In from three to six months a wounded lens will generally be absorbed, and nothing but some chalky-looking detritus remain in connection with the capsule. A very fine puncture of the lens is occasionally followed by nothing more than a small patch or narrow track of opacity, or by very slowly advancing general haze. Occasionally partial opacities of the lens caused by injury clear up entirely. The objects of *treatment* are to prevent iritis by atropine, and by leeching if there be pain ; it is usually safest to leave the wounded lens to become absorbed, but we must be prepared to extract it by linear operation or suction at any time, should glaucoma, iritis, or severe irritation arise. A *concussion* cataract, however, is seldom completely absorbed; the lens shrinks and may then become loosened, and fall either into the vitreous or aqueous chamber. I believe, therefore, that it is usually best to remove by operation a cataract following a blow. It will often be observed in both these forms of cataract that the opacity appears at the posterior surface of the lens quite early, whether the wound have penetrated deeply or not.

Dislocation of the lens in its capsule is usually caused by a blow on the eye, but may be spontaneous, or congenital ; in either case it is, as a rule only partial. The iris is often tremulous where its support is lost, and bulged forward at some other part where the lens rests against it ; by focal light, or by the ophthalmoscope, the free edge of the lens can be seen as a curved line passing across the pupil; more easily if the pupil be dilated. More rarely the dislocation is incomplete, either into the vitreous or into the anterior chamber. A full-sized lens dislocated into the anterior chamber causes acute glaucoma. Glaucoma, acute or chronic, may also follow at any time after a dislocation, either partial or complete, into the vitreous. Dislocated lenses often become opaque and shrunken, and then either remain loose or become adherent, and in either event are likely, sooner or later, to set up irritation and pain. Such a lens may sometimes be made to pass at will through the pupil by altering the position of the head. The edge of a transparent lens in the vitreous appears, by the mirror, as a dark line; when in the anterior chamber it appears as a bright line, by focal illumination. Congenital dislocation of the lens is often accompanied by other defects of development, such as coloboma.

For dislocation of lens beneath conjunctiva in rupture of eye, see p. 178.

CHAPTER XII

THE choroid is, next to the ciliary processes, the most vascular part of the eyeball, and from it the outer layers of the retina, certainly, and the vitreous humor probably, are mainly nourished. Inflammatory and degenerative changes often occur, some of them entirely local, as in myopia, others symptomatic of constitutional or of generalized disease, such as syphilis and tuberculosis. Choroiditis, unlike inflammation of its continuations, the ciliary body and iris, is seldom shown by external congestion or severe pain ; and as none of its symptoms are characteristic, the diagnosis rests chiefly on ophthalmoscopic evidence.

Blemishes or scars, permanent and easily seen, nearly always follow disease of the choroid, and such spots and patches are often as useful for diagnosis as cicatrices on the skin, and deserve as careful study. The retina lying over an inflamed choroid often takes on active changes, or becomes atrophied afterwards ; but in other cases, marked by equally severe changes, the retina is uninjured. Indeed, there is sometimes difficulty in deciding which of these two structures was first affected, especially as changes in the pigment epithelium, which is really part of the retina, are as often the result of deep-seated retinitis, or retinal hemorrhage, as of superficial choroiditis. Patches of accumulated pigment, though usually indicating spots of former choroiditis, are sometimes the result of bleeding, either from retinal or choroidal vessels, and their correct interpretation may therefore be difficult.

Appearances in health.—The choroid is composed chiefly
of bloodvessels and of cells containing dark-brown pigment.
The quantity of pigment varies in different eyes, and to
some degree in different parts of the same eye; it is scanty
in early childhood, and in persons of fair complexion; more
abundant in persons with dark or red hair, brown irides,
or freckled skin; more plentiful in the region of the yellow
spot than elsewhere. In old age the pigment epithelium
becomes paler. When examining the choroid we need to
think of four parts : (1) the retinal pigmented epithelium,
which is for ophthalmoscopic purposes choroidal, seen in
the erect image as a fine darkish stippling; (2) the capillary layer, chorio-capillaris, just beneath the epithelium,
forming a very close meshwork, the separate vessels of
which are not visible in life; (3) the larger bloodvessels,
often easily visible; (4) the pigmented connective-tissue
cells of the choroid proper, which lie between the larger
vessels.

In the majority of eyes these four structures are so toned
as to give a nearly uniform, full red color by the ophthalmoscope, blood-color predominating. In very dark races
the pigment is so excessive that the fundus has a uniform
slaty color. In very fair persons, and young children, the
deep pigment (4) is so scanty that the large vessels are
separated by spaces of lighter color than themselves, Fig.
34. In dark persons these same spaces are of a deeper hue
than the vessels, the latter appearing like light streams
separated by dark islands (*see* upper part of Fig. 70).
Near to the disc and y. s. the vessels are extremely abundant and very tortuous, the interspaces being small and
irregular; but toward and in front of the equator the veins
take a nearly straight course, converging toward the *venæ
vorticosæ*, and the islands are larger and elongated. The
veins are much more numerous and larger than the arteries,
Fig. 69, but we cannot often distinguish between them in

life. The vessels of the choroid, unlike those of the retina, present no light streak along the centre. The pigment epithelium and the capillary layer tone down the above contrasts, and so in old age, when the epithelium pigment is bleached, or if the capillary layer be atrophied after superficial choroiditis, Fig. 70, a and b, the above distinctions become very marked.

A vertical section of naturally injected human choroid is shown in Fig. 68; the uppermost dark line (1) is the pigment epithelium; next are seen the capillary vessels (2), cut across; then the more deeply-seated large vessels (3), and the deep layer of stellate pigment-cells of the choroid proper (4). Fig. 69 is from an artificially injected human choroid seen from the inner surface. The shaded portion is intended to represent the general effect produced by all the vessels and the pigment epithelium. The lower part shows the large vessels with their elongated interspaces, as may be seen in a case where the pigment epithelium and chorio-capillaris are atrophied, Fig. 70, b; in a dark eye the interspaces in Fig. 69 would be darker than the vessels.

FIG. 68.

Human choroid, vertical section. Naturally injected. × 20.

The middle part shows the capillaries without the pigment epithelium. Both figures are magnified about four times as much as the image in the indirect ophthalmoscopic examination.

OPHTHALMOSCOPIC SIGNS OF DISEASE OF THE CHOROID.

The changes usually met with are indicative of *atrophy*. This may be partial or complete: primary, or following inflammation or hemorrhage; in circumscribed spots and patches, or in large and less abruptly bounded areas. Secondary changes are often present in the corresponding

Fig. 69.

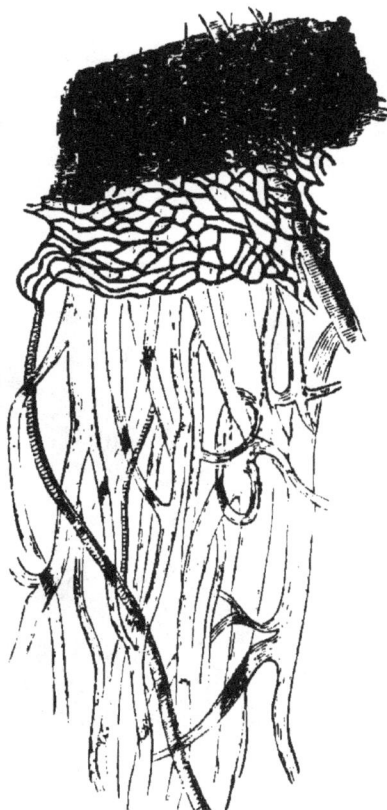

Vessels of human choroid artificially injected. Arteries cross-shaded. Capillaries too dark and rather too small. The uppermost shaded part is meant to represent the effect of the pigment epithelium. × 20.

parts of the retina. The chief signs of atrophy of the choroid are (1) the substitution of a paler color, varying from pale red to yellowish-white, for the full red of health, the subjacent white sclerotic being more or less visible

where the atrophic changes have occurred; (2) black pigment in spots, patches, or rings, and in varying quantity
upon or around the pale patches.   These pigmentations
result, 1st, from disturbance and heaping together of the
normal pigment; 2d, from increase in its quantity; 3d, from
blood-coloring matter left after extravasation.   Patches of
primary atrophy, *e.g.*, in myopia, are never much pigmented
unless bleeding have taken place.   The amount of pigmentation in atrophy following choroiditis is closely related
to that of the healthy choroid, *i. e.*, to the complexion of
the person.

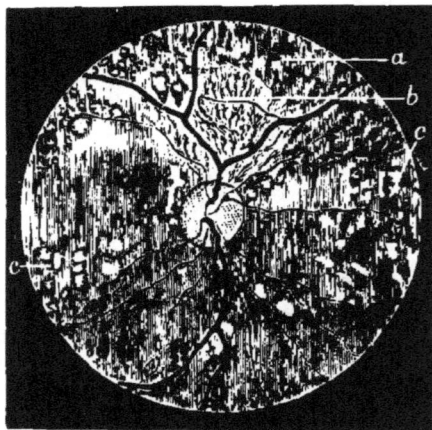

FIG. 70.

Atrophy after syphilitic choroiditis, showing various degrees of
wasting (Hutchinson). *a.* Atrophy of pigment epithelium. *b.* Atrophy
of epithelium and chorio-capillaris; the large vessels exposed. *c.* Spots
of complete atrophy, many with pigment accumulation.

Pigment at the fundus may lie in the retina as well as
in, or on, the choroid, and this is true whatever may have
been its origin, for in choroiditis with secondary retinitis
the choroidal pigment often passes forward into the retina.
When a spot of pigment is distinctly seen to cover over a

retinal vessel, that spot must be not only in, but very near the anterior (inner) surface of, the retina; and when the pigment has a linear, mossy or lace-like pattern, Fig. 81, it is always in the retina; these are the only conclusive tests of its position.

It is important, and usually easy, to distinguish between partial and complete atrophy of the choroid. In *superficial atrophy*, affecting the pigment epithelium and capillary layer, the large vessels are peculiarly distinct, Fig. 70, *a* and *b*. Such "capillary" or "epithelial" choroiditis often covers a large surface, the boundaries of which are sometimes well-defined, sinuous and map-like, but are as often

FIG. 71.

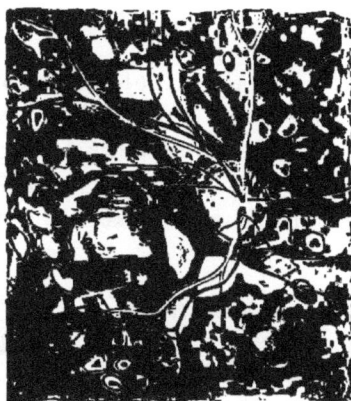

Atrophy after choroiditis. (Magnus.)

ill-marked; in the latter case we must carefully compare different parts of the fundus, and also make allowance for the patient's age and complexion. Complete atrophy is shown by the presence of patches of white or yellowish-white color of all possible variations in size, with sharply-cut, circular or undulating borders, and with or without pigment accumulations, Figs. 70, *c*, and 71. The retinal vessels pass unobscured over patches of atrophied choroid, proving that the appearance is caused by some change deeper than the surface of the retina.

If the patient comes with *recent choroiditis,* we also often see patches of palish color, but they are less sharply bounded and frequently of a grayer or whiter (less yellow) color than patches of atrophy; moreover, the edge of such

Fig. 72.

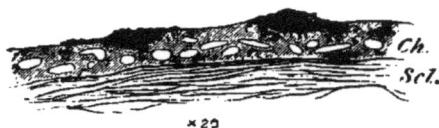

Minute exudations into inner layer of choroid in syphilitic choroiditis. Pigment epithelium adherent over the exudations, but elsewhere has been washed off. *Ch.* Choroid. *Scl.* Sclerotic.

a patch is softened, the texture of the choroid being dimly visible there, because only partly veiled by exudation. If the overlying retina be unaffected, its vessels are clearly seen over the diseased part; but if the retina itself is hazy or opaque, the exact seat of the exudation often cannot be

Fig. 73.

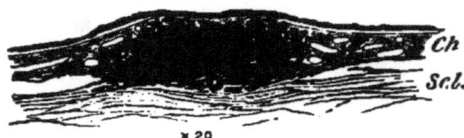

Section of miliary tubercle. Inner layers of choroid comparatively unaffected. The lighter shading, surrounding an artery in the deepest part of the tubercle, represents the oldest part, which is caseating; an artery is seen cut across in this part of the tubercle.

at once decided, and this difficulty is often increased by the hazy state of the vitreous.

Syphilitic choroiditis begins in, and is often confined to, the inner (capillary) layer of the choroid, Fig. 72, and

hence it often affects the retina. In miliary tuberculosis
of the choroid the overlying retina is clear, and the growth
is, for the most part, deeply seated, Fig. 73. After very
severe choroiditis, or extensive hemorrhage, absorption is
often incomplete; we find then, in addition to atrophy,
gray or white patches, or lines, which, in pattern and appearance, remind us of keloid scars in the skin, or of patches
and lines of old thickening on serous membranes.

Very characteristic changes are seen after *rupture of the
choroid* from sudden stretching caused by blows on the
front of the eye. These ruptures, always situated in the

FIG. 74.

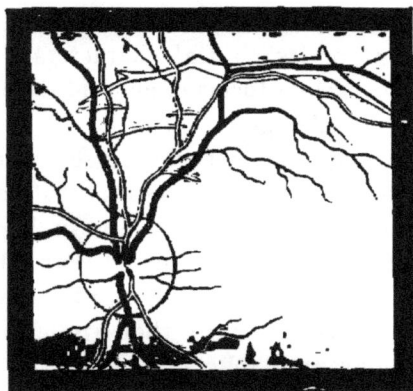

Ruptures of choroid. (Wecker.)

central region, occur in the form of long tapering lines of
atrophy, usually curved toward the disc, and sometimes
branched, Fig. 74; their borders are often pigmented. If
seen soon after the blow the rent is more or less hidden by
blood, and the retina over it is hazy.

The pathological condition known as "colloid disease"
of the choroid consists in the growth of very small nodules,
soft at first, afterward becoming hard like glass, from the

10

thin *lamina elastica*, which lies between the pigment epithelium and chorio-capillaris.   It is common in eyes excised for old inflammatory mischief, and in partial atrophy after choroiditis, Fig. 75.   But little is known of its ophthalmo-

FIG. 75.

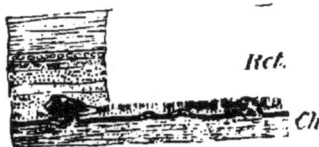

Ref.

Ch

Partial atrophy after syphilitic choroiditis.   Minute growths from inner surface of choroid, showing how they disturb the outer layers of the retina.   × 60.

scopic equivalent or its clinical characters.   Probably it may result from various forms of choroiditis, and may also be a natural senile change.

Hemorrhage from the choroidal vessels is not so often recognized as from those of the retina, but may be seen sometimes, especially in old people and in highly myopic eyes.   The patches are more rounded than retinal hemorrhage, and we can sometimes recognize the striation of the overlying retina.   Occasionally they are of immense size. Patches of atrophy may follow.

CLINICAL FORMS OF CHOROIDAL DISEASE.

(1.) Numerous discrete patches of choroidal atrophy, sometimes complete, as if a round bit had been punched out, in others incomplete, though equally round and well defined, are scattered in different parts of the fundus, but are most abundant toward the periphery ; or, if scanty, are found only in the latter situation.   They are more or less pigmented, unless the patient's complexion is extremely fair, Figs. 70, *c*, and 71.

(2.) The disease has the same distribution, but the patches are confluent ; or large areas of incomplete atrophy, passing by not very well defined boundaries into the healthy choroid around, are interspersed with a certain number of separate patches ; or without separate patches there may be a widely spread superficial atrophy with pigmentation. Fig. 70, *a* and *b*.

These two types of *choroiditis disseminata* run into one another, different names being used by authors to indicate topographical varieties. Generally both eyes are affected, though unequally ; but in some cases one eye escapes. The retina and disc often show signs of past or present inflammation.

Syphilis is by far the most frequent cause of symmetrical disseminated choroiditis. The choroiditis begins from one to three years after the primary disease, whether this be acquired or inherited ; occasionally at a later period.

The discrete variety, Fig. 70, *c*, where the patches, though usually involving the whole thickness of the choroid, are not connected by areas of superficial change, is the least serious form, unless the patches are very abundant. A moderate number of such patches confined to the periphery cause no appreciable damage to sight. The more superficial and widely-spread varieties, in which the retina and disc are inflamed from the first, are far more serious. The capillary layer of the choroid seldom again becomes healthy, and with its atrophy, even if the deeper vessels be not much changed, the retina suffers, passing into slowly progressive atrophy. The retina often becomes pigmented, Fig. 81, its bloodvessels extremely narrowed, and the disc passes into a peculiar hazy yellowish atrophy, "waxy disc," Hutchinson—" choroiditic atrophy," Gowers. The appearances may closely imitate those in true retinitis pigmentosa, and the patient, as in that disease, often suffers from marked night-blindness. Such patients continue to get slowly worse for many years, and may become nearly blind.

Syphilitic choroiditis generally gives rise, at an early date, to opacities in the vitreous ; these either form large, easily seen, slowly floating ill-defined clouds, or are so minute and numerous as to cause a diffuse and somewhat dense haziness, "dust-like opacities," Förster. (Chap. XVI.) Some of the larger ones may be permanent. In the advanced stages, as in true retinitis pigmentosa, posterior polar cataract is sometimes developed.

There are no constant differences between choroiditis in acquired and in inherited syphilis; in many cases it would be impossible to guess, from the ophthalmoscopic changes, with which form of the disease we had to do. But there is, on the whole, a greater tendency toward pigmentation in the choroiditis of hereditary than in that of acquired syphilis, and this applies both to the choroidal patches and to the subsequent retinal pigmentation.

In the treatment of syphilitic choroiditis we rely almost entirely on the constitutional remedies for syphilis—mercury and iodide of potassium. In cases which are treated early, sight is much benefited, and the visible exudations quickly melt away under mercury; but I believe that even in these complete restitution seldom takes place, the nutrition and arrangement of the pigment epithelium and bacillary layer of the retina being quickly and permanently damaged by exudations into or upon the chorio-capillaris, as in Fig. 72. In the later periods, when the choroid is thinned by atrophy, or its inner surface roughened by little outgrowths, Fig. 75, or adhesions and cicatricial contractions have occurred between it and the retina, nothing can be done. A long mercurial course should, however, always be tried if the sight be still failing, even if the changes all look old ; for in some cases, even of very long standing, fresh failure takes place from time to time, and mercury has a very marked influence. In acute cases rest of the eyes in a darkened room, and the employment of the artificial leech or of dry cupping at intervals of a few days, for some weeks, are useful. But it is often difficult to insure such functional rest, for the patients seldom have pain or other discomfort.

Disseminated choroiditis sometimes occurs without ascertainable evidence of syphilis, chiefly about the age of puberty. Such cases often differ in some of their ophthalmoscopic details from ordinary syphilitic cases, especially in the immunity of the retina and disc; and also in the absence of tendency to recur. It is but seldom that any definite cause, such as exposure to bright light, can be plausibly assigned.

In choroiditis from any cause iritis may occur.

(3.) The choroidal disease is limited to the central region. There are many varieties of such localized change.

In *myopia* the elongation which occurs at the posterior pole of the eye very often causes atrophy of the choroid contiguous to the disc, and usually only on the side next the yellow spot (see Myopia). The term *"posterior staphyloma"* is applied to this form of disease when the eye is myopic, because the atrophy is a sign of posterior bulging of the sclerotic. The term *sclerotico-choroiditis posterior* is often used, though we but seldom see evidence of exudative changes or hemorrhagic effusions at the fundus in myopia. A similar crescent, but seldom of great width, is very commonly seen, bounding the lower margin of the disc, in astigmatic eyes; its widest part nearly always corresponds with the direction of the meridian of greatest curvature of the cornea (Chap. XX.). A narrow and less conspicuous crescent, or zone, of atrophy around the disc is seen in some other states, notably in old persons and in glaucoma, Fig. 96. Separate, round patches of complete atrophy ("punched-out patches") at the central region may occur in myopia with the above-mentioned staphyloma, and must not then be ascribed to syphilitic choroiditis; in other cases of myopia ill-defined partial atrophy is seen about the y. s., sometimes with splits or lines running horizontally toward the disc.

Central senile choroiditis.—Several varieties of disease confined to the region of the y. s. and disc are seen, and chiefly in old persons. A particularly striking and rather rare form is shown in Fig. 76. In others a larger but less defined area is affected. Some of these appearances undoubtedly result from large choroidal or retinal extravasations, but the origin of the state shown in Fig. 76 is obscure. In these arcated forms the large, deep vessels are often much narrowed, or even converted into white lines and devoid of blood-column by thickening of their coats. In another form, Fig. 77, the central region is occupied by a number of small, white or yellowish-white dots, sometimes visible only in the erect image. This condition is very peculiar, and appears to be almost stationary; the discs are sometimes decidedly pale; when very abundant the spots coalesce, and some pigmentation is found; sometimes hemorrhages occur. The pathological anatomy and general relations of this disease are incompletely known; it was first described by Hutchinson and Tay, and is tolerably common. It is symmetrical and the changes may sometimes be mistaken for a slight albuminuric retinitis. No treatment seems to have any influence. Every case of immature cataract should, when possible, be examined for central choroidal changes.

(4.) **Anomalous forms of choroidal disease.**—Single, large patches of atrophy, with pigmentation, and not located in any particular part, are occasionally met with. Probably some of these have followed the absorption of tubercular growths in the choroid, while others are the result of large spontaneous hemorrhages; a blow by a

FIG. 76.

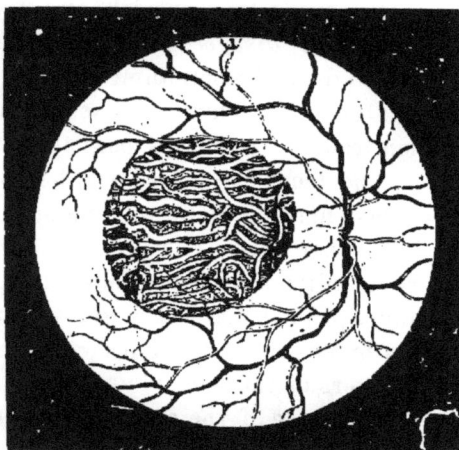

Central choroiditis.   (Wecker and Jaeger.)

FIG. 77.

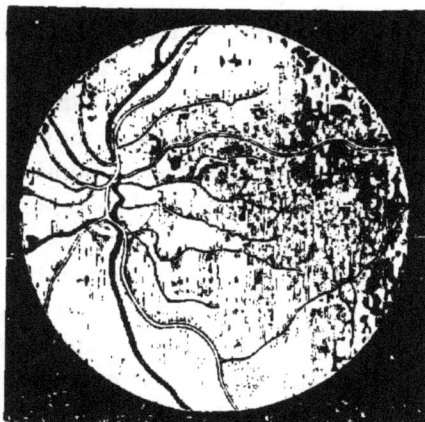

Central guttate senile choroiditis.

blunt object on the sclerotic causing local bleeding, or inflammation and subsequent atrophy, may account for such

a patch at the anterior part of the fundus. Single large patches of exudation are also met with, and are, perhaps, tubercular. *Choroidal disease* in disseminated patches seems sometimes to depend upon numerous scattered hemorrhages into the choroid, which may occur at different dates, and which lead to patches of partial atrophy with pigmentation. The local cause of such hemorrhages is obscure; the disease may occur in one eye or both, and in young adults of either sex. It may perhaps be called hemorrhagic choroiditis (compare Chapter XVI.). Although the changes produced are very gross, some of these patients regain almost perfect sight, a fact, perhaps, pointing to the deep layers of the choroid as the seat of disease. It is possible that over-use of the eyes or exposure to great heat or glare sometimes causes choroiditis.

Single spots of choroidal atrophy, especially toward the periphery, should, no less than abundant changes, always excite grave suspicion of former syphilis, and often furnish valuable corroborative evidence of that disease. The periphery cannot be fully examined unless the pupil be widely dilated. A few small scattered spots of black pigment on the choroid or in the retina, without evidence of atrophy of the choroid, often indicate former hemorrhages. Such spots are seen after recovery from albuminuric retinitis with hemorrhages, after blows on the eye, and sometimes without any relevant history.

Congestion of the choroid is not commonly recognizable by the ophthalmoscope. That active congestion does occur is certain, and it would seem that myopic eyes are especially liable to it, particularly when over-used or exposed to bright light and great heat. Serious hemorrhage may undoubtedly be excited under such circumstances. In conditions of extreme anæmia the whole choroid becomes unmistakably pale.

Coloboma of the choroid, congenital deficiency of the

lower part, is shown ophthalmoscopically by a large surface of exposed sclerotic, often embracing the disc, which is then much altered in form, and may be hardly recognizable, and extending downward to the periphery, where it often narrows to a mere line or chink. The surface of the sclerotic, as judged by the course of the retinal vessels, is often very irregular from bulging on its floor backward. The coloboma is occasionally limited to the part around the nerve, or may form a separate patch. Coloboma of the choroid is often seen without coloboma of the iris, and when both exist a bridge of choroidal tissue generally separates them in the region of the ciliary body. Cases of so-called coloboma of the choroid at the yellow spot are probably examples of severe fœtal or infantile inflammation of that part.

Albinism is accompanied by congenital absence of pigment in the cells of the epithelium and stroma of the whole uveal tract (choroid, ciliary processes, and iris). The pupil looks pink, because the fundus is lighted to a great extent indirectly through the sclerotic. Sight is always defective, and the eyes photophobic and usually oscillating. Many almost albinotic children become moderately pigmented as they grow up.

10*

CHAPTER XIII.

DISEASES OF THE RETINA.

OF the many morbid changes to which the retina is subject, some begin and end in this membrane, such as albuminuric retinitis and many forms of retinal hemorrhage ; in others the retina takes part in changes which begin in the optic nerve (neuro-retinitis), or in the choroid (choroido-retinitis); very serious lesions also occur from embolism or thrombosis of the central retinal vessels. The retina may be separated ("detached") from the choroid by serous fluid or blood. The retina may also be the seat of malignant growth (glioma), and probably of tubercular inflammation.

In health the human retina is so nearly transparent as to be almost invisible by the ophthalmoscope during life, or to the naked eye if examined immediately after excision. We see the retinal bloodvessels, but the retina itself, as a rule, we do not see. The main bloodvessels are derived from the *arteria* and *vena centralis*, which enter the outer side of the optic nerve, about 6 mm. behind the eye ; the veins and arteries are generally in pairs, the veins not being more numerous than the arteries ; all pass from or to the optic disc. Fig. 34. At the disc anastomoses, chiefly capillary, are formed between the vessels of the retina and those of the choroid and sclerotic. As no other anastomoses are formed by the vessels of the retina, the retinal circulation beyond the disc is terminal ; and further, as the vessels branch dichotomously, and the branches anastomose only by means of their capillaries, the circulation of each considerable branch is terminal also. The capillaries, which are not visible by the ophthalmoscope, are narrower than those of the choroid, and their meshes become much wider toward the anterior and less important parts of the retina.

At the y. s., Fig. 78, the only part used for accurate sight, the capillaries are very abundant (*compare* Fig. 69); but at the very centre of this region, *fovea centralis*, where all the layers except the cones and outer granules are excessively thin, there are no vessels, the capillaries forming fine, close loops just around it. The nerve-fibres in this part of the retina are finer than in other parts ; they seem also to be much more abundant, for Bunge has found that in a case of central scotoma, where only a very small part ($\frac{1}{40}$th) of the F. was lost, quite a large tract of fibres ($\frac{1}{4}$th of the whole) was atrophied in the optic nerve. The *fovea centralis* corresponds to an area at the centre of F., measuring only $1\frac{1}{2}°$ in diameter ; the part recognized as the *macula lutea* has an area, on the F., of about $7°$ (Bunge).

FIG. 78.

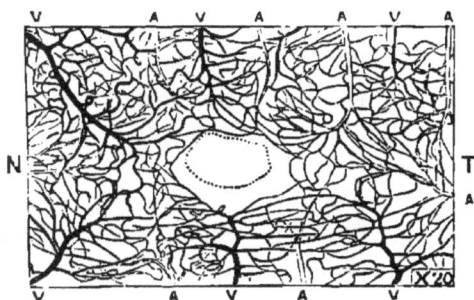

Bloodvessels of human retina at the yellow spot (artificial injection). The central gap corresponds to the Fovea centralis. A. Arteries ; v. Veins ; N. Nasal side (toward disc) ; T. temporal side. The meshes are many times wider at the periphery of the retina.

In children, especially those of dark complexion, a peculiar, white, shifting reflection, or shimmer, is often seen at the y. s. region, and along the course of the principal vessels. It changes with every movement of the mirror, and reminds one of the shifting reflection from "watered" and "shot" silk. Around the y. s. it takes the form of a ring or zone, and is known as the "halo round the macula." When the choroid is highly pigmented, even if this shifting reflection be absent, the retina is visible as a faint haze over the choroid like the "bloom" on a plum. Under the high magnifying power of the erect image the nerve-fibre layer is often visible near the disc, as a faintly marked radiating striation. The sheaths of the large central vessels at their emergence from the physiological pit, p. 72, show many variations in thickness and opacity.

In rare cases the medullary sheath of the optic nerve-fibres, which should cease at the lamina cribrosa, is continued through the disc into the retina, and causes the ophthalmoscopic appearance known as "opaque nerve-fibres." This congenital peculiarity may affect the nerve-fibres of the whole circumference of the disc, or only a patch or tuft of the fibres; it may only just overleap the edge of the disc or may extend far into the retina; and islands of similar opacity are sometimes seen in the retina quite separated from the disc. It is to be particularly noted that the central part, physiological pit, of the disc is not affected, because it contains no nerve-fibres. The affected patch is pure white, and quite opaque, its margin thins out gradually, and is striated in fine lines, which radiate from the disc like carded cotton-wool; the retinal vessels may be buried in the opacity, or run unobscured on its surface, and are of normal size. The deep layers of the affected parts of the retina being obscured by the opacity, an enlargement of the normal "blind spot" is the result. One eye, or both, may be affected. There is seldom any difficulty in distinguishing this condition from opacity due to neuro-retinitis.

OPHTHALMOSCOPIC SIGNS OF RETINAL DISEASE.

Congestion.—No amount of capillary congestion, whether passive or active, alters the appearance of the retina; and as to the large vessels, it is better to speak of the arteries as unusually large or tortuous, or of the veins as turgid or tortuous, than to use the general term congestion. Capillary congestion of the optic disc may undoubtedly be recognized, but even here caution is needed, and much allowance must be made for differences of contrast depending on variations in the tint of the choroid, for the patient's health and age, and for the brightness of the light used, or, what is the same thing, for the size of the pupil. Caution is also needed against drawing hasty inferences from the slight haziness of the outline of the disc, which may often be seen in cases of hypermetropia, and which is certainly not always morbid.

The only ophthalmoscopic proof of true *retinitis* is loss of transparency of the retina, and two chief types are soon recognized according as the opacity is diffused or consists chiefly of abrupt spots and patches. Hemorrhages are present in many cases of retinitis; but they may also occur without either inflammation or œdema. The state of the disc varies much, but it seldom escapes entirely in a case of extensive or prolonged retinitis. In a large majority of cases of recent retinitis the visible changes are limited to the central region, where the retina is thickest and most vascular.

(1.) The lessened transparency which accompanies *diffused retinitis* simply dulls the red choroidal reflex, and the term "smoky" is fairly descriptive of it. The same effect is given by slight haziness of any of the anterior media, but a mistake is excusable only where there is diffused mistiness of the vitreous from opacities which are too small to be easily distinguished, and the difficulty is then

increased because this very condition of the vitreous often
coexists with retinitis. A comparison of the erect and inverted images is often useful, for if the diffused haze noticed
by indirect examination be caused by retinitis, the direct
examination will often resolve what seemed a uniform
haze into a well-marked spotting or streaking. When the
change is pronounced enough to cause a decidedly white
haze of the retina, there is no longer any doubt. The
retinal arteries and veins are sometimes enlarged and tortuous in retinitis, and in severe cases they are generally
obscured in some part of their course. These forms of
uniformly diffused retinitis are usually caused either by
syphilis, embolism, or thrombosis.

(2.) Near the y. s. a number of small, intensely white,
rounded spots are seen, Fig. 79, either quite discrete or

FIG. 79.

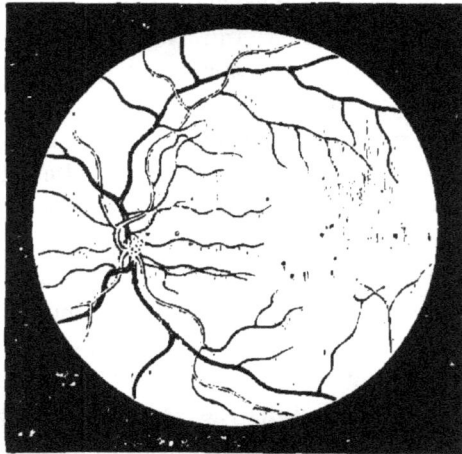

Renal retinitis at a late stage.   (Wecker and Jaeger.)

partly confluent. When very abundant and confluent they
form large, abruptly outlined patches, with irregular bor-

ders, some parts of these patches being striated, others
stippled.

(3.) A number of separate patches are scattered about
the central region, but without special reference to the y. s.
They are of irregular shape, white or pale buff, and sometimes striated, Fig. 80; they are easily distinguished from

FIG. 80.

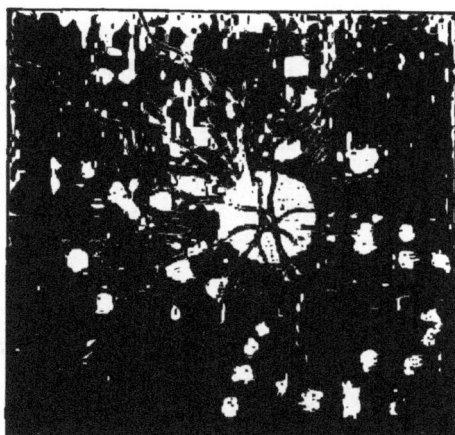

Recent severe retinitis in renal disease.   (Gowers.)

patches of choroidal atrophy by their color, the compara-
tive softness of their outlines, and the absence of pigmentation.

In types 2 and 3 some hemorrhages are usually
present; the retina generally may be clear, but more often
there is diffused haze and evidence of swelling.   The hemorrhages may be so numerous and large as to form the
chief feature, and then the retinal veins will be very tortuous and dilated.

Forms 2 and 3, which nearly always affect both eyes,
are generally associated with renal disease, but in rare

cases similar changes are caused by cerebral disease and other conditions.

(4.) Rarely a single large patch or area of white opacity is seen with softened, ill-defined edges, any retinal vessels that may cross it being obscured.   Such a patch of retinitis is usually caused either by subjacent choroiditis, or by local phlebitis or thrombosis.

Hemorrhage into (or beneath) the retina is known by its color, which is darker than that of an ordinary choroid, but redder and lighter than that of a very dark choroid. Blood may be effused into any of the retinal layers, and the shape of the blood patches is mainly determined by their position.   When effused into the nerve-fibre layer, or confined by the sheath of a large vessel, the extravasation takes a linear or streaked form and structure, following the direction of the nerve-fibres ; extravasations in the deeper layers are rounded.   Very large hemorrhages, many times as large as the disc, sometimes occur near the yellow spot, and probably all the layers then become infiltrated, while sometimes the blood ruptures the anterior limiting membrane of the retina and passes into the vitreous.

Retinal hemorrhages may be large or small, single or multiple ; limited to the central region or scattered in all parts ; linear, streaky, or flame-shaped, punctate or blotchy ; they may lie alongside large vessels, or have no apparent relation to them.   The hemorrhage may, as already mentioned, be the primary change, or may only form part of a retinitis or papillo-retinitis.   A hemorrhage which is mottled and of dark, dull color, is generally old.   The rate of absorption varies very much ; hemorrhage after a blow is very quickly absorbed, while effusions caused by the rupture of diseased vessels in old people, or accompanying retinitis from constitutional causes, often last for months, and leave permanent traces.

Pigmentation of the retina has been referred to in connection with choroiditis. Whenever pigment in the fundus forms long, sharply-defined lines, or is arranged in a mossy, lace-like, or reticulated pattern, we may safely infer that it is situated in the retina, and generally that it lies along the sheaths of the retinal vessels—compare Fig. 81 with Fig. 78. Pigment in or on the choroid never takes such a pat-

FIG. 81.

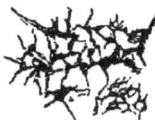

Study of pigment in the retina in a specimen of secondary retinitis pigmentosa, seen from the inner (vitreous) surface.

tern, being usually in blotches or rings. The two types, however, are often mingled in cases of choroiditis with secondary affection of the retina; indeed, whenever we decide that the retina is pigmented, the choroid must be carefully examined for evidences of former choroiditis.

Spots of pigment may be left after the absorption of retinal hemorrhages. Such spots can generally be distinguished from those following choroiditis by their more uniform appearance and by the absence of signs of choroidal atrophy.

Atrophy of the retina, of which pigmentation of the retina, when present, is always a sign, has for its most constant indication a marked shrinking of the retinal bloodvessels with thickening of their coats. When the atrophy follows a retinitis or choroido-retinitis, retinitis pigmentosa, syphilitic choroido-retinitis, etc., all the layers are involved, and the outer layers, those nearest the choroid, earlier than the inner; but when it is secondary to disease of the optic nerve, optic neuritis, progressive atrophy, and glaucoma, only the layers of nerve-fibres and ganglion cells are atro-

phied, the outer layers being found perfect, even after
many years. A retina atrophied after retinitis often does
not regain perfect transparency, and if there have been
choroiditis the retina remains especially hazy in the parts
where this has been most severe.

The disc after severe retinitis or choroido-retinitis always
passes into atrophy, often of peculiar appearance, being
pale, hazy, homogeneous-looking, and with a yellowish or
brownish tint.

Detachment (separation) of the retina.—As there is no
continuity of structure between the choroid and retina, the
two may be easily separated by effusion of blood or serous
fluid, the result of injury or disease, by morbid growths,
and by the traction of fibrous cords in the vitreous. Such
fibrous bands and strings develop in the vitreous in some
cases of irido-cyclitis, and perhaps in myopic eyes, without
signs of inflammation. Occasionally rents may be seen in
the separated retina. It has been suggested that such rents
occurring whilst the retina was still *in situ* might initiate
the detachment by allowing the intrusion of vitreous between the retina and choroid; and this explanation may
possibly hold good in very myopic eyes. The retina is
separated at the expense of the vitreous, which is proportionately absorbed, but always remains attached at the disc
and ora serrata, unless as the result of wound or great violence. The depth, area, and situation of the detachment
are subject to much variety. Fig. 82 shows a diagrammatic section of an eye in which the lower part of the
retina is separated. The pigment epithelium always remains on the choroid.

The separated portion is usually far within the focal
length of the eye; its erect image is, therefore, very easily
visible by the direct method, when it appears as a gray or
whitish reflexion in some part of the field, the remainder
being of the natural red color; the detached part is gray

or whitish, because the retina has become opaque. With
care we can accurately focus the surface of the gray reflection, see that it is folded, and see one or more retinal vessels
meandering upon it in a tortuous course; they appear small

FIG. 82.

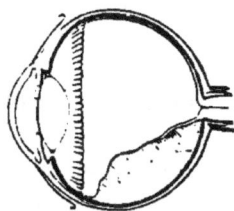

Section of eye with partial detachment of retina.

FIG. 83.

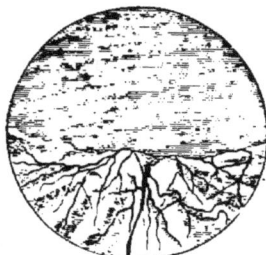

Ophthalmoscopic appearance of
detached retina (erect image).
(After Wecker and Jaeger.)

and of dark color. If the separation be deep the outline
of its more prominent folds, Fig. 83, can be seen standing
out sharply against the red background, and in some cases
the folds flap about when the eye is quickly moved. In
extreme cases we can see the detached part by focal light.
When the detachment is recent, especially if shallow, the
choroidal red is still seen through it; the diagnosis then
rests on the observation of whether the vessels in any part
become darker, smaller, and more tortuous, and upon
ophthalmoscopic estimation of the refraction of the retinal
vessels at different parts of the fundus, for the detached
part will be much more hypermetropic than the rest. In
very high myopia a shallow detachment may still lie behind
the principal focus, and therefore not yield an erect image
without a suitable concave lens; in such a case and in
others where minute rucks or folds of detachment are
present, examination by the indirect method leads to a
right diagnosis; the image of the detached portion is not

in focus at the same moment as its surrounding parts, *parallactic movement*[1] is obtained, and the vessels are tortuous. Deep and extensive detachment is often associated with opacities in the vitreous or lens, or with iritic adhesions; and any of these conditions interfere with the conclusive application of the above tests. In some cases of detachment, large patches and streaks of choroidal disease are to be found. The treatment of detachment of the retina is very unsatisfactory, improvement if obtained being seldom permanent, even when treatment is undertaken soon after the detachment has occurred. Puncture of the sclerotic over the detachment is occasionally followed by marked improvement, and the result is said to be better if the sclerotic be laid bare by dissecting up the conjunctiva before the puncture, and if the puncture be rather broad, about 2 to 4 mm., the subretinal fluid rapidly drains away. The conjunctival wound should be sutured. Profuse sweating and salivation, induced by pilocarpine (F. 38), have been recommended in recent cases. Mere rest in bed for some days in a subdued light and with the eyes tied up, is often followed for a time by decided improvement of sight. The best results seem to have been obtained by this means combined with scleral puncture, in recent cases.

Clinical Forms of Retinal Disease.

The symptoms of retinal disease relate only to the failure of sight which they cause, and this may be either general, or confined to a part of the field, according to the nature of the case. Neither photophobia nor pain occurs in uncomplicated retinitis.

[1] On closing one eye and viewing two objects, one beyond the other, but in the same line, one object seems to move over the other when the head is moved from side to side.

Syphilitic retinitis is generally associated with, and secondary to, choroiditis, but the retinitis may be primary. The vitreous in this disease, as in syphilitic choroiditis, is often hazy, and the opacities are sometimes seated deeply, just in front of the retina. The changes are those of diffuse retinitis, with slight "smoky" haze, often confined to the region of the yellow spot or disc; but in bad cases the haze passes into a whiter mistiness, and extends over a much larger region; sometimes long branching streaks or bands of dense opacity are met with, and hemorrhages may occur. The disc is always hazy, and at first too red, while the retinal vessels, both arteries and veins, are somewhat turgid and tortuous; rarely the disc becomes opaque and swollen. At a late period, in unfavorable cases, the vessels shrink slowly, almost to threads, the retina often becomes pigmented at the periphery, and the pigmented epithelium disappears.

Syphilitic retinitis is one of the secondary symptoms, seldom setting in earlier than six or later than eighteen months after the primary disease. It occurs in congenital as well as in acquired syphilis. It generally attacks both eyes, though often with an interval. Its onset is often rapid, as judged by its chief symptom, failure of sight, and it may be stated that as a rule the degree of amblyopia is much higher than would be expected from the ophthalmoscopic changes. Night-blindness is often a pronounced symptom. Its course is chronic, seldom lasting less than several months, and it shows a remarkable tendency for many months to repeated and rapid exacerbations after temporary recoveries, but with a tendency to get worse rather than permanently better. Amongst the early symptoms is often a "flickering" and micropsia; these with the history of variations lasting for a few days, and of marked night-blindness, often lead to a correct surmise before ophthalmoscopic examination. There is, however, nothing pathognomonic in any of the symptoms. An annular defect in the visual field, "ring scotoma," may often be found if sought; in the late stages the field is contracted.

Mercury produces most marked benefit, and when used early it permanently cures a large proportion of the cases; but in a number of cases, perhaps in those where there is most choroiditis, the disease goes slowly from bad to worse for several years in spite of very prolonged mercurial treatment. Of the efficacy of prolonged disuse of the eyes and of local counter-irritation or depletion, strongly recommended by many authors, I have had but little experience.

Albuminuric retinitis (papillo-retinitis).—The changes are strongly marked, and so characteristic that it is possible in most cases to say from an ophthalmoscopic examination alone that the patient is suffering from kidney disease.

The *earliest change,* the stage of œdema and exudation, is a general haze of grayish tint in the central region of the retina, mostly with some hemorrhages and soft-edged whitish patches, and with or without haze and swelling of the disc. In this stage the sight is often unimpaired and so the cases are seldom seen by ophthalmic surgeons till a few weeks later, when the translucent, probably albuminous exudations in the swollen retina have passed into a state of fatty or fibrinous degeneration, a change which affects both the nerve-fibres and connective tissue.

In this, the *second stage,* we find a number of pure white dots, spots, or patches in the hazy region, and especially grouped around the yellow spot. Their peculiarity is their sharp definition and pure, opaque, white color; indeed, when small and round they are almost glistening. When not very numerous they are generally confined to the yellow-spot region, from which they show a tendency to radiate in lines, Fig. 79; when very small and scanty they may be overlooked, unless we examine the erect image; but frequently large patches are formed by the confluence of small

spots, and the borders of these patches are striated, crenated, or spotted. At this stage the soft-edged patches,
Fig. 80, have often to a great extent disappeared or become
merged into more general opacity of the retina; the disc is
hazy and somewhat swollen, especially just at its margin,
and the retina, as judged by the undulations of its vessels,
and confirmed by post-mortem examination, is much thickened. Hemorrhages are generally still present and occasionally they constitute the most marked feature; they are
usually striated. Sometimes an artery is seen sheathed by
a dense white coating.[1] In another group papillitis is the
most marked change, though some bright white retinal spots
are always to be found by careful examination.

The usual tendency is toward subsidence of the œdema
and absorption of the fatty deposits and extravasations,
generally with improvement of sight—the *third stage*, or
stage of absorption and atrophy.

In the course of several months the white spots diminish
in size and number, until only a few very small ones are
left near the yellow spot, with, perhaps, some residual haze;
the blood-patches are slowly absorbed, often leaving small
round pigment spots, and the retinal arteries may be
shrunken. In cases of only moderate severity almost perfect sight is restored. But when the optic disc suffers
severely, severe papillitis, or if the retinal disease be excessive and attended by great œdema, sight either improves
very little, or, as the disc passes into atrophy and the retinal
vessels contract, it may sink to almost total blindness.
Such a condition may be mistaken for atrophy after cerebral neuritis; but the presence of a few minute bright dots
or of some superficial disturbance of the choroid at the
yellow spot, or of some scattered pigment spots left by ex-

---

[1] Illustrations of this are given in Gowers' Medical Ophthalmoscopy,
pl. xii., fig. 1, and in Trans. Ophth. Soc., vol. ii. pl. ii.

travasations, will generally lead to a correct inference. In the cases attended by the greatest swelling and opacity of retina and disc, death often occurs before retrogressive changes have taken place. In extreme cases the retina may become deeply detached from the choroid.

Albuminuric retinitis is almost invariably symmetrical, but seldom quite equal in degree or result in the two eyes.

The kidney disease in the malady under consideration is nearly always chronic. The retinitis may occur in any chronic nephritis, and in the albuminuria of pregnancy. Whatever be the form of the kidney disease, the retinitis usually occurs with other symptoms of active kidney mischief, such as headache, vomiting, loss of appetite, and often anasarca; but occasionally the retinitis is the first recognizable sign. The quantity of albumen varies very much. In the absence of anasarca the symptoms are often put down to "biliousness," and as in such cases the failure of sight is the most troublesome symptom, the ophthalmoscope often leads to the correct diagnosis. A second attack of retinitis sometimes occurs in connection with a relapse of renal symptoms. Many of the best marked cases of albuminuric retinitis occur in the albuminuria of pregnancy, and the prognosis for sight is good in many of these if the symptoms come on sufficiently late in the pregnancy to permit of the cause being removed by the induction of artificial labor; but some of them (probably cases of old kidney disease) do very badly, and pass into atrophy of the nerves.

Though the diagnosis of renal disease, based on the presence of the symmetrical retinal changes above described, will usually be verified by the physician, we do unquestionably now and then meet with cases of similar retinitis in which no kidney disease can be clinically proved. Trousseau describes several cases of this sort in which albumen appeared later.[1] Such cases need further attention. The cases of cerebral neuro-retinitis mentioned at p. 255, and rare cases of retinitis, exactly like renal retinitis, but confined to one eye, have also to be allowed for. Retinal changes more or less like those above described are also found in other chronic general diseases, e. g., diabetes, pernicious anæmia, and leucocythæmia (Chapter XXIII.).

The term *retinitis hæmorrhagica* has been given to cases characterized by very numerous linear or flame-shaped retinal hemorrhages, chiefly of small size, all over the fundus, sometimes with extreme venous engorgement and retinal œdema, but in other cases without these features. It usually occurs in only one eye at a time, and comes on rapidly. The patients are often gouty, or the subjects of disease of cardiac valves, or of the arterial system. Thrombosis of the trunk of the *vena centralis retinæ* is probably the determining cause of the condition[2] when there is much venous distention and retinal œdema; multiple disease of minute retinal vessels, when these symptoms are absent. Retinitis hæmorrhagica, of whichever type, is not common.

Other cases are seen where extravasations, varying much in size, number, and shape, are scattered in different parts of the fundus of one or both eyes. Some of them are probably allied to the above, but often the nature of the case is obscure, or the hemorrhages are related to senile degeneration of vessels. Such cases have been called *retinitis apoplectica*.

Lastly, in an important group, a single very large extravasation occurs from rupture of a large retinal vessel, probably an artery. The hemorrhage is generally in the yellow-spot region; in process of absorption it becomes mottled, the densest parts remaining longest, and if seen in

---

[1] Bull. de l'Hôpital des Quatre-vingts, iv. 4, 173.
[2] Hutchinson ; Michel, Graefe's Arch. f. Ophth., xxiv. 2.

that condition for the first time, the case may be taken for one of multiple hemorrhages. These large extravasations cause great defect of sight, which comes on in an hour or two, but not with absolute suddenness. Absorption, in the several groups of cases just mentioned, is very slow.

Hemorrhages may occur from blows on the eye. They are usually small, and quickly absorbed, differing in the latter respect very much from the cases before described.

Embolism of the central artery of the retina, or of one or more of its main divisions, gives rise to a characteristic retinitis, the cause of which can in most cases be recognized at once if it be recent; whilst in old cases the appearances, taken with the history, lead to a right diagnosis. *Thrombosis* of the artery causes similar changes.

The leading symptom of embolism is the occurrence of an instantaneous defect of sight, which is found on trial to be limited to one eye; sometimes the feeling is as if one eye had suddenly become "shut," the blindness being as sudden as that from quickly closing the lids; but whether the defect amounts to absolute blindness or no, depends on the position and size of the plug. Many of the patients have evidence of cardiac disease. Chorea has been present in a few. In any case, owing to the temporary establishment of collateral circulation by the capillary anastomoses at the disc, the patient sometimes notices an improvement of sight a few hours after the occurrence. This improvement, however, is but slight, the collateral channels being quite insufficient to meet the demand; nor is it often permanent, because the retina suffers very quickly from the almost complete stasis, œdema and inflammation rapidly setting in and leading to permanent damage.

If the case be seen within a few days of the occurrence, the red reflex of the choroid around the yellow spot and disc is quite obscured, or partially dulled, by a diffused and uniform white mist. The opacity is greatest just around the centre of the yellow spot, where the retina is very vascular, Fig. 78, and where its cellular elements, ganglion and granule layers, are more abundant than elsewhere; but at the very centre of the white mist a small, round, red spot is generally seen, so well defined that it may be mistaken for a hemorrhage; it represents the *fovea centralis*, where the retina is so thin that the choroid continues to shine through it when the surrounding parts are opaque; it is spoken of by authors as the "cherry-red spot at the macula lutea." This appearance is very seldom seen except after sudden arrest of arterial blood supply, by embolism or thrombosis of the arteria centralis and perhaps by hemorrhage into the optic nerve compressing the vessels; and of these causes embolism appears to be the commonest. The haze surrounds, and generally affects, the disc also, which soon becomes very pale. The small veins in the yellow-spot region often stand out with great distinctness, being enlarged by stasis, and conspicuous from contrast with the white retina. Small hemorrhages are often present. The larger retinal vessels, both arteries and veins, are more or less diminished at or near the disc, the arteries in the most typical cases being reduced to mere threads; both arteries and veins are, however, sometimes observed to increase in size as they recede from the disc. The arteries, however, are not always extremely shrunken in cases of retinal embolism, the variations depending upon the position and size of the plug, *i. e.*, upon whether the occlusion is complete or not. The sudden and complete failure of supply to a single branch of a retinal artery is sometimes followed by its emptying and shrinking to a white cord almost immediately. In other cases the branch may for a time be little, if at all, altered in size, and yet its bloodcolumn be quite stagnant, as is proved by the impossibility of producing pulsation in it by the firmest pressure on the globe, whilst the other branches respond perfectly to this test. Sometimes this pressure test, which showed blockage of some or all branches shortly after the onset, again produces pulsation a few days later without visible evidence of collateral circulation, thus proving the re-establishment of the main channel.

In from one to about four weeks the cloudiness clears off, and the disc passes into moderately white atrophy; the arteries, or some of them, according to the position of the plugging, are either reduced to bloodless white lines or simply narrowed.

Sight is almost always lost, or only perception of large objects retained, whatever be the final state of the blood-vessels. In the rare cases where an embolus passes beyond the disc, and is arrested in a branch at some distance from it, the changes are confined to the corresponding sector of the retina, and a limited defect of the field is the only permanent result. It is scarcely necessary to say that no treatment can be of any use in cases of lasting occlusion of the retinal arteries. It will be obvious, too, that these lesions will be limited to one eye, though a similar accident is occasionally seen afterwards in the other.

In a few cases sudden simultaneous blindness of *both* eyes has occurred with extremely diminished retinal arteries, *ischæmia retinæ*, and iridectomy has been followed by return of sight; lower tension causing re-establishment of circulation. See also Quinine-blindness.

Retinitis pigmentosa is a very slowly progressive symmetrical disease, leading to atrophy of the retina, with collection of black pigment in its layers and around its bloodvessels, and secondary atrophy of the disc. The earliest symptom is inability to see well at night, or by artificial light, night-blindness, nyctalopia. Concentric contraction of the visual field soon occurs, Fig. 84. These defects may reach a high degree whilst central vision remains excellent in bright daylight. The symptoms are noticed at an earlier stage by patients in whom the choroid is dark, and absorbs much light.

Ophthalmoscopic examination, where these symptoms have been present for some years, shows—(1) at the equator or periphery a greater or less quantity of pigment arranged in a reticulated or linear manner, Fig. 81, often with some small, separate dots; (2) in advanced cases, evidence of removal of the pigment epithelium, but no patches of

FIG. 84.

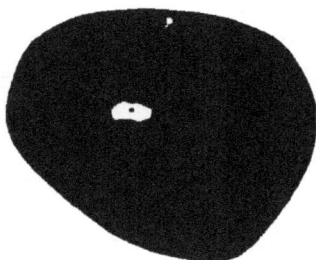

Extreme concentric contraction of field of vision (R.) in a case of advanced retinitis pigmentosa. The central dot shows the fixation point. The black shows the part lost.

choroidal atrophy; (3) the pigment arranged in a belt, which is generally uniform, the pattern being most crowded at the centre, and thinning out towards the borders of the belt; (4) that the changes are always symmetrical, and the symmetry very precise. These appearances are quite characteristic of true retinitis pigmentosa. In addition, we find (5) diminution in size of the retinal bloodvessels, the arteries in advanced cases being mere threads; (6) a peculiar hazy, yellowish, "waxy" pallor of the optic disc; (7) sometimes the pigmented parts of the retina are quite hazy; (8) posterior polar cataract and disease of the vitreous are often present in the later stages. The latter changes (5 to 8), however, are found in many cases of late retinitis consecutive to choroiditis, and are not peculiar to the present malady.

The disease begins in childhood or adolescence, progresses slowly but surely, and, as a rule, ends in blindness some time after middle life. A few cases of apparently recent origin are seen in quite aged persons, and a few are considered to be truly congenital. The quantity of pigment visible by the ophthalmoscope varies much in cases of apparently equal duration, and is not in direct relation to the defect of sight; cases even occur, which certainly belong to the same category, in which no pigment is visible during life, the retina being merely hazy, though microscopical examination reveals abundance of minutely divided pigment (Poncet). The pathogenesis of the disease is not finally settled; it is at present doubtful whether there is from the first a slow sclerosis of the connective-tissue elements of the retina, with passage inwards of pigment from the pigment epithelium, or whether the disease begins in the superficial layer of the choroid and the pigment epithelium. Its cause is obscure. It is undoubtedly strongly heritable, and many high authorities believe that it is really produced by consanguinity of marriage, either between the parents or near ancestors of the affected persons. Some of its subjects are full of mental and bodily vigor; but many are badly grown, suffer from progressive deafness, and are defective in intellect. Although want of education, as a consequence of defective sight and hearing, may sometimes account for this result, we cannot thus explain the various defects and diseases of the nervous system which are not infrequently noticed in kinsmen of the patients. That the subjects of this disease should be discouraged from marrying is sufficiently evident. In a few cases galvanism has been followed by improvement both of vision and visual[1] field,

---

[1] Gunn, Ophth. Hosp. Reports, x. 161, and others.

but no other treatment has any influence. Complications such as cataract and myopia are not uncommon, and must be treated on general principles.

It is sometimes very difficult to distinguish widely-diffused and superficial choroiditis, with pigmentation of retina and atrophy of the disc, from true retinitis pigmentosa. The question will generally relate to cause, as between retinitis pigmentosa and choroido-retinitis from syphilis.

Retinal disease from intense light.—A number of cases have now been observed in which blindness of a small area at the centre of the field has been caused by staring at the sun, usually during an eclipse. Corresponding to this functional defect, ophthalmoscopic evidences of choroiditis or choroido-retinitis have been found at the yellow spot. The defect often lasts for months, if not permanently.[1] *Compare* blindness from snow, electric light, etc.

---

[1] For accounts of cases and experiments on this affection see Lond. Med. Record, October, 1883; also Ophthalmic Review, April and May.

CHAPTER XIV

THE optic nerve is often diseased in its whole length, or in some part of its course, either within the skull, in the orbit, or at its ocular end.

The effect of disease of the optic nerve in producing (1) ophthalmoscopic changes in its visible portion (the optic disc, or *papilla optica*), and (2) defect of sight, varies greatly according to the seat, nature, and duration of the disease. The appearance of the disc may be entirely altered by œdema and inflammation, without the nerve-fibres losing their conductivity, and, therefore, without loss, or even defect, of sight; on the other hand, inflammatory or atrophic changes, causing destruction of the nerve-fibres, may arise in the nerve at a distance from the eye, and, whilst producing great defect of sight, cause little or no immediate change at the disc. Although we are here concerned chiefly with the ophthalmoscopic and visual sides of the question, a few words are needed as to the morbid changes in the nerve.

The pathological changes to which the optic nerve is liable include those which affect other nerve-tissues. Inflammation varying in seat, cause, and rapidity, and resulting in recovery or atrophy, may originate in the nerve itself, may pass down it from the brain (descending neuritis), or may extend into it from parts around; atrophy may occur from pressure by tumors, or distention of neighboring cavities, e. g., the third ventricle, or from laceration of the nerve or its central vessels in the orbit, or damage from fracture of the optic canal; and the optic nerve is very subject to the change known as "gray degeneration" or "sclerosis."

Lastly, the optic nerve being surrounded by a lymphatic space, "subvaginal space," which is continuous through the optic foramen with the meningeal spaces in the skull, and is bounded by a tough, fibrous "outer sheath," is liable to be affected by morbid processes going on in that space. This subvaginal or inter-sheath space, bounded externally by the outer sheath of the optic nerve, is lined internally by the inner sheath which is closely adherent to the nerve itself, Fig. 37. Fluid retained or secreted in the subvaginal space is often found there *post-mortem*, in cases of the optic neuritis about to be described as so commonly associated with intracranial disease, and has been held to explain the occurrence of this neuritis. Recent microscopical researches, however, have shown that inflammatory changes can usually be traced along the whole course of the optic nerves from their intracranial part to the eye. The occurrence of *optic papillitis*[1] in intracranial disease is probably, therefore, explained by an extension of inflammation from the brain or its membranes either along the interstitial connective tissue of the nerve or down the inner nerve-sheath, or perhaps, in some cases, along the intrinsic bloodvessels of the optic nerve. This explanation by "descending neuritis" has always been accepted for the papillitis caused by meningitis; but other hypotheses which have been, or seem likely to be, given up, have until lately been held by most authorities to be more applicable to the papillitis caused by cerebral tumor, because in this form the signs of inflammation, as distinguished from œdema and degeneration, in

---

[1] "Papillitis" has been proposed by Leber instead of "neuritis" to designate the ophthalmoscopic appearances of the inflamed or swollen *disc*, without reference to theories of causation, or to the state of the *nerve-trunk*.

the nerve above the disc and in the membranes at the base
of the brain, are so slight as to have eluded discovery until
sought carefully by modern microscopical methods.   The
part taken by the fluid which, as stated above, is often
present in the subvaginal space of the nerve and in greatest
quantity close to the eye, is not yet known.   It may act in
either or both of two ways : mechanically, by compressing
the nerve and hindering return of blood from the retina,
and thus complicating an already existing neuritis; or
vitally, by carrying inflammatory germs from the cranial
cavity to the optic nerve.   It is not yet fully known how
cerebral tumors set up descending optic neuritis when the
absence of fluid in the sheath precludes any appeal to its
influence ; but many facts point to the probability that
they do so by lighting up irritation with increase of cell-
growth in the surrounding brain substance, and local
meningitis.   Nor is it fully understood why the other
cranial nerves are so seldom damaged, at least permanently.[1]

As already stated in previous chapters, inflammation
may extend into the disc from the retina or choroid near
to it, and may occur in consequence of the sudden arrest
of the blood-current caused by embolism and thrombosis
of the central retinal vessels, in their course through the
nerve.

The ophthalmoscopic signs of papillitis are caused by
varying degrees of œdema, congestion, and inflammation

[1] For a full and masterly statement of this difficult subject, enriched
with many new facts, the reader is referred to Dr. Gowers's Manual
and Atlas of Medical Ophthalmoscopy. In recent careful papers Drs.
Edmunds and Lawford maintain that meningitis is probably always the
starting-point of optic neuritis, even in cases of cerebral tumor, and that
the inflammation usually travels down the inner sheath of the optic
nerve, Trans. Ophth. Soc., 1883-1886. See also the papers by Drs.
Stephen Mackenzie, Brailey, and others, in the first volume of the same
Trans., 1881, and in the Trans. Internat. Med. Congress, 1881.

of the disc.   It is no longer useful to maintain the old
ophthalmoscopic distinction between "swollen disc," or
" choked disc," and "optic neuritis "   The latter term was
formerly reserved for cases showing little œdema but much
opacity, changes which were supposed especially to indicate
inflammation passing down the nerve from the brain ; but
if œdema and venous engorgement predominated, " choked
disc," the changes were attributed to compression of the
optic nerve by fluid in its sheath-space, or with less reason
to pressure on the ophthalmic vein at the cavernous sinus.
The changes are often mixed, or vary at different stages of
the same case.   The terms "neuritis" and "papillitis" will
be here used to the exclusion of "choked disc."

The most important early changes in optic papillitis are
blurring of the border of the disc by a grayish opalescent

FIG. 85.

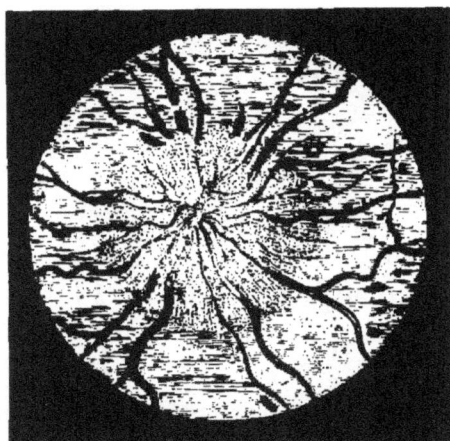

Ophthalmoscopic appearance of severe recent papillitis.   Several
elongated patches of blood near border of disc.   (After Hughlings
Jackson.)   Compare with Fig. 86.

haze, distention of the large retinal veins, and swelling of
the disc above the surrounding retina.   Swelling is shown

by the abrupt bending of the vessels, with deepening of
their color and loss of their light streak—they are, in fact,
seen foreshortened; also by noticing that slight lateral movements of the observer's head, or lens, cause an apparent
movement of the vessels over the choroid behind, because
the two objects are on different levels ("parallactic test,"
p. 235). The patient may die, or the disease may, after a
longer or shorter time, recede at this stage. But further
changes generally occur, the haziness becomes decided
opacity, which more or less obscures the central vessels,
and covers and extends beyond the border of the papilla,
Fig. 85, so that the disc appears enlarged ; its color becomes
a mixture of yellow and pink with gray or white, and it
looks striated or fibrous, appearances due to a whitish
opacity of the nerve-fibres mingled with numerous small
bloodvessels and hemorrhages. The veins become larger

FIG. 86.

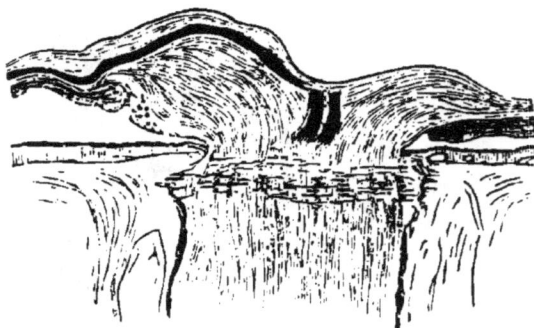

Section of the swollen disc in papillitis, showing that the swelling is
limited to the layer of nerve-fibres (longitudinal shading); other retinal
layers not altered in thickness. (Compare with Fig. 37.)   × about 15.

and more tortuous, even kinked or knuckled ; the arteries
are either normal or somewhat contracted ; there may be
blood-patches.   The swelling of the disc may be very great,

and is appreciated either by the above-mentioned foreshort-
ening of the vessels, by the parallactic test, or by ophthalmoscopic measurement

Such changes may disappear, leaving scarcely a trace;
or a certain degree of atrophic paleness of the disc, with
some narrowing of the retinal vessels and thickening of
their sheaths, or other slight changes, may remain. But
in many cases the disc gradually, in the course of weeks or
months, passes into a state of "post-papillitic" or "consecutive" atrophy; the opacity first becomes whiter and
smoother-looking, "woolly disc;" then it slowly clears off,
generally first at the side next the yellow spot, and the
retinal vessels simultaneously shrink to a smaller size,
though they often remain tortuous for a long time, Fig. 87.

FIG. 87.

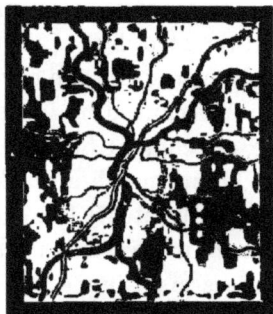

Atrophy of disc after papillitis. Upper and lower margins still hazy;
veins still tortuous; arteries nearly normal; disturbance of choroidal
pigment at inner and outer border. Sight in this case remained fairly
good. The disc is not represented white enough.

As the mist lifts, the sharp edge, and finally the whole surface of the disc, now of a staring white color, again comes
into view. A slight haziness often remains, and the
boundary of the disc is often notched and irregular; but
upon these signs too much reliance must not be placed.

Sight is seldom much affected[1] until marked papillitis has existed some little time. If the morbid process quickly cease, often no failure occurs; or sight may fail, may even sink almost to blindness, for a short time, and recovery take place, if the changes cease before compression of the nerve-fibres has given rise to atrophy. Early blindness in double papillitis may be due to pressure on the chiasma or tracts, rather than to the changes we see in the eyes. Gradual failure late in the case, when retrogressive changes are already visible at the disc, is a bad sign. The sight seldom changes, either for better or worse, after the signs of active papillitis have quite passed off, and though the relations between sight and final ophthalmoscopic appearances vary, it is usually true (1) that great shrinking of the central retinal vessels indicates a high grade of atrophy and great defect of sight, and is generally accompanied by extreme pallor, with some residual haziness, of the disc, advanced post-papillitic atrophy; (2) that considerable pallor and other slight changes, such as white lines bounding the vessels, or streaks caused by increase of the connective tissue of the disc, are compatible with fairly good sight, if the central vessels be not much shrunken.

Advanced atrophy, undoubtedly following papillitis, does not, however, always show signs of the past violent inflammation; the appearances may, indeed, be indistinguishable from those caused by primary atrophy.

Papillitis is double in the great majority of cases. If single, it generally indicates disease in the orbit. It is true that single papillitis from intracranial disease is occasionally met with, and that in many double cases inequalities

---

[1] Dr. Hughlings Jackson was the first to notice and insist upon the frequency of papillitis without failure of sight. The discovery was of immense value, for double papillitis, without other changes in the eye, is one of the most important objective signs we possess of the existence of tumor or inflammation within the skull.

are often seen between the two eyes as to time of onset, degree, and final result.

The changes are not always limited strictly to the disc and its border, pure papillitis, for in some cases a wide zone of surrounding retina is hazy and swollen, exhibiting hemorrhages and white plaques, or lustrous white dots, *papilloretinitis*. It is not always easy to say, in such a case, whether the changes are due to renal disease, with great swelling of the disc, or to some intracranial malady. In renal cases there is albuminuria, the patient is seldom a young child, and the cases with more severe neuro-retinitis, where the differential diagnosis is most important, occur in an advanced stage of the kidney disease ;[1] in the cases of neuro-retinitis most closely resembling renal cases, but caused by cerebral disease, there is no albumin, and the white deposits are seldom arranged quite as in renal retinitis, Fig. 79, whilst the papillitis is greater than is usual in renal cases.

Etiology (compare Chap. XXIII.). Papillitis occurs chiefly in cases of irritative intracranial disease—viz., in meningitis, both acute and chronic, and in intracranial new-growths of all kinds, whether inflammatory (syphilitic gummata), tubercular, or neoplastic. It is very rare in cases where there is neither inflammation nor tissue growth, as in cerebral hemorrhage and intracranial aneurism. Further, it must be stated that no constant relationship has been proved between papillitis and the seat, extent, or duration of the intracranial disease. Papillitis has occasionally been found without coarse disease, but with widely diffused minute changes, in the brain. Thus, the occurrence of papillitis, although pointing very strongly to organic disease within the skull, and especially to intracranial tumor, is not of itself either a localizing or a differentiating

[1] Gowers, p. 187.

symptom. Inflammation about the sphenoidal fissure, and tumors, nodes, and inflammations in the orbit, are occasional causes of papillitis, which is then usually one-sided, and often accompanied by extreme œdema and venous distention ; in some of these there is protrusion of the eye with affection of other orbital nerves, and the exact seat and nature of the disease may be obscure.   Optic neuritis from intracranial disease very seldom recurs after subsidence.[1]

Other occasional causes of double papillitis, with or without retinitis, are lead-poisoning, the various exanthemata (including recent syphilis), sudden suppression of menses, simple chronic anæmia, rapid copious loss of blood, especially from the stomach, and, perhaps, exposure to cold. In a few cases, well-marked double papillitis occurs without other symptoms, and without assignable cause.

Certain cases of failure of sight, usually single, with slight neuritic changes at the disc, followed by recovery or by atrophy, must be referred to a local, primary, optic neuritis some distance behind the eye, *retro-ocular neuritis*. The changes are, clinically, very different from those above described.

Syphilitic disease within the skull is a common cause of papillitis, but the eye-changes alone furnish no clue to the cause, nor to its mode of action, which may be (1) by giving rise to intracranial gummata, not in connection with the optic nerves, but acting as any other tumor acts (see above) ; (2) by direct implication of the chiasma or optic tracts in gummatous inflammation ; (3) in rare cases neuritis, ending in atrophy and blindness, occurs in secondary syphilis, with head symptoms pointing to meningitis ; (4) there are few cases of double papillitis in late secondary syphilis, without either head symptoms or signs of ocular

---

[1] A well-marked case has, however, been recorded by Dr. James Anderson in the Ophthalmic Review for May, 1886.

disease other than in the discs; these may properly be called "syphilitic optic neuritis."

The condition of the pupil in neuritic affections depends partly on the degree and partly on the rapidity of failure of vision. As a rule, in amaurosis from atrophy of the discs after papillitis, the pupils are, for a time, rather widely dilated and motionless; after a while they often become smaller, and, unless the blindness be complete, they regain a certain amount of mobility to light.

ATROPHY OF THE OPTIC DISC.

By this is meant atrophy of the nerve fibres of the disc and of the capillary vessels which feed it. The disc is too white; milk-white, bluish, grayish, or yellowish, in different cases. Its color may be quite uniform, or some one part

FIG. 88.

FIG. 89.

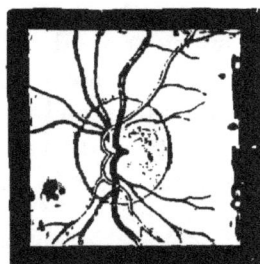 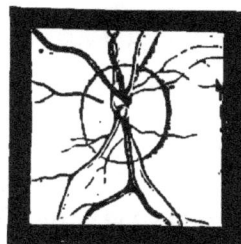

Simple atrophy of disc. Stippling of lamina cribrosa exposed. (Wecker.)

Atrophy of disc from spinal disease. Lamina cribrosa concealed. Vessels normal. (Wecker.)

may be whiter than another; the stippling of the *lamina cribrosa* may be more visible than in health, or, on the other hand, entirely absent, as if covered, or filled up by white paint, Figs. 88 and 89. The central retinal vessels may be shrunken or of full size, and their course natural

or too tortuous; both these points bear upon the diagnosis
of cause and the prognosis. The choroidal boundary may
be too sharply defined, or, as in Fig. 87, too hazy; it may
be even and circular, or irregular and notched. The sclerotic ring is often seen with unnatural clearness, exposed
by wasting of the overlying nerve fibres. Mere pallor of
the disc, such as we see in extreme general anæmia, must
not be mistaken for atrophy: the change is then one of
color only, without unnatural distinctness, loss of transparency, or disturbance of outline.

Varieties.—(1.) The nerve fibres undergo atrophy during
the absorption and shrinking of the new connective tissue
formed in severe neuritis (post-papillitic atrophy, p. 253;
embolism, p. 242).

(2.) When the disc participates secondarily in inflammation of the retina or choroid it also participates in the suc-
ceeding atrophy.

(3.) Atrophy of any part of the optic nerve or chiasma
from pressure—as by a tumor or by distention of the third
ventricle in hydrocephalus—from injury or local inflammation, leads to secondary atrophy, which sooner or later
reaches the disc. Such cases often show the condition of
pure atrophy, without adventitious opacity or disturbance
of outline, and often without change in the retinal vessels.
They are not very common.

(4.) The optic nerves are liable to chronic sclerotic
changes, with thickening of the connective-tissue framework
and atrophy of the nerve-fibres, without the occurrence of
papillitis. The change in these cases appears often to begin
at the disc, but the exact order of events in this large and
important group is not fully known. Groups 3 and 4
furnish the cases which are known clinically as "primary"
or "progressive" atrophy of the optic disc.

Clinical aspects of atrophy of the discs.—As in optic
neuritis, so in atrophy and pallor of the disc, there is no

invariable relation between the appearance, especially the color, of the disc and the patient's sight. A considerable degree of pallor, which it may be impossible to distinguish from true atrophy, is sometimes seen with excellent central

FIG. 90.

L.   R.

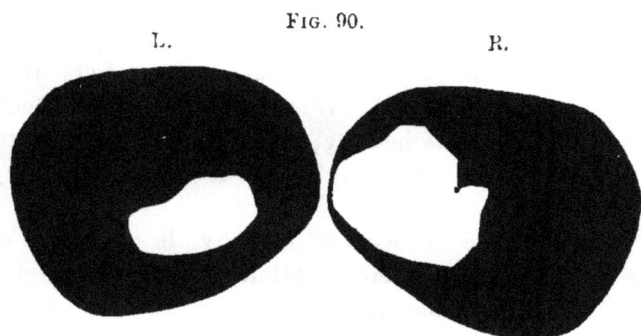

Irregular contraction of fields of vision in a case of progressive atrophy of optic nerves. The loss is symmetrical, but more advanced in the L., where it has extended over the fixation point : in the R. it has just reached the fixation point at one place. The black represents the parts lost.

FIG. 91.

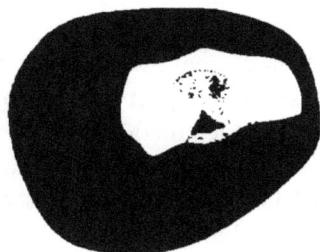

Irregular contraction, with central loss of L. visual field, from progressive atrophy of optic nerve in locomotor ataxy. The black represents the blind parts ; the shading shows partial loss of vision.

vision, though usually accompanied by some defect of the visual field. Again, the discs often look alike, although the sight is much better in one than the other.

Patients with atrophy of the disc come to us because they cannot see well or are quite blind. There are usually no other local symptoms except such as may be furnished by the pupils. In post-papillitic atrophy the pupils are generally too large and sluggish or motionless to light; in most cases of primary progressive atrophy they are of ordinary size, or smaller than usual, and act very imperfectly. (Chap. XXIII.) When only one eye is affected, the other being quite healthy, the pupil of the amaurotic eye has no direct action to light, and is often a little larger than its fellow.

The visual field, in cases of atrophy, is generally contracted, or shows irregular invasions or sector-like defects, Figs. 90 and 91. Color-blindness is a marked symptom in nearly all cases, but is not always proportionate to the loss of visual acuteness, being in some much greater and in others much less than the state of central vision would lead us to expect. Green is the color lost soonest in nearly all cases, and red next.

A. Cases in which *both discs are atrophied* may be conveniently classified as follows in regard to diagnosis and prognosis:

(1.) If the changes point decidedly to recently past papillitis there is some prospect of improvement; but on the other hand, sight may for a time get worse. The case must, of course, be investigated most carefully as to the cause of the neuritis. If sight have been stationary for some months further change is unlikely.

(2.) If the retinal arteries are much shrunken, whether neuritis have occurred or not, the prognosis is bad.

(3.) If we cannot decide after careful examination whether or no papillitis have preceded, inquiry should be made as to former symptoms of intracranial disease, since consecutive cannot always be distinguished from primary atrophy. But in a large number of those cases which present no ophthalmoscopic evidence of previous papillitis, the history will be quite negative as to cerebral symptoms; —and these will, for the most part, fall into the two following groups.

(4.) There are symptoms of chronic disease of the spinal cord, usually of locomotor ataxy; or much more rarely symptoms of general paralysis of the insane.

(5.) No cause can be assigned for the atrophy. These are less common than has been supposed.

The sclerosis leading to atrophy of the discs in locomotor ataxy (4) usually comes on early in that disease, often before well-marked spinal symptoms have appeared. The optic atrophy always becomes symmetrical, though it generally begins some months sooner in one eye than in the other; it always progresses, though sometimes not for years, to complete, or all but complete, blindness. The discs are usually characterized by a uniformly opaque, gray-white color, the lamina cribrosa being often concealed, although neither the central vessels nor the disc margins are obscured in the least, Fig. 89. The central vessels are often not materially lessened in size, even when the patient is quite blind.

Cases of progressive atrophy are seen which resemble the above, but where no signs of spinal-cord disease are present, even though the patient have been long blind (5). It is known that in some of these patients ataxic symptoms come on sooner or later, and it is highly probable that, could the cases be followed up for a sufficient number of years, this termination would be found to be common.[1]

[1] I have found decided spinal symptoms in 58 of a series of 76 consecutive cases of progressive atrophy, and of the remaining 18, several showed one or more symptoms which were probably of spinal origin. Peltesohn finds about 40 per cent. of all cases of non-neuritic progressive optic atrophy, in Hirschberg's clinic, to be associated with spinal or cerebro-spinal disease. Knapp's Arch., xvi. 142.

Indeed, pre-ataxic optic atrophy is now a recognized method of onset of the disease. Cases of Classes 4 and 5 are far commoner in men than women. In a few the atrophy is caused by the pressure of a tumor which compresses the chiasma, without setting up papillitis.

In making the prognosis of cases of progressive, uncomplicated amblyopia or amaurosis, with more or less atrophy of discs, special attention is to be paid to whether or not the failure was synchronous, and whether it is now equal in the two eyes. The state of the field of vision in cases seen early is also of much importance; peripheral contraction, as distinguished from central defect, is a bad sign, for progressive atrophy seldom begins with defect in the centre of the field. In cases of gradual, uncomplicated failure of sight, where the symptoms have, from the beginning, been equally symmetrical, the atrophic changes are usually but slight in comparison with the defect of sight.

B. *Single amaurosis with atrophy of the disc*, in a majority of the cases, indicates former embolism of the central artery, some local affection of the trunk of the optic nerve, "retroocular neuritis," or pressure on the nerve by tumor just in front of the chiasma. But here it must be remembered that in cases of progressive atrophy, accompanying or preceding spinal disease, a very long interval occasionally separates the onset of the disease of the two eyes,[1] and we may see the first eye before the commencement of the disease in the second.

Blindness of one eye following immediately after a fall or blow on the head, and leading in a few weeks to atrophy, indicates damage to the nerve from fracture of the optic canal. The blow has generally been on the front of the head, and on the same side as the affected eye. A similar

[1] This interval may be three or four years, and an interval of from one to two years is not very rare.

condition follows wound or rupture of the nerve in the orbit, by a thrust, stab, or gunshot injury. Laceration of the central retinal vessels alone, behind the point at which they enter the nerve, is said to cause appearances like those due to embolism and thrombosis. In cases of injury to the optic nerve improvement is rare.

CHAPTER XV.

THE term amblyopia means dulness of sight, but its use is generally restricted to cases of defective acuteness of sight, short of blindness, in which there is little or no ophthalmoscopic change. Amaurosis indicates a more advanced affection, complete blindness without visible changes. These terms, then, refer to the patient's symptoms, whilst papillitis and atrophy imply changes seen by the observer. Amblyopia may depend upon disease in the retina, in any part of the optic nerve or tract, or in the optic centres; and it may be temporary or permanent. It is always most important to distinguish single from symmetrical cases.

Two common and important forms of unsymmetrical amblyopia may be considered first.

(1.) **Amblyopia from suppression of image** ("*congenital amblyopia*").—It is well known that many children with convergent squint see badly with the squinting eye; that this defect varies in degree, and may be so great that fingers can hardly be counted; that, at any rate in the higher grades, the defect is chiefly, or only, present in that part of the visual field which is common to both eyes, Fig. 23, and is irremediable, whilst in the lower degrees the defect may be more or less removed by separate practice of the defective eye.[1] It has been assumed by one school that this amblyopia is due to a congenital defect, presumably of the visual centre, which determines the incidence of the squint, just

---

[1] Of such improvement I have myself had very little experience.

as defect due to an ulcer of the cornea may do. Another view supposes that the child, born with two good eyes, but being obliged to squint owing to hypermetropia, learns to suppress the consciousness of the image in the squinting eye in order to avoid the inconvenience of double vision, and that this habit, if begun very early in life, causes permanent amblyopia of the eye, or rather loss of perception in the corresponding centre. For the former view it is urged, that no one has ever watched the onset of this amblyopia, since it is always present at the youngest age when tests can be applied; that we meet with cases of unexplained defect of one eye without squint; and that this supposed power of suppression cannot be learnt in later life, as is shown by the permanence of diplopia in all cases of paralytic squint acquired after childhood. In favor of the suppression theory we may argue, that whilst such defect might be acquired early, it could not be expected to come on late, after the visual centre in question had been educated; precisely as want of training of the ocular muscles in early infancy, from defective sight due to disease, leads to incurable nystagmus (Chap. XXI.) much more frequently than do similar defects of sight acquired after the muscles have been got into harmonious use; that in many of the cases of defect without squint a history of previous squint can be obtained;[1] and that if the defect were congenital it would involve the whole field equally, not only that part which is common to the two eyes. In alternating concomitant squint, whether convergent or divergent, there is no diplopia, although the vision of each eye is as a rule equally good; the patient has the power of instantaneously suppressing the consciousness of the image in whichever happens to be the squinting eye, a fact in favor, so far as it

---

[1] I believe that the spontaneous disappearance of hypermetropic squint, which is not uncommon, has received too little attention.

12

goes, of the suppression theory., On the other hand, it is true that in cases of anisometropia great variations are encountered in the degree of perfection to which the more ametropic eye can be raised by glasses, a fact perhaps in favor of the congenital amblyopia theory.

(2.) **Amblyopia from defective retinal images.**—In cases of high hypermetropia or astigmatism, when clear images have never been formed, the correction of the optical defect by glasses at the earliest practical age often fails, at any rate for a time, to give full acuteness of sight. Want of education in the appreciation of clear images is probably the chief cause, though defective development of the retina may also come into play. We may explain in the same way the common cases in which, with anisometropia (Chap. XX.), the sight of the more ametropic eye, even when corrected by the proper glasses, remains defective, although no squint have ever existed ; and in some degree also the defect often observed after perfectly successful operations for cataract in children. Amblyopia of this kind when discovered late in life is seldom altered by correcting the optical error, but in children the sight often improves when suitable glasses are constantly worn.

Great defect of one eye, from the cause just mentioned, or gradual painless failure from disease, often exists unknown for years, until accidentally discovered by closing the sound eye, or by trying the sight of each eye separately, e. g., in an examination for the army or other public service. The patient in such cases is naturally concerned at what he thinks is a recent defect, but caution is needed in accepting his views, unless he have previously been in the habit of "sighting" objects with the eye in question, as in rifle-shooting. But *sudden* failure of one eye is, as a rule, dated correctly.

In cases of amblyopia not belonging to the above categories, a definite date of onset will generally be given.

Two principal divisions may be formed, according as the amblyopia affects one eye or both.

(3.) Cases of recent failure of one eye with little or no ophthalmoscopic change occur rather rarely, and generally in young adults; the onset is often rapid, with neuralgic pain, sometimes very severe, in the same side of the head. There may be pain in moving the eye, or tenderness when it is pressed back into the orbit. The degree of amblyopia varies much, but is often especially marked at the centre of the field. The disc of the affected eye is sometimes hazy and congested. The attack is often attributed to exposure to cold. Most of the cases recover under the use of blisters and iodide of potassium, but in a certain number the defect is permanent, and the disc becomes atrophied. A *retroocular neuritis*, often slight and transient, most likely occurs, and the cases are perhaps analogous to peripheral paralysis of the facial nerve.

(4.) Much commoner is a progressive and equal failure in both eyes, often amounting in a few weeks, or months, to great defect (14 or 20 Jaeger, or V. from $\frac{1}{5}$ to $\frac{1}{10}$), with no other local symptoms except perhaps a little frontal headache, but often with nervousness, general want of tone, and loss of sleep and appetite. Ophthalmoscopic changes, never pronounced, may be quite absent: at an early period the disc is often decidedly congested, and slightly swollen and hazy, but these changes are all so ill-marked that competent observers may give different accounts of the same case; later, the side of the disc near the y. s., and, finally, in bad cases, the whole papilla, become pale, and the diagnosis of incomplete atrophy is given. The defect of sight is described as a "mist," and is usually most troublesome in bright light and for distant objects, being less apparent early in the morning and toward evening. The pupils are normal, or at most rather sluggish to light. The defect of V. is limited to, or most intense at, the central part of the

field, *central scotoma*, occupying an oval patch which extends from the fixation point (corresponding to the y. s.)
outward, toward, and often as far as, the blind spot, corresponding to the optic disc.   The affected area is also
found to be color-blind for red and green ; but this loss of
color-perception being usually incomplete, alike in degree
and superficial extent, Fig. 92, will often escape detection

FIG. 92.

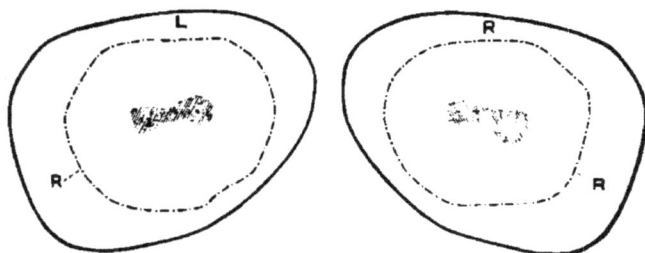

R. right, L. left, visual field in a case of central amblyopia from
tobacco-smoking.   The shaded area is the part over which acuteness of
vision and color-perception are lowered (relative central scotoma), no
part of the field being absolutely blind.   The dotted line marked R.
shows the boundary of the field for red (see Fig. 22).

if large color-tests be used; whilst it will readily be found
by using a small colored spot of from 5 to 15 mm. square.
The patient, closing one eye, "fixes" the finger or nose of
the observer, who then removes the colored spot from the
fixation point in various directions toward the periphery ;
the color, instead of appearing brightest at the centre of the
field, will be dull or unrecognizable there, becoming brighter
and easily recognized toward the periphery.   There is no
contraction of the field, and thus, since surrounding objects
are seen as well as ever, and the patient has no difficulty
in going about, his manner differs from that of one with
progressive atrophy, who finds difficulty in guiding himself,
because his visual field is contracted.

AMBLYOPIA. 269

The patients are, almost without exception, males, and at or beyond middle life. With very rare exceptions they are smokers, and have smoked for many years, and a large number are also intemperate in alcohol. The exceptions occur chiefly in a very few patients to whom a similar kind of amblyopia is hereditary, is liable to affect the female as well as the male members, and may come on much earlier in life. The etiology of such cases is obscure, and in some few of them there is no evidence of heredity.

In the common cases it is now generally agreed that tobacco has a large share in the causation, and in the opinion of an increasing number of observers it is the sole excitant. The direct influence of alcohol, and of the various causes of general exhaustion, such as anxiety, underfeeding, and general dissipation, is still to some extent an open question (see Chap. XXIII., Diabetes). My own opinion, based on the examination of a large number of cases, is that tobacco is the essential agent, and that the disuse, or greatly diminished use, of tobacco is the one essential measure of treatment. It is important to remember that the disease may come on when either the quantity or the strength of the tobacco is increased, or when the health fails and a quantity which was formerly well borne becomes excessive. Hence, cases of *double central amblyopia* may, as a rule, except in the rare form above mentioned, be named *tobacco amblyopia*. The symmetry of tobacco amblyopia is not always precise, and it appears, in very rare cases, to be delayed.[1]

The prognosis is good if the patient come early, and if the failure have been comparatively quick. In such cases really perfect recovery may occur, and very great improvement is the rule. In the more chronic cases, or cases where already the whole disc is pale, a moderate improvement, or

---

[1] J. Hutchinson, Jr., Ophth. Hosp. Reports, xi., 1886.

even an arrest of progress, is all we can expect. If smoking be persisted in, no improvement takes place, and the amblyopia increases up to a certain point, but complete blindness very seldom, if ever, occurs. In the treatment, disuse of tobacco is the one thing essential. Relapse sometimes occurs if smoking be resumed. Drink should, of course, be moderated. It is usual to give strychnia, subcutaneously or by mouth, for a considerable period, but whether any medicine acts otherwise than by improving the general tone is doubtful; subcutaneous injections of strychnia, carefully carried out, have not given definite results in my own cases. Others believe that the constant current is useful. There is reason to believe that the disease depends on a chronic inflammation of the central bundles of the optic nerve, beginning at, or at a short distance behind, the eye.[1]

Hemianopia, usually called *hemiopia*, denotes loss of half the field of vision. When uniocular, the defect is seldom quite regular, and generally depends upon detachment of the retina or a very large retinal hemorrhage. It is usually binocular, and then indicates disease at or behind the optic chiasma. In the great majority of cases the R. or L. lateral half of each field is lost. Sometimes only a quarter of each field is lost. The line of separation between the blind and seeing halves is usually sharply defined and nearly straight, only deviating a degree or two at the fixation point so as just to leave central vision intact over an area about corresponding to the fovea centralis, Fig. 93. In other cases the separating line is undulating and a comparatively large central area of the field remains intact. The boundary between sight and blindness in hemianopia, though usually abrupt, is sometimes gradual. The retention of central vision over a considerable central area has

---

[1] Trans. Ophth. Soc., vol. i. p. 124, and iii. p. 160.

been explained on the assumption that the v. s. area receives nerve-fibres from both optic tracts, and Bunge and
others have lately found microscopical evidence that such
is really the case ; in cases like Fig. 93, the apparent deviation of the dividing line may perhaps be explained by the

Fig. 93.

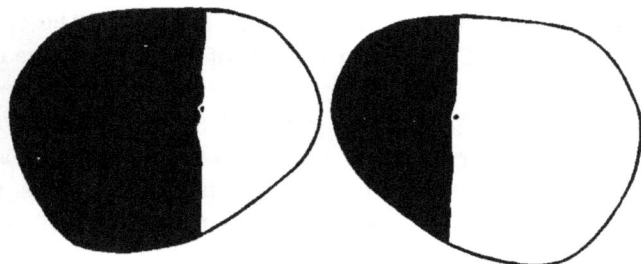

Fields of vision in a case of L. homonymous lateral Hemianopia.
The dividing line comes within one or two degrees of the fixation point
(shown by the central dot) in each eye. The lesion causing this hemianopia is probably in the optic tract, or not higher than the corpora
geniculata.

difficulty which the patient has in keeping the eye perfectly
fixed when the test object comes close to the centre.
Loss of the R. half of each *field*, meaning loss of function
of the L. half of each *retina*, points to disease of the L.
optic tract[1] or its continuations, or of some part of the L.
occipital lobe or angular gyrus. Loss of the two nasal
halves is extremely rare. Loss of the two temporal halves,
temporal hemianopia, points to disease at the anterior part
of the chiasma. Even when hemianopia has lasted for
years the optic discs seldom show any change. When the
lateral hemianopia coexists with hemiplegia, the loss of
sight is on the paralyzed side; "the patient cannot see

[1] Because the L. optic tract consists chiefly of fibres which supply
most of the L. half of each retina, those of them destined for the R.
eye crossing over at the optic commissure.

to his paralyzed side" (Hughlings Jackson). If double
hemiopia occurs the patient is totally blind in both eyes.
Another less common affection of sight, crossed amblyopia,
is believed to be due to a lesion of a higher centre in the
angular gyrus which presides in some degree over the
whole of both fields of vision, but chiefly over that of the
opposite eye. A unilateral lesion of this kind produces
amblyopia with great contraction of the field of the opposite eye, and with some contraction of the field of the eye
on the same side. The symptoms are much like those of
hysterical amblyopia in one eye. If such a lesion were
double it would presumably produce a high degree of amblyopia, with contraction of the fields in both eyes, the
activity of the pupils being retained. A few cases of hemianopia for colors alone have been recorded.[1]

Hysterical amblyopia and amaurosis take various forms,
and real defect may be mixed up with feigning. In hysterical hemianæsthesia the eye on the affected side is sometimes defective or quite blind. In other cases of hysteria
both eyes are defective, but one worse than the other;
there is concentric contraction of the visual fields, sometimes with and sometimes without color-blindness, a varying degree of defective visual acuteness, and sight is often
disproportionately bad by feeble light (hence the term
" anæsthesia of the retina" is sometimes used). There
may, however, be in addition irritative symptoms—watering, photophobia, and spasm of accommodation—and then
the term " hyperæsthesia retinæ," or " oculi," seems more
appropriate. Amblyopia with the above characters has
been known to follow a blow upon the eye affected which
was so slight as not to cause the least ophthalmoscopic
change ; again, when one eye has been suddenly lost by
wound or embolism a condition indistinguishable from hys-

[1] See an exhaustive paper by Mackay, Brit. Med. Journ., Nov. 10, 1888.

terical blindness may rapidly come on in the other. It is important to note that in hysterical amblyopia, even of high degree and long standing, the reflex action of the pupil, direct as well as indirect, is fully preserved, and the ophthalmoscopic appearances quite normal. The prognosis is nearly always good, though recovery is sometimes slow, and relapses may occur. In some of the worst cases I have seen there has been considerable ametropia.

True hysterical amblyopia seems allied, from the ophthalmic standpoint, with a much larger and more important class, best epitomized by the term *asthenopia*, in which photophobia, irritability, and want of endurance of the ciliary muscle, *accommodative asthenopia*, or sometimes of the internal recti, *muscular asthenopia*, with some conjunctival irritability, are the main symptoms, acuteness of sight being usually perfect, and the refraction nearly or quite normal. Of the retinal, conjunctival, and muscular factors, any one may be more marked than the others, and it would seem that, given a certain state of the nervous system, which may be described as impressionable or hyperæsthetic, over-stimulation of any one is liable to set up an over-sensitive state of the other two. These patients often complain also of dazzling, pain at the back of the eyes, and headache or neuralgia in the head. All the symptoms are worse after the day's work, and sometimes on first waking in the morning, and they are liable to vary much with the health. Artificial light always aggravates them, because it is often flickering and insufficient, but especially because it is hot. The symptoms often last for months or years, causing great discomfort and serious loss of time.

CAUSATION.—The patients are seldom children or old people. Most are women, either young or not much past middle life, often very excitable, and often with feeble circulation. If men, they are emotional, fussy, and often hypochondriacal. Some cause, such as prolonged and

12*

intense application at needlework or reading, can often be traced, and in such cases the symptoms may come on so suddenly that the patient becomes within a few hours or a day or two quite incapacitated for reading. Sometimes bright colors, glittering things, or exposure to kitchen fire, seems especially injurious. Or, again, there is a history of phlyctenular ophthalmia, or superficial ulcers, which have left the fifth nerve permanently unstable. Accommodative asthenopia with hypermetropia or astigmatism is at the bottom of nearly all the cases in which vision is supposed to have been injured by railway and other accidents; the lowered tone caused by the shock is often more apparent in the ciliary muscle because this muscle is in almost constant action and has no substitute.

TREATMENT.—The refraction and the state of the internal recti should always be carefully tested, and any error corrected by lenses, which may often be combined with prisms, with their bases toward the nose. Plain colored glasses are sometimes useful. But glasses will not cure the disease, and we must not promise too much from their use. The patient may be assured that there is no ground for alarm, and that the symptoms will probably pass off sooner or later. He should be discouraged from thinking about his eyes, and he need seldom be quite idle. The artificial light used should be sufficient and steady, not flickering, and should be shaded to prevent the heat and light from striking directly on the eyes. Bathing the eyes freely with cold water, and the occasional employment of weak astringent lotions, are useful, and cold air often acts beneficially. The eyes are often much better after a day or two. Outdoor exercise, and only moderate use of the eyes, therefore, should be enjoined. General measures must be taken according to the indications, especially in reference to any ovarian, uterine, or digestive troubles, or to sexual exhaustion in men.

FUNCTIONAL DISEASES OF THE RETINA.

Functional night-blindness (endemic nyctalopia) is caused by temporary exhaustion of the retinal sensibility from prolonged exposure to diffused, bright light. The circumstances under which it occurs usually imply not only great exposure to bright light, but lowered general nutrition, and probably some defect in diet. It often co-exists with scurvy. Sleeping with the face exposed to bright moonlight is believed to bring it on. It is commonest in sailors after long tropical voyages under bad conditions, and in soldiers after long marching in bright sun. In some countries it prevails every year in Lent when no meat is eaten, and again in harvest-time. It is now but rarely endemic in our country, but scattered cases occur, especially in children,[1] and it still occasionally prevails in large schools.

In this malady two little dry films, consisting of fatty or sebaceous matter and epithelial scales, often form on the conjunctiva at the inner and outer border of the cornea. Their meaning is obscure. There are no ophthalmoscopic changes. This night-blindness is soon cured by protection from bright light and improvement of health, and especially by cod-liver oil. That the affection is local in the eye is shown by the fact that darkening one eye, with a bandage, during the day, has been found to restore its sight enough for the ensuing night's watch on board ship, the unprotected eye remaining as bad as ever. *Snow-blindness* or *ice-blindness* is essentially the same disease, with the addition of congestion, intense pain, photophobia, contraction of pupils, and sometimes of conjunctival ecchymoses. These

---

[1] Snell reports numerous cases from near Sheffield. Transactions of the Ophthalmological Society, vol. i., 1881. Since Mr. Snell drew attention to this subject I have seen several cases, all of them (as were most of Snell's) in the spring or early summer.

peculiarities doubtless depend chiefly on powerful and prolonged stimulation of the whole retina, leading to congestion of its own vessels and those of the choroid, and subsequently of the whole eyeball ; something may also be due
to the effect of the reflected heat upon the conjunctiva.
Snow-blindness is effectually prevented by wearing smoke-
colored glasses.   Attacks, apparently identical with snow-
blindness, but of shorter duration, sometimes occur in men
engaged in trimming powerful electric lights.   The symptoms do not come on until several hours after exposure to
the light.[1]

Hemeralopia (day-blindness) occurs in certain cases of
congenital amblyopia.

Colored vision is sometimes complained of, and red is
the color usually noticed.   Red vision (Erythropsia) is
most common some time after extraction of senile cataract,
and is associated with fatigue ; everything looks rosy red,
" as if there was a most beautiful sunset," as one patient
said.   Overworked, anxious, neurotic children sometimes
complain that after reading or sewing "everything turns
red" or "red and blue."   I have not heard green or yellow
mentioned.   It has also been seen in women much exhausted
by fasting.

Micropsia.   Patients sometimes complain that objects
look too small.   When not due to insufficiency of accommodative power it is generally a symptom of disease of the
outer layers of the retina, especially in the central region,
and syphilitic retinitis is the commonest cause.   Both
micropsia and its opposite, megalopsia, are sometimes seen
in hysterical amblyopia.

By **muscæ volitantes** are understood small dots, rings,
threads, etc., which move about in the field of vision, but
do not actually cross the fixation point, and never interfere

---

[1] Ophthalmic Review, April, 1883.

with sight. They are most easily seen against the sky, or
a bright background such as the microscope field. They
depend upon minute changes in the vitreous, which are
present in nearly all eyes, though in much greater quantity
in some than others. They vary, or seem to vary, greatly
with the health and state of the circulation, but are of no
real importance. They are most abundant and troublesome in myopic eyes.

Diplopia, see Chap. XXI.; also pp. 60 and 195 for Uniocular Diplopia.

For affections of sight in Megrim and Heart Disease,
see Chap. XXII.

Malingering. Patients now and then pretend defect or
blindness of one or both eyes, or exaggerate an existing
defect, or sometimes secretly use atropine in order to dim
the sight. The imposture is generally evident enough from
other circumstances, but detection is occasionally very difficult. Malingering and intentional injuries of the eye are
very rare here, but common in countries where the con-
scription is in force.

The pretended defect of sight is usually confined to one
eye. If the patient be in reality using both eyes, a prism
held before one, by preference the "blind" one, will produce double vision. The stereoscope, and also colored
glasses, may be made very useful. Another test, when only
moderate defect is asserted, is to try the eye with various
weak glasses, and note whether the replies are consistent;
very probably a flat glass or a weak concave may be said
to "improve" or "magnify" very much. Again, atropine
may be put into the *sound* eye, and when it has fully acted
the patient be asked to read small print; if he reads easily
with both eyes open the imposture is clear, for he must be
reading with the so-called "blind" eye. If absolute blindness of one eye be asserted, the state of the pupil will be
of much help, unless the patient have used atropine; for

if its direct reflex action be good, the retina and nerve cannot be much diseased.

Pretended defect of both eyes is more difficult to expose, and, indeed, it may be impossible absolutely to convict the patient if he be intelligent and instructed. The state of the pupils, of the visual fields, and of color perception are amongst the best tests.

Color-blindness may be congenital or acquired. When acquired it is symptomatic of disease of the optic nerve, or as, for example, in hysterical amblyopia, of some affection of the visual centre.

Congenital color-blindness is not often found unless looked for. According to recent and extended researches in various countries, a proportion varying from about 3 to 5 per cent. of the males are color-blind in greater or less degree, and it appears to be more common in the lower than in the upper classes. These facts show the importance of carefully testing all men whose employment renders good perception of color indispensable, such as railway signalmen and sailors. Color-blindness is usually partial, i. e. for only one color or one pair of complementary colors, but is occasionally total. The commonest form is that in which pure green is confused with various shades of gray and of red (red-green blindness); blindness for blue and yellow is very rare. The blindness may be incomplete, perception of very pale, or very dark, red or green, i. e., being enfeebled, whilst bright red and green are well recognized; or it may be complete for all shades and tints of those colors. Congenital color-blindness is very often hereditary, but nothing further is known of its cause. It is very rare in women (0.2 per cent.). The acuteness of vision, i. e., perception of form, is normal. Both eyes are affected.[1]

[1] But on this point further research is needed.

The detection of color-blindness, either congenital or acquired, is easy, if, in making the examination, we bear in mind the two points already referred to at p. 47, viz.: (1) Many persons with perfect color *perception* know very little of the *names* of colors, and appear color-blind if asked to name them; (2) the really color-blind often do not know of their defect, having learned to compensate for it by attention to differences of shade and texture. Thus, a signalman may be color-blind for red and green; yet he may, as a rule, correctly distinguish the green from the red light, because one appears to him "brighter" than the other. The quickest and best way of avoiding these sources of error has been mentioned at p. 47. A certain standard color is given to the patient without being named, and he is asked to choose from the whole mass of skeins of wool all that appear to him of nearly the same color and shade (no two being really quite alike). If, for example, he cannot distinguish green from red, he will place the green test-skein side by side with various shades of gray and red. Wilful concealment of color-blindness is impossible under this test if a sufficient number of shades be used.

As it is necessary to detect slight as well as high degrees, the first or preliminary test should consist of very pale colors, and a pale pure green is to be taken as the test No. I. (see plate in the Appendix); Nos. 1 to 5 are liable to be confused with this color. For ascertaining whether the defect be of higher degree or not, stronger colors are then used; a bright rose color, *e. g.*, II. *a*, may be confused with blue, purple, green, or gray of corresponding depth (Nos. 6 to 9); and a scarlet, II. *b*, with various shades and tints of brown and green (Nos. 10 to 13).

It may here be noted that the visual field is not of the same size for all colors, Fig. 22, green and red having the smallest fields, and that the perception of all colors is, like perception of form, sharpest at the centre of the field.

With diminished illumination some colors are less easily perceived than others, red being the first to disappear, and blue persisting longest, *i. e.*, being perceived under the lowest illumination; but in dull light the colors are not confused, as in true color-blindness.   In congenital color-blindness, as we have seen, red-green blindness is the commonest form; and in cases of amblyopia from commencing atrophy of the optic nerve, green and red are almost always the first colors to fail, blue remaining last.

THE vitreous humor is nourished by the vessels of the ciliary body, retina, and optic disc, and is probably influenced by the state of the choroid also; and in most cases disease of the vitreous is associated with, and dependent on, disease of one or other of the structures named.

Thus, in connection with various surrounding morbid processes, the vitreous may be the seat of inflammation, acute or chronic, general or local, and of hemorrhage. It may also degenerate, especially in old age; its cells and solid parts undergoing fatty change, become visible as opacities, whilst its general bulk becomes too fluid. The only alteration that we can directly prove in the vitreous during life is loss of transparency, from the presence of opacities moving, or more rarely fixed, in it, but according as such opacities move quickly or slowly we infer that the humor itself is, or is not, more fluid than in health.

Opacities in the vitreous may take the form of large dense masses, or of membranes, like muslin, crape, "bees' wings" of wine, bands, knotted strings, or isolated dots; and they may be either recent or the remains of long antecedent exudation, hemorrhage, or degeneration, or newly-formed bloodvessels. Again, the vitreous may become uniformly misty, owing to the diffusion of numberless dots, "dust-like" opacities, which need careful focussing by direct examination with a convex lens (about + 12 D.) behind the mirror to be separately seen.

Opacities in the vitreous are usually detected with great

case by direct ophthalmoscopic examination at about 12″ from the patient, but are generally situated too far forward, i. e., too far within the focus of the lens system, to be seen clearly at a very short distance without a + lens behind the mirror. If the patient move his eye sharply and freely from side to side and from above downward, the opacities will be seen against the red ground as dark figures which continue to move after the eye has come to rest; they are thus at once distinguished from opacities in the cornea or lens, or from dimly seen spots of pigment at the fundus which stop when the eye stops. The opacities in the vitreous move just as solid particles and films move in a bottle after the bottle has been shaken; the quickness and freedom of their movement in the one case, as in the other, depending very much on the consistence of the fluid. When the opacities pass across the field quickly and make wide movements, we may be sure that there is *synchysis* or fluidity of the vitreous humor; if they move very lazily, its consistence is probably normal; if only one or two opacities be present, they may only come into view now and then. Moving opacities in the vitreous obscure the fundus both to the direct and indirect ophthalmoscopic examination, in proportion to their size, density, and position; a few isolated dots scarcely affect the brightness of the ophthalmoscopic image.

The opacities may lie quite in the cortex of the vitreous and be anchored at the fundus, so as to have but little movement. Such opacities, generally single, are found lying over or near to the disc, and may be the result either of inflammation or of hemorrhage; they are often membranous, more rarely globular, and not perfectly opaque. Such an opacity should be suspected when, by indirect ophthalmoscopic examination, a localized haze or blurring of some part of the disc or its neighborhood is noticed. The opacity must then be searched for by the direct method, the patient's eye being at rest; by altering the distance from the patient, or by turning on various convex lenses (or concave, if the eye be very highly myopic), the opacity will come sharply into view. The patient's refraction must be approximately known in order to make this examination properly. Densely opaque white membranes may also form over the disc or upon the retina, the nature and situation of which are diagnosed in the same way.

Diffused haziness of the vitreous causes a corresponding degree of dimness of outline and darkening of the details of the fundus as if these were seen through a thin smoke. The disc in particular appears red, without really being so. Much the same appearances are caused by diffused haze of the cornea or lens, but the presence of these changes will, of course, have been excluded by focal illumination. There are even cases of vitreous disease where no details can be seen, even by careful examination, though plenty of light reaches and returns from the fundus. In these the light is scattered by innumerable little particles, each of which is transparent, so that the light, without being absorbed, is distorted and broken up, as in passing through ground-glass or white fog or a partial mixture of fluids of different densities, such as glycerine and water. This fine general haze is found chiefly in syphilitic choroido-retinitis, in which infiltration of the vitreous with cells is known to occur. It is not always easy, nor indeed possible, to distinguish with certainty between diffuse haze of the vitreous and diffuse haze of the retina.

Crystals of cholesterin sometimes form in a fluid vitreous and are seen with bright illumination as minute, dancing, golden spangles, when the eye moves about, *sparkling synchysis*. They proportionately obscure the fundus. Large opacities just behind the lens may be seen by focal light in their natural colors. In rare cases of choroido-retinitis, minute growths consisting chiefly of bloodvessels, form on

the retina and project into the vitreous; they are rather
curiosities than of practical importance.

Parasites (cysticercus cellulosæ) occasionally come to
rest in the eye, and in development penetrate into the vitreous; they are rarely seen in England, but are comparatively common in some parts of Germany. Very rarely a
foreign body may be visible in the vitreous.

The following are the conditions in which disease of the
vitreous is most commonly found:

(1.) Myopia of high degree and old standing; the opacities move very freely, showing fluidity of the humor, and
are sharply defined. They are often the result of former
hemorrhage.

(2.) After severe blows, causing hemorrhage from the
vessels of the choroid or ciliary body. When recent, and
situated near the back of the lens, the blood can often be
seen by focal light; if very abundant it so darkens the
interior of the eye that nothing whatever can be seen with
the mirror.

(3.) After perforating wounds. The opacity will be
blood if the case be quite recent. Lymph or pus in the
vitreous gives a yellow or greenish-yellow color, easily seen
by focal light, or even by daylight, and usually most dense
toward the position of the wound.

(4.) In rare cases large hemorrhages into the vitreous
occur spontaneously in healthy eyes, with hemorrhages into
the retina (not to be confused with retinitis hæmorrhagica).
Relapses often occur, and detachment of retina may ensue.
The subjects are generally young adult males liable to
epistaxis, constipation, and irregularity of circulation
(Eales); gout may have some influence (Hutchinson).
This affection seems sometimes to be related with the form
of choroiditis referred to at p. 222.

In all of the above cases detachment of the retina is

likely to occur sooner or later, and if both be present the differential diagnosis may be difficult.

(5.) Syphilitic choroiditis and retinitis. There is often diffuse haze in addition to large, slowly floating opacities. The change here is due to inflammation, and the opacities may entirely disappear under treatment. These are the cases in which new vessels in the vitreous are most common.

(6.) Some cases of cyclitis and cyclo-iritis. The opacities are inflammatory.

(7.) In the early stage of sympathetic ophthalmitis. The opacities are inflammatory.

(8.) In various cases of old disease of choroid, usually in old persons, and without proof of syphilis. No doubt many of these indicate former choroidal hemorrhages.

(9.) Cases occur in which no cause, either local or general, can be assigned for the presence of opacities in the vitreous.

CHAPTER XVII.

GLAUCOMA.

IN this peculiar and very serious disease the character-istic objective symptom is increased tightness of the eye-capsule, sclerotic and cornea, "increased tension;" all the characteristic features of the disease depend upon this. The disease is much commoner after middle life, when the sclerotic becomes less distensible than before; and it is commoner in hypermetropic eyes, where the sclerotic is too thick, than in myopic eyes, where it is thinned by elongation of the globe.

Glaucoma may be primary, coming on in an eye appa-rently healthy, or the subject of some disease, such as senile cataract, which has no influence on the glaucoma; or it may be secondary, caused by some still active disease of the eye, or by conditions left after some previous disease, such as iritis. It is always important, and seldom difficult, to distinguish between primary and secondary glaucoma.

Glaucoma differs in severity and rate of progress from the most acute to the most chronic and insidious form; but in every form it is a progressive disease, and unless checked by treatment goes on to permanent blindness. The disease is very often symmetrical, attacking the second eye after an interval which varies.

It is customary and useful to speak of glaucoma as either acute, subacute, or chronic. But many intermediate forms are found, and the same eye may, at different stages in its history, pass through each of the three conditions. We may, indeed, here observe that acute and subacute outbursts are generally preceded by a so-called "premonitory" stage, in which the symptoms are not only chronic and mild, but remittent; the intervals of remission becoming shorter and shorter, till at length the attacks become continuous, and the glaucomatous state is fully established. Rapid increase of presbyopia (Chap. XX.), shown by the need for a frequent change of spectacles, is a common premonitory sign, though often overlooked.

Chronic glaucoma sets in with a cloudiness of sight, or "fog," varying in density, and often clearing off entirely for days and even weeks, "premonitory stage." But, in some cases, according to the patient, the failure progresses without remissions from first to last. During the attacks of "fog," artificial lights are seen surrounded by colored rings, "rainbows" or "halos," due to haze of the cornea, which are to be distinguished from those due to mucus on the cornea. The attacks of fog are often noticed only after long use of the eyes, as in the evening or when exhausted, the sight being better in the early part of the day and after food. Even when the sight has become permanently cloudy, complete recovery no longer occurring between the attacks, variations of sight still form a marked feature. There is no congestion, and pain of neuralgic character, though not uncommon, is often entirely wanting. The disease has to be distinguished from incipient nuclear cataract, disease of the optic nerve, syphilitic retinitis, and attacks of megrim.

If we see the patient during one of the brief early fits of cloudy sight, or after the fog has settled down permanently, the following changes will be found. A greater or less defect of sight in one eye, or if in both, more in one than the other, and not remedied by glasses; the pupil a little larger and less active than normal; the anterior chamber may be shallow, and there is usually slight dulness of the eye from steaminess of cornea, or haze of the aqueous

humor, and some engorgement of the large perforating
vessels at a little distance from the cornea; the tension
somewhat increased, usually about $+$ 1, p. 43; and the
field of vision may be contracted, especially on the nasal
side.   The optic disc will be found normal, pale, or sometimes congested, in early cases; pale and cupped all over
at a later stage.   There may be spontaneous pulsation of
all the vessels on the disc; or the arteries, if not pulsating
spontaneously, will do so on *very slight* pressure on the eyeball.   In old standing cases the tension will often be much
increased, the pupil dilated and sluggish, though not motionless, the lens hazy, the field of vision much contracted,
Fig. 94, acuteness of vision extremely defective, the cornea
sometimes clear, in other cases dull.   In nearly all cases of
glaucoma the temporal part of the field, nasal part of the
retina, retains its function longest; and in advanced cases
the patient will often show this by his manner or state-
ments; occasionally the field becomes extremely contracted
before central vision fails.   In some few cases of simple
glaucoma scotomata appear at the central part of the
field without contraction.

An eye in which the above symptoms have set in may
progress to total blindness in the course of months or
several years without a single "inflammatory" symptom,
without either pain or redness—*chronic painless glaucoma*
(*glaucoma simplex*); and since the lens often becomes partially opaque, and of a grayish or greenish hue, cases
of chronic glaucoma are sometimes mistaken for senile
cataract.

But more commonly, in the course of a chronic case,
periods of pain and congestion occur, with more rapid
failure of sight; or the disease sets in with "inflammatory"
symptoms at once.   In these cases of *subacute glaucoma*,
besides the symptoms named above, we find dusky, reticulated congestion of the small and large episcleral vessels in

the ciliary region, with pain referred to the eye, the side of
the head or of the nose, and rapid failure of sight.   The
increase of tension, steaminess, and partial anæsthesia of the
cornea, enlarged and sluggish pupil, and shallowness of the
anterior chamber, are all more marked than is usual in
chronic cases, and the media are too hazy to allow a good
ophthalmoscopic examination.

FIG. 94.

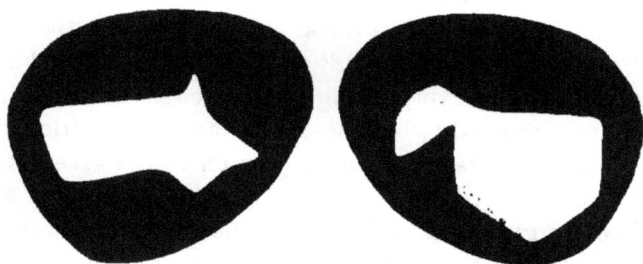

Irregular contraction of R. and L. fields of vision in chronic glaucoma;
from two different cases.   The black parts show complete loss ; the
shaded area shows partial loss.   Each field remains best in the outer
part.   (Compare with Figs. 90 and 91.)

These symptoms, ending after a few weeks or months in
complete blindness, may remain at about the same height
for months after that event, with slight variations, the eye
gradually settling down into a permanent state of severe,
but chronic, non-inflammatory glaucomatous tension.
Short attacks of subacute glaucoma, with intervals of
perfect recovery, sometimes occur, *remittent glaucoma ;*
permanent glaucoma usually supervenes.

Acute glaucoma differs from the other forms only in
suddenness of onset, rapidity of loss of sight, and severity
of congestion and pain.   The congestion, both arterial and
venous, is intense ; in extreme cases the lids and conjunctiva are swollen, and there is photophobia, so that the case
may be mistaken for an acute ophthalmia.   All the specific

signs of glaucoma are intensified; the pupil considerably
dilated and motionless to light, the cornea very steamy, the
anterior chamber very shallow, and tension + 2 or 3.
Sight will fall in a day or two down to the power of only
counting fingers, or to mere perception of light, and if
the case have lasted a week or two, even p. l. is usually
abolished. The pain is very severe in the eye, temple,
back of the head, and down the nose; not unfrequently it
is so bad as to cause vomiting, and many a case has been
mistaken for a "bilious attack" with a "cold in the eye,"
for "neuralgia in the head," or "rheumatic ophthalmia."
Some cases, however, though very acute, are mild and
remit spontaneously; but these, like the ones mentioned in
the preceding paragraph, often pass on to the severe type
now described.

Absolute glaucoma is glaucoma that has gone on to permanent blindness. Such an eye continues to display the
tension and other signs of the disease, and remains liable
to attacks of pain and congestion for varying periods, but
in many "absolute" cases, especially when the original
attack was acute, changes occur sooner or later, leading to
staphylomata, cataract, atrophy of iris, and finally to softening and shrinkage of the globe.

As a rule, glaucoma runs the same course in the second
eye as in the first, but sometimes it will be chronic in one
and acute or subacute in the other.

EXPLANATION OF THE SYMPTOMS.—The causes which
produce the temporary attacks or "premonitory symptoms"
lead, if continued, to atrophy of the inner layers of the
retina and of the disc, and to consequent blindness. The
increase of tension damages the retina both by direct compression and by impeding its circulation, the latter being
probably the more important factor in the early stages. If
the media be clear enough to allow a good view, the retinal
arteries are seen to be narrow, and often pulsating spontane-

ously, and the veins engorged. The periphery of the retina
suffers soonest and most from this lowering of arterial blood
supply, and hence probably the contraction of the visual
field ; but the inner layers of the retina, over its whole extent, suffer if the pressure be kept up—(1) from this same
insufficiency of arterial blood, and the changes, including
hemorrhage, which follow impeded venous outflow ; (2)
from direct compression of the retina ; (3) from stretching
and atrophy of the nerve-fibres on the disc. The floor of
the disc, *lamina cribrosa*, being the weakest part of the eye-
capsule, is slowly pressed backward, the nerve-fibres being
dragged upon, displaced, and finally atrophied ; the direct
pressure on the nerve-fibres, as they bend over the edge of
the disc, helps in the same process. Hence finally the disc
becomes not only atrophied, but hollowed out, Fig. 95, into

FIG. 95.

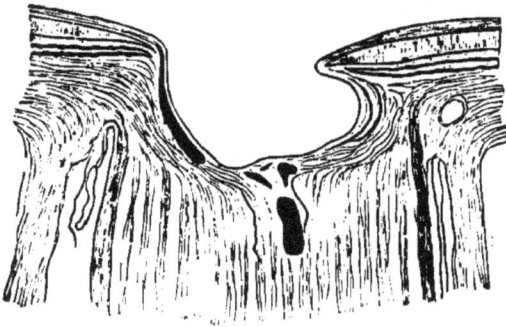

Section of very deep glaucoma cup. (Compare Fig. 35.)

the well-known " glaucomatous cup." This cup, when
deep, has an overhanging edge, because the border of the
disc is smaller at the level of the choroid than at the level
of the *lamina cribrosa ;* its sides are quite steep even when
the cup is shallow, Fig. 97.

With the ophthalmoscope this cupping is shown by a

sudden bending of the vessels just within the border of the disc, where they look darker because foreshortened, Fig.

FIG. 96.

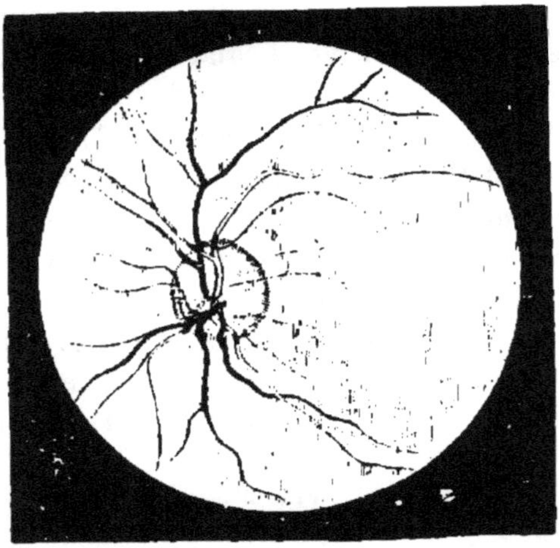

Ophthalmoscopic appearance of slight cupping of the disc in glaucoma. The disc is surrounded by a narrow, irregular zone of atrophied choroid. (Wecker and Jaeger.) × 7.

FIG. 97.

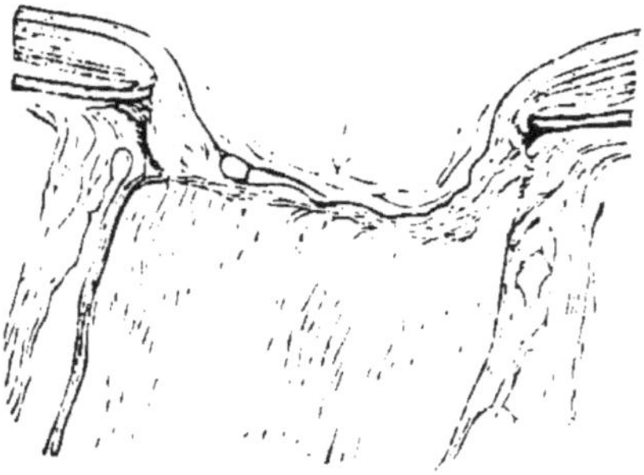

Section of less advanced glaucoma cup.

96; if the cup be deep they may disappear beneath its edge to reappear on its floor, where they have a lighter shade,

Fig. 98. The vessels seldom all bend with equal abrupt-
ness, some parts of the disc being more deeply hollowed
than others, or some of the vessels spanning over the interval instead of hugging the wall of the cup. Increase of
tension must be maintained for several months to produce

FIG. 98.

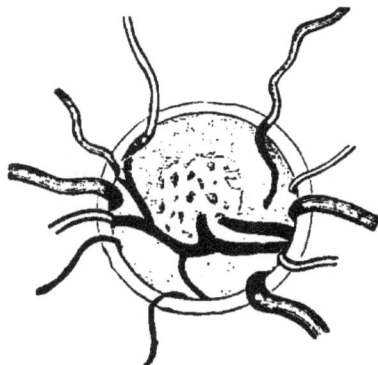

Ophthalmoscopic appearance of deep cupping of the disc in glaucoma.
(Altered from Liebreich.) ✕ about 15.

cupping recognizable by the ophthalmoscope. When recent acute glaucoma has been cured by operation, the disc,
though not cupped, often becomes rather hazy and very
pale. Although usually the excavation extends from the
first over the whole surface of the disc, it appears sometimes
to begin at the thinnest part (the physiological pit), and
spread centrifugally toward the border. A deep cup is
sometimes partly filled up by fibrous tissue, the result of
chronic inflammation, and its true dimensions are not then
appreciable by the ophthalmoscope.

The shallowness of the anterior chamber is probably due
to advance of the lens; it is by no means a constant symptom. Compression of the ciliary nerves accounts, in early

cases, for the sluggish and usually dilated pupil, and for the corneal anæsthesia. In old-standing cases the iris is often atrophied and shrunken to a narrow rim ; in uncomplicated glaucoma iritic adhesions are never seen. · The corneal changes depend partly on "steaminess" of the epithelium, partly upon haze of the corneal tissue from œdema (Fuchs). In recent cases, especially if acute, the aqueous humor and the lens appear to become somewhat turbid. In old cases, as already stated, the lens often becomes slowly cataractous. There is some doubt whether or not the vitreous becomes hazy in glaucoma ; it is certainly very seldom so when the cornea and lens are clear, and the point cannot be settled when these media are hazy. The internal pressure tends, in acute cases, to make the globe spherical, by reducing the curvature of the cornea to that of the sclerotic ; it also in all cases weakens the accommodation, at first by pressing on the ciliary nerves, later by causing atrophy of the ciliary muscle ; these facts together explain the rapid decrease of refractive power (*i. e.*, rapid onset or increase of presbyopia) which is sometimes noticed by the patient. The choroidal circulation is obstructed by the increase of pressure, and in severe glaucoma, especially of old standing, the *anterior ciliary veins* (forming the episcleral plexus), as well as the arteries, become very much enlarged.

MECHANISM OF GLAUCOMA.—The increased tension is due to excess of fluid in the eyeball. Impeded escape is probably the chief cause of this excess, and recent research has proved that changes are present in nearly all glaucomatous eyes, which must lessen, or prevent, the normal outflow. But increased secretion, and internal vascular congestion, undoubtedly play an important part in certain cases. Some authorities have attributed the phenomena of glaucoma to vaso-motor changes in the size of the blood-vessels, but such hypotheses are wanting in proof. Both conditions would have most effect when the sclerotic was most unyielding, *i. e.*, in old age, and in hypermetropic eyes. It is probable that there is a constant movement of fluid from the vitreous humor through the suspensory ligament of the lens, and also from the anterior part of the ciliary processes, into the anterior chamber, as shown by the dotted line in Fig. 99. The fluid escapes from the anterior chamber into the lymphatics and perhaps into the veins

FIG. 99.

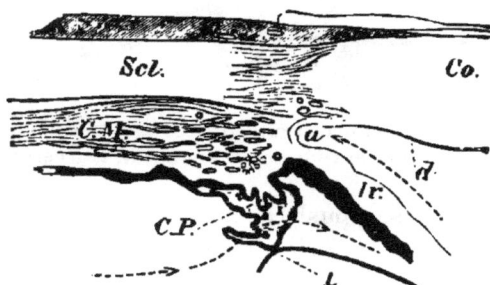

Section through the ciliary region in a healthy human eye. *Co.*, cornea; *Scl.*, sclerotic; *C. M.*, ciliary muscle; *C. P.*, two ciliary processes, one larger than the other ; *Ir.*, iris ; *L.*, the marginal part of the crystalline lens ; *a*, angle of anterior chamber ; *d*, membrane of Descemet, which ceases (as such) before reaching the angle *a*. The dotted line shows the course probably taken by fluid fro n the anterior part of the vitreous into the posterior aqueous chamber, where it is augmented by aqueous humor secreted by the anterior part of the ciliary process, thence through the pupil (not shown) into the anterior aqueous chamber, to the angle *a*. Suspensory ligament of lens not shown. × 10.

of the sclerotic, through the meshes of the *ligamentum pectinatum* (*Fontana's spaces*), which close the angle *a*; and it has been proved that very little fluid can pass through any other part of the cornea. In glaucoma the angle *a* is nearly always closed, in recent cases by contact, in old cases by permanent cohesion, between the periphery of the iris and the cornea, Figs. 100 and 101. No complete explanation

of this advance of the iris has yet been given. Dr. Adolf
Weber holds that the ciliary processes, becoming swollen

FIG. 100.

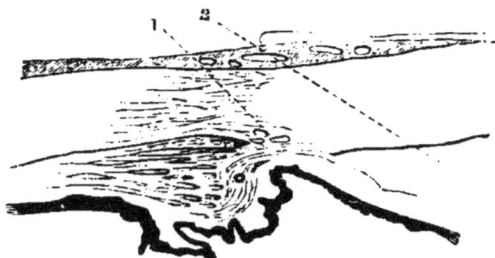

Ciliary region from a case of acute glaucoma of one month's duration
(1 and 2, situations of iridectomy wounds in two cases) × 10.

from various causes, push the iris forward, and so start the
glaucomatous state. Priestley Smith[1] believes that the primary obstruction is at the narrow chink between the edge
of the lens and at the tips of the ciliary processes ("circum-
lental spaces"), and that the block may depend upon one

FIG. 101.

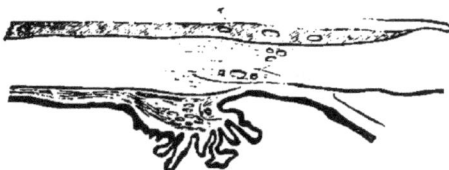

Ciliary region in chronic glaucoma of three years' standing. × 10.

or more of three factors—increase in the size of the lens
due to advancing years,[2] abnormal smallness of the ciliary

[1] Priestley Smith, Trans. of Ophth. Soc., vol. vi., 1886.
[2] The increase in the size of the lens as age advances has been proved
beyond doubt by Priestley Smith's researches. Ibid., vol. iii. (1883).

area as in hypermetropia, and abnormal enlargement of the
ciliary processes. Obstruction of this space leads to rise of
pressure in the vitreous, followed by advance of the lens
and ciliary processes against the base of the iris and consequent closure of the angle. Brailey holds that a chronic
inflammation of the ciliary muscle and processes, and of the
iris, quickly passing on to atrophic shrinking, leads to narrowing of the angle and initial rise of tension ;[1] in a later
paper, however, he agrees to some extent with the view of
Weber, above referred to.[2] Cases of chronic glaucoma
have been seen in which the iris was congenitally absent.

But there are cases which show that thé matter is not
always so simple. Stilling, of Strasbourg, has lately (1885)
contended that the waste fluids escape by the central canal
of the vitreous into the optic nerve, and partly also by fil-
tration through the circum-papillary portion of the sclerotic,
and that a sclerosis of these parts, by diminishing their
permeability, leads to glaucoma ; Brailey[3] states from pathological research that inflammation of the optic nerve is
always present quite early in glaucoma, and that it precedes
the increased tension ; and ophthalmoscopic examination in
certain cases lends support to this statement.[4] It may be
added, in support of these views, that glaucoma may occur
after removal of the lens, that in some cases of glaucoma
the angle of the anterior chamber remains freely open, and
that the ophthalmoscopical appearances of glaucoma are
occasionally seen without increase of T. (For other causes
see Secondary Glaucoma.)

An over-supply of fluid affects the tension differently in
different cases. Congestion and ordinary inflammations of
the retina and uveal tract do not cause glaucoma, and dila-

[1] Brailey, Ophth. Hosp. Reports, x., pp. 14, 89, 93 (1880).

[2] Brailey, ibid., p. 282 (1881).

[3] Brailey, ibid., pp. 86, 277, 282.

[4] Nettleship, St. Thomas's Hosp. Rep., vol. xiv.

tation of the arteries by vaso-motor paralysis is said to be
accompanied by diminished tension. But tumors in, and
even upon, the eye often give rise to secondary glaucoma,
and probably the active congestion and transudation of
fluid and small cells which occur near to a quickly growing tumor are the chief factors ; certainly the glaucoma
stands in no constant relation either to the size or position
of the tumor. A relation is observed in some cases between
glaucoma and neuralgia of the fifth nerve ; and T. is said
to be lowered in paralysis of this nerve. Probably the
pain acts by causing associated congestion, and thus setting
up glaucoma in a predisposed eye.

GENERAL AND DIATHETIC CAUSES.—In an eye predisposed, by the changes above mentioned in the ciliary
region, any cause of congestion may precipitate an acute
attack. Congestion of the eyes in connection with disturbances of the general circulation from heart disease,
bronchitis, or portal engorgement, or due to loss of sleep
from gout, neuralgia, worry, etc., or caused by the over-use
of presbyopic eyes without suitable glasses, or by a blow,
or prolonged ophthalmoscopic examination, or exposure to
cold wind, may all bring it about. Atropine has sometimes
caused an attack, because, by lessening the width, it increases the thickness of the iris, and so crowds it into the
angle of the anterior chamber. Iridectomy on one eye
occasionally sets up acute glaucoma in the other, probably
by causing general excitement and disturbance, and it is
now customary to use eserine as a preventive in the second
eye after iridectomy in the first. Glaucoma is uncommon
before the age of forty, and is most frequent between fifty-
five and sixty-five ;[1] the rare cases seen in young adults and
children are generally chronic and often associated with

---

[1] Statistics of 1000 cases collected by Priestley Smith, loc. cit. (1886).
Gallenga (Turin), in 330 cases, finds the frequency greatest between 60
and 70.

other changes in the eyes, particularly myopia. Acute
cases are often dated from a period of overwork of the eyes,
or want of sleep, as from sitting up, nursing, etc. Patients
who have had glaucoma in one eye should be emphatically
warned as to the danger of over-using the eyes, or of working without proper glasses, and against dietetic errors.
Primary glaucoma is, according to the newest statistics,[1] as
a whole, rather commoner in women than men; and whilst
the acute congestive forms are much commoner in women,
very chronic glaucoma is rather commoner in men.

TREATMENT.—Iridectomy, or an equivalent operation,
is, with very few exceptions, the only curative treatment.
Eserine or pilocarpine (gr. $\frac{1}{2}$-ij to $\bar{3}$j) used locally, however, diminishes the tension in acute glaucoma, and a few
attacks seem to have been permanently cured by it. But
although seldom really curative, eserine is of great temporary value in cases where an operation has to be deferred.
It has little or no effect on the tension unless it causes
marked contraction of the pupil. Eserine acts (1) by
stretching the iris and drawing it away from the angle
of the anterior chamber; (2) by the contraction of the
ciliary muscle which it causes, the meshes of the tissue
bounding this angle are more widely opened. Eserine
causes congestion of the ciliary processes, and probably
this explains why, if it do not soon relieve, it sometimes
aggravates, the symptoms. It is of use chiefly in recent,
and especially in acute, cases; a solution of half a grain
or a grain of the sulphate to the ounce is to be used about
every two hours and continued if relief be obtained. If
in a few hours it increases the pain and do not lessen the T.
it should be abandoned. The pain in acute cases may be
much relieved by leeching, warmth to the eye, derivative

[1] Priestley Smith, loc. cit. (1886); in 1000 cases 569 women and 431
men.

treatment such as purgation and hot foot-baths, and sopo-
rifics. Cocaine is used with the eserine by some surgeons,
and seems to increase its efficacy.

Iridectomy cures glaucoma by permanently reducing the
tension to the normal or nearly normal degree. It is found
that the best results are obtained—(1) if the path of the
incision lie in the sclerotic from 1 to 2 mm. from the apparent corneal border, Fig. 100; (2) if the wound be large,
allowing removal of about a fifth of the iris; (3) if the iris
be removed quite up to its ciliary attachment, which is best
done by first cutting one end of the drawn-out loop of iris,
then tearing it from its ciliary attachment along the whole
extent of the wound, and cutting through the other end
separately. (See Operations.) Evacuation of the aqueous
humor by paracentesis of the anterior chamber gives only
temporary relief.

A mere wound in the sclerotic, differing but little in position and extent from that made for iridectomy, is sufficient
to relieve $+$ T., and to cure some cases of glaucoma permanently, and this operation, *subconjunctival sclerotomy*,
was largely adopted by some operators a few years ago.
Iridectomy, however, has held its ground as the more
effectual operation. Sclerotomy is open to objection—(1)
because the position and length of the wound are not perfectly under control; if too far forward and too short it
is ineffectual, if too far back and too long there is risk of
wounding the ciliary processes and getting hemorrhage
into the vitreous; even shrinking of the operated eye and
sympathetic inflammation of the other have occurred; (2)
because the iris may prolapse into the wound, and need
removal, and the operation then becomes an iridectomy;
(3) when the anterior chamber is very shallow sclerotomy
cannot be supposed to aid the exit of fluid so much as the
removal of a piece of the iris.

Several other operations, the principle of which is to

make a puncture at the sclero-corneal junction, or through the sclerotic near the equator, have been tried, but have not gained general confidence.

Whichever operation be employed in glaucoma, the formation of the operation scar in the sclerotic is certainly a most important factor.

Iridectomy in acute glaucoma no doubt acts, at first, by removing a portion of the iris from the blocked angle, Fig. 100, and thus allowing the normal escape of fluid. Some high authorities, hold, however, that its permanent effect is due to the formation, at the seat of the wound, of a layer of tissue more pervious to the eye-fluids than the sclerotic, "filtration-scar;" an iridectomy for glaucoma which heals slowly is at any rate believed to be more favorable than one which heals immediately, i. e., with no new tissue, and a slight bulging of the scar is held by some surgeons to be rather desirable than otherwise. That a mere sclerotomy may be sufficient points in the same direction. Such a porous scar never forms if the incision be in the cornea.

An operation, usually iridectomy, is to be done in all cases of acute and subacute glaucoma, whether there be great pain or not, so long as some sight still remains, and even if all p. l. be lost, provided that the blindness be of only a few days' duration. Even if the eye be permanently quite blind, iridectomy or sclerotomy, or perhaps stretching the infra-trochlear nerve is sometimes preferable to excision of the globe, for the relief of pain.

Chronic ("simple") glaucoma should, in my opinion, always, if possible, be operated upon early, as soon as the diagnosis is certain and before the field is much damaged; the prognosis is then fairly good. In advanced chronic glaucoma, when the field has become much contracted, visual acuteness usually much lowered, and the disc pale and considerably cupped, the rule is less clear, for it is well known that the effect of operation in such cases is far from constant. But as no other treatment is of use, and iridectomy is certainly often beneficial, it should usually be performed, especially if the disease affect both eyes. The patient's prospect of life must be allowed for in chronic glaucoma ; if he be old and feeble, life may end before the disease have progressed to blindness.

There is often difficulty in deciding upon the best course in the so-called "premonitory" stage, which consists, in truth, of transient attacks of slight glaucoma. When it is clear that attacks of temporary mistiness and rainbows are glaucomatous, and that they are getting more frequent, iridectomy should seldom be deferred ; but if the patient can be seen at short intervals, eserine should have a fair trial before operation is resorted to. It is to be remembered that iridectomy done when sight is still good may, by allowing spherical aberration and causing corneal astigmatism, increase the defect; and this, though not of necessity a contra-indication, must be taken into account.

THE PROGNOSIS after operation is, in general terms, better in proportion as the disease is acute and recent. If operated on within a few days of the onset of acute symptoms, provided that fingers can still be counted at the time of operation, sight is often restored to the state in which it was at the onset, i. e., if the disease be recent, nearly perfect sight will be restored. Even in cases combining the maximum of acuteness and severity, in which vision has for the last few days been reduced to mere p. l., the operation is often successful in restoring some degree of useful sight. But the prognosis is not always so favorable in acute glaucoma, especially if the patient's health be much broken down ; and if there be, as is by no means uncommon, evidence that sight had been already damaged by chronic glaucoma before the acute attack set in, the prognosis must be guarded. In simple chronic glaucoma we can only hope, as a rule, to stop the disease where it is and prevent the sight from getting worse.

The full effect of the operation is not seen for several weeks, though a marked immediate effect is produced in acute cases. In cases of long standing T. may remain permanently rather $+$ after operation, without bad effect, provided it be very much less than before the operation; the eye tissues can in some degree adapt themselves to increased pressure.

A second iridectomy in the opposite direction, or a sclerotomy, should be done if T., having been reduced to normal, or very slightly $+$, after the first operation, rise definitely and be accompanied by a return of other symptoms; but several weeks should generally elapse, for slight waves of glaucomatous tension may occur before the eye has fully recovered from the first operation, and these may often be relieved by other means. Cases which relapse definitely, or which steadily get worse after the first operation, are always very grave, and the second operation must not be confidently expected to succeed. If, after iridectomy in acute glaucoma, the symptoms are not relieved, even for a time, or become worse, some complication is to be suspected, such as hemorrhage from the retina or choroid, or a tumor. (See Secondary Glaucoma.)

OTHER TREATMENT.—If we are obliged to delay the operation, the other means mentioned at p. 299 should be prescribed, including eserine. The diet should, as a rule, be liberal, unless the patient be plethoric. It is very important to insure sound sleep and mental calm. After the operation, until the eye has become quiet, all causes likely to induce congestion must be carefully avoided, such as use of the eyes, stooping or straining, and prolonged ophthalmoscopic examination. Atropine must never be used. We should be on the alert for the earliest symptoms in the

second eye after operation on the first, and the use of
eserine may be advisable as a prophylactic.

In a few cases of very chronic or subacute character,
with great increase of T., iridectomy seems to aggravate
the disease, being followed, not even by temporary benefit,
but by persistence of + T., increased irritability, and still
further deterioration of sight (*"glaucoma malignum"*).
Perhaps the tilting forward of the lens, which sometimes
follows iridectomy, may account for the result.

Glaucoma may occur independently in cataractous eyes,
and in eyes from which the lens has been extracted, with
or without iridectomy.

Secondary glaucoma may be acute or chronic, according as it is a consequence of active disease or of sequelæ.
It may be caused by circular iritic synechia with bulging
of the iris. Various forms of chronic irido-keratitis and
irido-choroiditis, especially in the sympathetic form, are
liable to be accompanied by it; in the former it may be
due to choking of the spaces of Fontana by inflammatory
products, and perhaps to excessive secretion from the
ciliary processes; in the sympathetic disease, to total posterior synechia. It may follow perforation of the cornea
with large anterior synechia. The eye often becomes temporarily glaucomatous in the course of traumatic cataract
from the pressure of the swollen lens on the iris and ciliary
processes, especially in patients past middle life. In none
of these cases is there much danger of mistaking secondary
for idiopathic glaucoma.

But secondary glaucoma may result from various deeper
changes. When the lens is dislocated, either behind or in
front of the iris, it often sets up glaucoma, sometimes of
very severe type, apparently by pressing on the ciliary processes or iris. There is generally the history of a blow;
and in posterior dislocation, even if the edge of the displaced lens cannot be seen, the iris is usually tremulous,

and its surface concave or flat at one part, whilst bulging
or prominent at another. If we are sure that a lens dislocated into the vitreous is causing the symptoms, it should
be extracted with a scoop (see Operations), and if lying in
the anterior chamber should also usually be removed. If
the eye become glaucomatous immediately after a severe
blow the condition of the lens may not be ascertainable,
and then an iridectomy must be done and the eye be
watched: vitreous is very likely to escape at the operation
if there be dislocation of the lens, for the latter condition
implies rupture of the suspensory ligament. Hemorrhage
into an eye whose retina is detached, e. g., in high degrees
of myopia, may give rise to acute glaucoma with severe
pain. A glaucomatous attack generally occurs during the
growth of an intra-ocular tumor. It is often impossible to
distinguish such a case, in an adult, from one of idiopathic
glaucoma of the same severity and standing; for even if
the lens be not opaque, and it often is so, the other media
will probably be too hazy to allow an ophthalmoscopic
examination, the growth itself is usually of a dark color,
and both idiopathic glaucoma and choroidal sarcoma are
diseases of advanced life. In almost every case, however,
the glaucoma will be "absolute," and will be known to
have been so for weeks or months, and there will also be
the negative fact that the fellow-eye shows no signs of
glaucoma. If a glaucomatous eye, which has been absolutely blind for several months, remain painful and congested, and its media too opaque for ophthalmoscopic
examination, it should be excised as likely to contain a
tumor. Tumors in the eyes of children also cause secondary
glaucoma, but there is seldom any difficulty in making the
diagnosis; the patient is far below the age for primary
glaucoma, and the growth is usually conspicuous from its
whitish color. Secondary glaucoma now and then supervenes in cases of albuminuric retinitis, and of embolism or

thrombosis of the retinal vessels, and in cases of retinal
hemorrhage from other causes, *hemorrhagic glaucoma.* In
glaucoma with hemorrhage the diagnosis can sometimes be
completed only after an unsuccessful operation has shown
that the case is not a simple one.

CHAPTER XVIII.

TUMORS AND NEW-GROWTHS OF THE EYEBALL AND CONJUNCTIVA.

A. Tumors and Growths of the Conjunctiva and Front of the Eyeball.

Cauliflower warts, with narrow pedicles like those on the glans penis, but flattened like a cock's comb by pressure, are sometimes seen on the ocular and palpebral conjunctiva. Each wart, with a small portion of healthy conjunctiva around its pedicle, must be snipped off, or the growth is likely to recur.

Lupus occasionally extends from the skin of the eyelid to the palpebral, and later to the ocular, conjunctiva. The part affected is very vascular, irregularly thickened, and ulcerated. It may also appear independently on the palpebral conjunctiva, the skin of the eyelid being healthy. It is usually limited to a part of one eyelid. There may be co-existent lupus, either of skin or oral mucous membrane. There seems much doubt whether any distinction can be made between the rare cases that have been described as *tubercle of the conjunctiva* (ocular or palpebral), and what most surgeons call lupus.[1] Conjunctival lupus is much benefited by the usual local treatment.

The eyelid, and especially the tarsus, is now and then the seat of diffused gummatous inflammation in the tertiary

---

[1] Consult Hirschberg, Trans. Internat. Med. Cong. 1881, 3, 117; Benson, Trans. Oph. Soc., v. 41 and 51 (1885) ; Mules, Oph. Rev., iv. 3 (1885).

stage of syphilis. The infiltration gives rise to a hard, indolent swelling of the whole lid, *syphilitic tarsitis*. Chancres and tertiary syphilitic ulcers may occur on the lids.

Pinguecula, a yellowish spot, looking like adipose tissue, in the conjunctiva close to the inner or outer edge of the cornea, consists of thickened conjunctiva and subconjunctival tissue, and contains no fat. It is commonest in old people, and in those whose eyes are exposed to local irritants. Though of no consequence, advice is often asked about it.

Pterygium is a triangular patch of thickened ocular conjunctiva, the apex of which encroaches on the cornea ; it is almost always seated on the exposed part of the eye. It varies much in area, thickness, and vascularity, and, though usually stationary, may be progressive. It is to be distinguished from opacity of the cornea and from the cicatricial band, symblepharon, which often forms between lid and globe after burns or wounds of the conjunctiva. It is rarely seen except in those who have spent some years in hot countries. The best treatment is, after dissecting up the growth, to double it inward upon itself, drawing its apex into the chink between sclerotic and conjunctiva by means of a deep suture, which is brought out again near the caruncle ; or to transplant the growth into a cleft in the conjunctiva below the cornea ; excision or ligature is less effectual. Adhesion of swollen conjunctiva to a marginal ulcer of cornea is the starting-point of pterygium.

Small thin cysts, sometimes elongated and beaded, with clear watery contents, are not uncommon in the ocular conjunctiva near to one of the canthi. They are formed by distention of valved lymphatic trunks.

Dermoid tumors (*solid*) of the eyeball are much scarcer than the cystic dermoids of the eyebrow. They are whitish, smooth, hemispherical, and firm. They generally lie in the palpebral fissure, and are either wholly conjunctival and movable, or partly corneal and fixed. They are solid, and hairs may grow from their surface. They may be combined with other congenital anomalies of the eye or lids. The corneal portion of such a tumor cannot always be perfectly removed.

The swelling in some cases of *episcleritis*, syphilitic or not, may be mistaken for a tumor. A few cases of innocent tumor on the edge of the cornea have been described as fibroma; it is not certain that some of these may not have been chronic gummata.

A congenital *fibro-fatty growth* sometimes occurs in the form of a yellowish, lobulated, tongue-like protrusion between the lid and the globe, and usually at the outer and upper side of the orbit.

Cystic tumors may be met with beneath the palpebral conjunctiva. The very rare form known as *Dacryops* is a bluish tumor caused by occlusion and distention of a duct of the lachrymal gland; but other cystic conjunctival tumors are met with which cannot be so explained. *Fibrous*, and even *bony, tumors* are occasionally seen in the substance of the upper lid, perhaps starting from the tarsus; in one case a tooth was removed from the lower lid by Carver (Nagel, p. 423); and soft *polypoid growths* have been met with in the sulcus between lid and globe.

Malignant tumors arise much less commonly on the front of the eye than in the choroid or retina. They may be either epithelial or sarcomatous. An injury is often stated to be the cause of the growth.

Epithelioma may begin on the ocular conjunctiva, in which case it remains movable, or at the sclero-corneal junction, when it quickly encroaches on the cornea, infiltrates its superficial layers, and becomes fixed. It may be pigmented. When such a growth is not seen until late it may perhaps be as large as a walnut, may cover or sur-

round the cornea and present a papillary or lobulated
surface.   The glands in front of the ear may be enlarged.

Sarcoma in this region may or may not be pigmented.
It generally arises at the sclero-corneal junction, and when
small the conjunctiva is traceable over the growth.   But
in advanced cases it may be impossible from the clinical
features to diagnose the nature of a tumor in this part.

Movable tumors, epithelioma, not involving the cornea,
may be cut off, but are very likely to recur; and recurrence is still more likely in the case of growths fixed to
the cornea or sclerotic.   Removal of the eyeball at an
early date, especially in the case of sarcomata, is the best
course in the majority of cases.

The lachrymal sac is occasionally the seat of new-growth,
which may be mistaken for chronic mucocele.

B. Intra-ocular Tumors.

By far the commonest forms are glioma of the retina
and sarcoma of the choroid.

Glioma of the retina is a disease of infancy or early
childhood, the patients being generally under three years
old when first brought for treatment; it may, however, be
present at birth, and is said occasionally to begin as late
as the eleventh or twelfth year.   Glioma is very soft, composed of small round cells which grow from the granule
layers of the retina, and it either grows outward, causing
detachment of the retina, or inward into the vitreous;
often several more or less separate lobules are present.   It
often fills the eyeball in a few months and then spreads by
contact to the choroid, and to the sclerotic and orbit.   It
is especially prone to travel back along the optic nerve
to the brain; and it may cause secondary deposits in the
brain and in the scalp, and more rarely in distant parts.
If the eye be removed before either the optic nerve or the

orbital tissues are infiltrated the cure is radical, but in the more numerous cases, where the patient is not seen till what may be called clinically the second stage (see below), a fatal return in the orbit or within the skull is the rule. Glioma sometimes occurs in both eyes and in several children of the same parents.

The earliest symptom is a shining whitish appearance deep in the eye, and the eye is soon noticed to be blind; as there is neither pain nor redness, advice is seldom sought at this stage. T. is n. or rather —. When the peculiar appearance has become very striking, or the eye becomes painful, the child is brought. In this (the second) stage there is generally some congestion of the scleral vessels, and a white, pink, or yellowish reflection from behind the lens (which remains clear), steaminess of the cornea, mydriasis, T. +, anterior chamber shallow and of uniform depth; there may be enlargement or prominence of the eyeball. On examination by focal light, some vessels can generally be seen on the whitish background, and white specks, indicating degeneration, are sometimes present.

In young children the above appearances are sometimes simulated by inflammatory changes in the vitreous, with detachment of the retina, the result of spontaneously arrested severe irido-choroiditis. The differential diagnosis is occasionally very difficult. In these cases of *pseudo-glioma* iritic adhesions are usually present, T. is —, the eye somewhat shrunken, the anterior chamber deep at its periphery, whilst absent or shallow at the centre. There is often the history of some illness with a definite inflammation of the eye before the change was seen in the pupil. When in doubt the eye should be excised, for there is reason to think that exceptionally a true glioma may inflame and shrivel for a time, and the nature of the case be thus obscured until too late,[1] when growth has again set in.

[1] See two cases in point by Snell and Brailey, Trans. Oph. Soc., iv. 49, *et seq.* (1884).

Sarcoma of the choroid and ciliary body is a growth of late or middle life, being rarely seen below the age of thirty-five. The majority of these tumors are pigmented, melanotic, some being quite black, others mottled or streaked. A few are free from pigment. Some are spindle-celled or mixed, others composed of round cells ; some are truly alveolar, but in many specimens there is very little connective-tissue stroma, and no very defined arrangement of the cells. These tumors are moderately firm but friable ; some are very vascular, and hemorrhages often occur into them. The tumor grows from a broad base, and usually forms a well-defined rounded prominence, pushing the retina before it ; blood or serous fluid is effused round its base, so that the retinal detachment is more extensive than the tumor. These tumors often grow slowly so long as they are wholly contained within the eye, and several years may elapse before the growth passes out of the eye and invades the orbit. Orbital infection does not usually occur till the globe is filled to distention by the growth ; but it may happen much earlier, the cells travelling out along the sheaths of the perforating bloodvessels and producing large extra-ocular growths, while the primary intra-ocular tumor is still quite small.   The lymphatic glands do not enlarge, but there is great danger of secondary growths in distant parts, especially in the liver, a risk not entirely absent even when the eye tumor is small.   Hence early removal of the globe is of the utmost importance, and a good, though not too confident, prognosis may be given when the optic nerve and tissues of the orbit show no signs of disease.

Metastatic growths.--In nearly every case malignant tumor of the choroid is primary, but it is important to know that growths may occur here secondary to those in other parts of the body ; in one case, quoted by Manz, both eyes were affected, the original growth being cancer of the breast.

SYMPTOMS AND COURSE.—If the case be seen early,
when defect of sight is the only symptom, the tumor can
often be seen and recognized by its well-defined rounded
outline, some folds of detached retina often being visible
near it; the pupil, cornea, and tension will probably be
natural. When the tumor originates in the central region
the sight is immediately affected, and the patient seeks advice very early; the differential diagnosis then lies between
localized plastic choroiditis and tumor. In tumor there is
often some detachment of the retina at or near the area of
the disease, but there is no evidence of retinitis, and no
patches of black pigment about the swelling. By ophthalmoscopic estimation the diseased area is found to be more
or less raised. An inflammatory exudation of similar size
commonly causes haze of the neighboring retina, and opacities in the vitreous; if of some weeks' duration, part of it
will usually have become absorbed, leaving exposed sclerotic with accumulations of pigment. But sooner or later
the tumor in its growth sets up symptoms of acute or subacute glaucoma, sometimes iritis; subsequently secondary
cataract forms. It is in this glaucomatous (second) stage
that relief is usually sought. Unless some part of the
tumor happens to be visible outside the sclerotic, or project
into the anterior chamber, a positive diagnosis will often
now be impossible, owing to the opacity of the media;
although by exclusion we may often arrive at great probability. If the eye be left alone, or iridectomy be performed,
glaucomatous attacks and pain will recur, and the eye will
enlarge and gradually be disorganized by the increasing
growth, which will then quickly fill the orbit and fungate.
But sometimes a deceptive period of quiet follows the glaucomatous attack; even decided shrinking and softening of
the eye may occur; but the growth will sooner or later
make a fresh start and become apparent. It is chiefly in
very old patients that this slow course is noticed. Sarcoma

14

is especially likely to form in eyes previously injured, or already shrunken from disease.

Thus it is apparent that in a majority of cases of choroidal tumor we can only guess at the truth. We suspect a tumor and urge excision in the following cases: (1) When an eye that has been for some time failing or blind from deep-seated disease becomes painful, congested, and glaucomatous, there being no glaucoma of the other eye, and particularly if there be secondary cataract. (2) Similar eyes with normal or diminished tension are best excised as possibly containing tumor. (3) In extensive detachment of retina confined to one eye, without history of injury or evidence of myopia, the patient should be warned, or the eye excised, according to circumstances.

In all cases of suspected glioma or sarcoma the eye should be opened at once, and, if a tumor be found, the cut end of the optic nerve of the excised eye should be carefully looked at; if this be pigmented or thickened, another piece should be at once removed, and the orbit searched by the finger for evidence of growth; the surface of the eye should also be carefully examined for external growths. When infection of the nerve or orbit is suspected the orbit should be cleared out and chloride of zinc paste applied.

Tumors of the iris are rare. Melanotic as well as unpigmented sarcomata are occasionally met with.[1] The definite development of melano-sarcoma of the iris has been known to be preceded for many years by an apparently innocent pigmented spot on the iris. In eyes blind and degenerated after irido-cyclitis, the uveal pigment may increase in amount, and creep round the pupillary border to the anterior surface of the iris; these areas of new pigment might be mistaken for melanotic growths. Sebaceous

[1] A well reported case, with numerous references, is given by Little, in Trans. Ophth. Soc., vol. iii., 1883.

or epithelial tumors are also seen; they are nearly always the result of transplantation of epithelium, or of a hair, into the iris through a perforating wound of the cornea. In rare cases cystic tumors with thin walls are formed between the layers, or connected with the posterior surface of the iris, particularly in eyes which have been operated on or otherwise injured.

Diffuse sarcoma of iris.—Sarcoma of the iris may be white or pigmented; it usually takes the form of a single large prominent growth. A melanotic tumor of the iris has been seen to develop from what appeared to be a natural pigment spot. I have twice seen a sarcoma of the iris take the form of a diffused thickening, with a mottled or tortoise-shell aspect; such a diffuse form is more difficult to diagnose, and probably more dangerous, if left alone, than a definite tumor.

Cases of disease of the iris are seen from time to time, the special feature of which is the presence of one or more nodular growths, usually of small size; iritis is generally present. It is often impossible to determine the nature of the growth until the case has been watched, or microscopical examination or inoculation experiments have been made. These cases, which have often been described as granuloma of the iris, are certainly sometimes tubercle, sometimes chronic gummata, sometimes part of a severe so-called serous iritis, and sometimes the nature of the growth is doubtful. Inoculation of lupous material into the anterior chamber of rabbits has repeatedly been followed by the formation of multiple nodules, similar in appearance to those in some of these cases, and some of the growths in human cases have given the microscopical reactions of true tubercle. The disease is probably tubercular when the growths are multiple, non-vascular, and gray, especially when accompanied by enlarged glands in the patient, or a family history of tubercle.

Large masses of confluent tubercle occasionally form in the choroid or other parts of the uveal tract, leading to disorganization of the eye, with mixed symptoms of intra-ocular growth and inflammation. As it is probable that this ocular tubercle may be a source of general tuberculosis, excision of the eye is the best course in any doubtful case, where it is clear that the eye is lost.

The cornea is much less liable to tubercular infiltration than the iris, but small growths have been observed in it, both as the result of inoculation, and in the course of spontaneous tubercle of the iris.

C. Tumors of the Orbit, see Chap. XIX.

CHAPTER XIX.

INJURIES, DISEASES, AND TUMORS OF THE ORBIT.

(1.) **Contusion and concussion injuries.** — *Bruising* of the eyelids from direct blows ("black eye") may usually with care be distinguished from the deeper extravasation following fracture of the walls of the orbit. In ordinary "black eye" the ecchymosis comes very quickly and remains superficial, and, if it affect either the palpebral or ocular conjunctiva, does not pass far back. The ecchymosis following fracture of the orbital plate of the frontal bone comes more gradually, is deep-seated, often entirely beneath, rather than in, the skin and conjunctiva, diminishes in density toward the front and borders of the lids, and when considerable causes proptosis. But if a fracture involve the rim of the orbit, the above characters are likely to be mixed and therefore misleading. Wasting of the adipose tissue of the orbit, and consequent sinking back of the eye, sometimes follow severe blows, with much extravasation of blood.

Fracture of the inner wall of the orbit into the nose, the sinuses opening into it, or the nasal duct, is often followed by *emphysema of the orbital cellular tissue.* This can occur only when the mucous membrane is torn. The emphysema comes on quickly from "blowing the nose," and is shown by a soft, whitish, doughy swelling of the lids, which crepitates finely under the finger; the globe is more or less protruded and its movements limited. The emphysema disappears in a few days if the lids be kept bandaged. These fractures are usually caused by blows over the inner angle of the orbit, but occasionally by blows on the malar region.

Partial ptosis is an occasional result of blows upon the upper lid. It is generally accompanied by paralysis of accommodation and dilatation of the pupil, and it seldom lasts more than a few weeks. Ocular paralysis following injury to the head (see Chap. XXI.).

(2.) **Orbital abscess** and **orbital cellulitis** may follow injuries, but are often of apparently spontaneous origin. Cellulitis may spread to the orbit from the face in erysipelas, from the throat in severe tonsillitis, or from the socket of an inflamed tooth. Diffused acute inflammation of the cellular tissue is difficult to distinguish from acute orbital abscess, since in both there are the signs of deep inflammation, with displacement of the eye, and limitation of its movements, chemosis of the conjunctiva, and brawny swelling and redness of the lids. An acute abscess soon points between the globe and some part of the rim of the orbit, but even in cellulitis the swelling may be greater at some one part, and give rise to a feeling deceptively like fluctuation.

Orbital abscess may be so chronic as to simulate a solid tumor until the pus nears the surface; even then an exploratory incision may be needed to set the question at rest. Abscess of the orbit, whether acute or chronic, is very often the result of periostitis, and a large surface of bare bone is often found with the probe.

In acute cases, as soon as fluctuation is certain, an incision is to be made with a narrow, straight knife, generally through the skin, or, if practicable, through the conjunctiva. As the pus is often curdy, it is best not to use a grooved needle. Chronic cases of doubtful nature may be watched for a time. It may be necessary to go deeply into the orbit, either with the knife, probe, or dressing-forceps, before matter is reached. A drainage-tube should be inserted if the abscess be deep. The proptosis does not always disappear when the abscess is opened, for in addition to hemorrhage caused by the operation, there may be much thickening of the tissues. Sight may be injured or lost by stretching of, or pressure on, the optic nerve, and the cornea may lose sensation, and ulcerate, from damage to the ciliary nerves behind the globe.

Thrombosis of the cavernous sinus, which may result from several causes, produces local symptoms which it is difficult, often impossible, to distinguish from those of cellulitis beginning in or limited to the orbit. The thrombosis, however, often spreads to the other cavernous sinus, and the other orbit; and in any case it produces the gravest head symptoms, which, as a rule, end fatally in a short time.[1] Cases taking this course are not ophthalmic.

The lachrymal gland is but seldom the seat of inflammation or abscess. In chronic cases the enlarged gland is distinctly felt projecting, and can generally be recognized by its well-defined and lobulated border; but the enlargement cannot always be distinguished from that caused by a morbid growth in the gland or corresponding part of the orbit. In acute inflammation there are the usual signs, local heat, tenderness, and pain, with swelling, which may obscure the boundaries of the gland. If the enlargement be great, the eyeball is displaced, and the oculo-palpebral fold of the conjunctiva in front of the gland is pushed downward, and projects more or less between the lid and the eye. When an abscess forms, it usually points to the skin, and should seldom be opened from the conjunctival surface. If it be allowed to burst spontaneously through the skin, a troublesome fistula may follow. A little abscess sometimes forms in one of the separate anterior lobules of

---

[1] An able paper on this little-known subject has been communicated o the Ophthalmological Society by Dr. Sidney Coupland (Oct. 1886).

the gland.   There is limited swelling and tenderness of the
lid at the upper outer angle, not passing back beneath the
orbital rim.   The abscess points through the conjunctiva,
above the outer end of the tarsal cartilage, and is thus distinguished from a suppurating Meibomian cyst.

(3.) **Wounds.**—Wounds of the *eyelids* need no special
treatment, beyond very careful apposition by sutures,
sometimes with a small harelip pin, so as to secure primary
and accurate union.   Lacerated wounds of the ocular conjunctiva, if extensive, need a few fine sutures, and they
seldom lead to any deformity.   When a rectus tendon has
been torn through I have never succeeded in getting the
ends to unite.

Penetrating wounds through the lids or conjunctiva,
which pass deeply into the orbit, may be much more serious than they appear at first sight, since the wounding body
may have caused fracture of the orbit, and damage to the
brain membranes, or a piece of the wounding instrument
may have been broken off and lie embedded in the roomy
cavity of the orbit, without at first exciting disturbance or
causing displacement of the eye.   Some extraordinary cases
are on record,[1] in which very large foreign bodies have
lain in the orbit for a long time undetected.   The optic
nerve is occasionally torn across without damage to the
globe.   Every wound of the eyelids or conjunctiva should,
therefore, be carefully explored with the probe, and, whenever possible, the instrument which caused the wound
should be examined.

When a foreign body is suspected or known to be firmly
embedded, and is not removable through the original
wound, it is generally best to divide the other canthus, and
prolong the incision into the conjunctiva ; in some cases an
incision through the skin over the margin of the orbit, at

[1] In Mr. Lawson's well-known treatise and elsewhere.

the situation of the foreign body, will be preferable. Single shot, corns, embedded and causing no symptoms, should not be interfered with unless they can be easily reached.

Wounds of the orbit, by gunshot or other explosives, when extensive and caused by numerous shots or fragments of sand, gravel, etc , driven into the tissues, are of course serious, particularly if the eyeball itself be injured. Such injuries may cause tetanus.

TUMORS OF THE ORBIT.

A tumor of any notable size in the orbit always causes protrusion of the eye (proptosis), with or without lateral displacement and limitation of its movement. As a rule there are no inflammatory symptoms. An exact diagnosis of the seat, attachments, and nature of an orbital tumor is, of course, often impossible before operating; and it may be further observed that there has occasionally been great difficulty in deciding whether the symptoms pointed to a tumor or to some form of chronic hypertrophy of cellular tissue or quiet gummatous inflammation.

A tumor in the orbit may originate in some of the loose orbital tissues, in the lachrymal gland, in the periosteum, upon or within the eyeball, or from the optic nerve ; or it may have encroached upon the orbit from one of the neighboring cavities. Fluctuating tumors in the orbit may be cystic or ill-defined, and may or may not pulsate. Solid tumors in the orbit may be movable, or be fixed by broad attachments to the wall of the cavity. Sight is often damaged or destroyed in the corresponding eye by compression or infiltration in the optic nerve.

(1.) **Distention of the frontal sinus** by retained mucus causes a well-marked, fixed, usually very chronic swelling, not adherent to the skin, at the upper inner angle of the orbit above the *tendo oculi*. Hard at first, it fluctuates when the bony wall has been absorbed. Its course is usually slow, but acute suppuration may supervene, and the swelling be mistaken for a lachrymal abscess. There is generally a remote history of injury. The aim of treatment is to re-establish the opening, closed probably as the result of fracture, between the floor of the sinus and the nose. The most prominent part of the swelling is freely opened; a finger is then passed up the nostril and the floor of the sinus perforated on the finger by a scissor or trocar passed from above through the incision. A seton or drainage-tube is then passed through the hole, brought out at the nostril, and must be worn for several weeks or months.

(2.) Pedunculated *ivory exostoses* sometimes grow from the walls of the same sinus or its neighborhood; beginning early in life they increase very slowly, cause absorption of their containing walls, and often in the end undergo spon-taneous necrosis and fall out. Their removal while still fixed is very difficult and dangerous, owing to the prox-imity of the dura mater.

(3.) Tumors encroaching on one or both orbits from the base of the skull, the antrum, the nasal cavity, or the tem-poral fossa, generally admit of correct diagnosis.

The suspicion of tumor on the inner or lower wall of the orbit should always lead to an examination of the palate, pharynx, and teeth, of the permeability of each nostril, of the functions of the cranial nerves, of the state of the glands behind the jaw on both sides, and to an inquiry as to epi-staxis or discharge from the nose.

(4.) **Pulsating tumors of the orbit and cases of proptosis with pulsation** are in most cases due to arterio-venous in-ter-communication in the cavernous sinus, in consequence of which the ophthalmic vein and its branches become greatly distended with partially arterialized blood. In a large proportion the symptoms follow rather gradually after

a severe injury to the head. In others they come on suddenly with pain and noises in the head, without apparent
cause, and these idiopathic cases are usually in senile persons.   In several examples of both forms a communication
has been found, *post mortem*, between the internal carotid
artery and the cavernous sinus, the result of wound from
fracture of the base of the skull in the traumatic cases,
and of rupture of an aneurism in the idiopathic ones.   The
typical symptoms are proptosis, with chemosis, pulsation of
the eyeball, paralysis of orbital nerves, a soft pulsating
tumor under the inner part of the orbital arch, and a bruit.
A bruit with proptosis and conjunctival swelling may be
present without demonstrable tumor of pulsation.   Ligature of the common carotid has been practised with good
results in a large number of cases ; subsequent excision of
the eye and evisceration of the orbit for a dangerous return
of symptoms in one or two.   An unruptured aneurism of
the internal carotid does not cause the symptoms just
described.   Aneurism of the intra-orbital arteries and
arterio-venous communications in the orbit, if they occur,
are excessively rare.   Erectile tumors, well defined and
separable, but not causing decided pulsation, are sometimes met with in the orbit, and can be dissected out.

(5.) A fluctuating tumor which does not pulsate, is not
inflamed, and not connected with the frontal sinus, may be
a chronic orbital abscess, a hydatid, or a cyst containing
bloody or other fluid and of uncertain origin.   An exploratory puncture should be made after sufficiently watching
the case, and the further treatment must be conditional.
Perfectly clear, thin fluid probably indicates a hydatid, and
in this case the swelling is likely to return after a puncture,
and the cyst will need removal through a free opening.
The echinococcus hydatid often contains daughter-cysts,
some of which escape puncture.   Suppuration may take
place around any species of hydatid.

(6.) Examination leads to the diagnosis of a *solid tumor limited to the orbit.* We must try to determine whether the growth began in the eyeball or optic nerve, or in some of the surrounding tissues. We therefore examine the globe for symptoms of intra-ocular tumor.

Solid growths independent of the eyeball may arise as follows: (*a*) From the *periosteum;* these are firmly attached by a broad base, are generally malignant, and seldom admit of successful removal. (*b*) The *lachrymal gland* may be the seat of various morbid growths, including carcinoma; a great part of the growth is in the position of the gland, and can be explored by the finger. Although such a growth is often attached firmly to the orbital wall, its position, lobulated outline, and well-defined boundary will often lead to a correct diagnosis. Tumors of the lachrymal gland should always be removed if they are increasing, for we can never feel sure that they are innocent. (*c*) Solid tumors originating in some of the softer orbital tissues, especially the form known as cylindroma, or plexiform sarcoma, occur more rarely. (*d*) Tumors of the optic nerve, usually myxomatous, occur, though rarely;[1] they generally cause neuro-retinitis and blindness, but no absolutely pathognomonic symptoms; they may sometimes be extirpated without removing the globe.

When an orbital tumor is found during operation to be adherent to bone or to infiltrate the soft parts, chloride of zinc paste (F 21) should be applied on strips of lint, either at once or the next day when oozing has ceased. If the periosteum be affected it is to be stripped off, and the paste applied to the bare bone. Hemorrhage from the depth of the orbit can always be controlled by perchloride of iron and a firm, graduated compress.

In every case of suspected primary orbital tumor the

---

[1] For references see Knapp's Archives of Ophthalmology, xii. 292.

question of syphilis must be carefully gone into; although neither periosteal nor cellular nodes are common in the orbit, both are known to occur, and disappear under proper treatment.

Nævus may occur on the eyelids and in the orbit, and implicate the conjunctiva, both of the lids and eyeball. Deep nævi may degenerate and become partly cystic. Some cases of nævus of the face are associated with nævus of the choroid; in such, the eyes are generally very defective.

Dermoid tumors (*cystic*) are not uncommon at the outer end of the eyebrow; more rarely they occur near the inner canthus. Lying deeply, beneath the orbicularis, they are not adherent to the skin, like sebaceous cysts; the subjacent bone sometimes is hollowed out. They often grow faster than the surrounding parts, and should then be extirpated, the thin cyst-wall being carefully and completely removed through an incision parallel with, and situated in, the eyebrow. They usually contain sebaceous matter and short hairs; occasionally, clear oil.

CHAPTER XX.

As stated at p. 38, § 19, when the length of the eye is normal, and the accommodation relaxed, only parallel rays are focussed on the retina, and, conversely, pencils of rays emerging from the retina are parallel on leaving the eye,

FIG. 102.

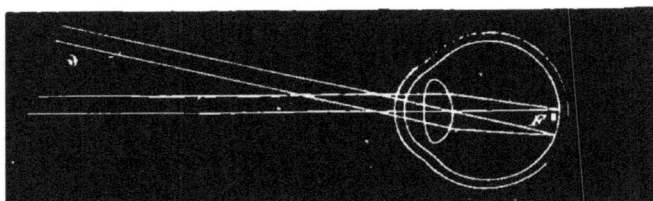

Pencils of parallel rays entering or emerging from an emmetropic eye.

Fig. 102, and this, the condition of the normal eye in distant vision, is called emmetropia (E.). All permanent departures from the condition in which, with relaxed accommodation, the retina lies at the principal focus, are known collectively as ametropia.

In E., rays from any near object, e. g., divergent rays from *Ob*, Fig. 103, are focussed behind the retina at CF, every conjugate focus being beyond the principal focus. Reaching the retina before focussing, such rays will form a blurred image, and the object *Ob* will therefore be seen dimly. But by using accommodation the convexity of the crystalline lens can be increased and its focal length shortened, so as to make the conjugate focus of *Ob* coincide

exactly with the retina (CF, Fig. 104). Under this condition the object *Ob* will be clearly seen, whilst the focus

FIG. 103.

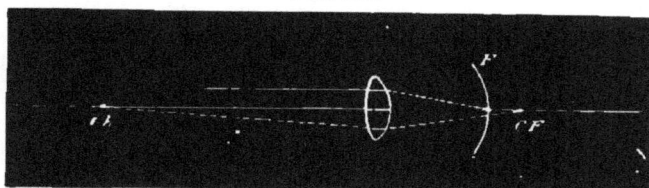

Emmetropia. Distant objects (parallel rays) focussed on retina ; near
objects (divergent rays) focussed behind retina.

of a distant object, formed in Fig. 103 on the retina,
will now lie in front of it (F, Fig. 104), and the distant

FIG. 104.

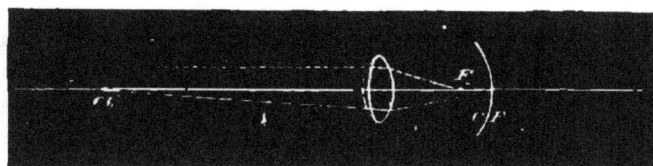

Eye during accommodation. Near objects (divergent rays) focussed
on retina ; distant objects (parallel rays) focussed in front of retina.
The dotted line in front of the lens shows its increase of convexity.

object will appear indistinct. The nearest point of distinct vision (*p*) and the farthest (*r*) have been defined at
p. 49.

MYOPIA (M.).

In Fig. 103, if the retina were at CF instead of at F, a
clear image would be formed on an object at *Ob* without
any effort of accommodation, whilst objects farther off
would be focussed in front of the retina. This state, in
which the posterior part of the eyeball is too long, so that,
with the accommodation at rest, the retina lies at the con-

jugate focus of an object at a comparatively small distance,
is called Short-sight or Myopia (M.), *Axial Myopia.*

In Fig. 105 the inner line at R is the retina, and F the
principal focus of the lens-system, *i. e.,* the position of the
retina in the normal eye. Rays emerging from R will, on
leaving the eye, be convergent, and, meeting at the conju-

FIG. 105.

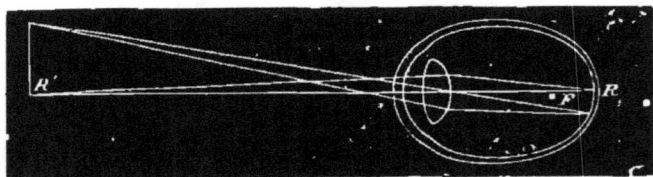

Myopia. Retina beyond principal focus, hence only near objects
(divergent rays) focussed on retina.

gate focus R′, will form a clear image in the air. Conversely, an object at R′ will form a clear image on the
retina (R). The image of every object at a greater distance than R′ will be formed more or less in front of R,
and every such object must, therefore, be seen indistinctly.
But objects nearer than R′ will be seen clearly by exerting
accommodation, just as in the normal eye, Figs. 103 and
104.

In M. the indistinctness of objects beyond the far point
(*r*) is lessened by partially closing the eyelids. This habit
is often noticed in short-sighted people who do not wear
glasses, and from it the word myopia is derived.

The distance of *r* (R′, Fig. 105) from the eye will depend
on the distance of its conjugate focus R, *i. e.,* upon the
amount of elongation of the eye. The greater the distance
of R beyond F, the less will be the distance of its conjugate
focus R′ ($=r$); in other words, the higher will be the M.,
and the more indistinct will distant objects be. If the
elongation of the eye be very slight, R nearly coinciding

with F, R′ (= r) will be at a much greater distance, and distant objects will be less indistinct. As the retinal images formed in a myopic eye are larger than normal, myopic persons can distinguish smaller objects at the same distance as those with normal eyes.

SYMPTOMS OF M.—In low degrees the patient's complaint is that he cannot see distant objects clearly; in moderate and high degrees it is rather that he can see distinctly only when things are held very close, for objects a few feet off are so indistinct that many such persons neglect them. Adults often tell us that their distant sight was good till about eight or ten years of age, that it then began to shorten, and that the defect, after increasing for several years, at length became stationary.

In high degrees of M. the patient is apt to complain of special difficulty in seeing at night, probably because—(1) the mobility of the eye being below normal, the field of fixation is diminished, and (2) the elongation of the eye by altering the position of the retina leads to some narrowing of the field of indirect vision.[1]

In many cases no other complaint is made, but in a certain number complications are present. There is often intolerance of light, an additional cause for the half-closed lids and frowning expression so often noticed. Aching of the eyes is a very common and troublesome symptom, and is especially frequent if the M. is increasing; it is often brought on, and always made worse, by over-use of the eyes, but sometimes it is very troublesome when quite at rest, and even in bed at night. One or both internal recti often act defectively, so that convergence of the optic axes for near vision becomes difficult, painful, or impossible, and various degrees of divergent strabismus result;

[1] Wecker and Landolt, Traité, T. 1, i. p. 595. Landolt, Refraction and Accommodation of the Eye, p. 425.

this occurs oftenest, but by no means only, in the higher degrees of M., where *r* is so near that binocular vision involves a strong effort of convergence. When this "muscular asthenopia," or "insufficiency of the internal recti," is slight or intermittent it causes indistinctness or "dancing" of the print, sometimes actual diplopia, beside the other discomforts mentioned ; but diplopia is seldom present when a constant divergent squint has been established.

This tendency to divergence in M. is also partly due to the natural association between relaxation of the ciliary muscles and of the internal recti—the converse of convergent squint in H.

The lower degrees of M. are sometimes accompanied by involuntary contraction of the ciliary muscle, "spasm of accommodation," by which M. is temporarily increased ; and the habitual approximation of objects which thus becomes necessary is one cause of still further elongation of the eye and increase of the structural M.

Floating specks, *muscæ volitantes*, are especially common and troublesome in myopia.

FIG. 106.

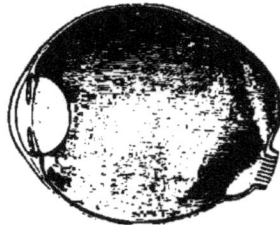

Section of a highly myopic eyeball. The retina has been removed.

OBJECTIVE SIGNS AND COMPLICATIONS.—In high degrees of M the sclerotic is enlarged in all directions, Fig. 106 ; the eye being too large often looks too prominent, and its movements are somewhat impeded. But apparent prominence of the eye may depend on many other causes.

The existence of M. is made certain by the ophthalmoscope in four different ways: (1.) By direct examination,
the image of the fundus formed in the air, Fig. 105, is
clearly visible to the observer if he be not nearer to it than
his own near point. The image is inverted and magnified,
the enlargement being greater the further it is formed from
the patient's eye, *i. e.*, the lower the M. For very low degrees this test is not easy to use, because of the great distance (3' or 4', *e. g.*) that must intervene between observer
and patient; but it is easily applied if the image be not
more than 2' in front of the patient.

(2.) By indirect examination the disc in M. appears
smaller than usual. If now the object lens be gradually
withdrawn from the patient's eye, the disc will seem to
grow larger. This appearance, which depends on a real
increase in the size of the aërial image, is less evident the
lower the M., Fig. 108, C.

(3.) By direct examination no clear view of the fundus
is obtained if the distance between the patient and observer

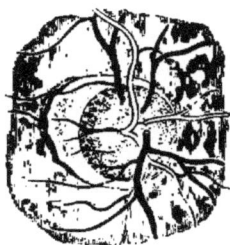

Myopic crescent or small posterior staphyloma. (Wecker and Jaeger.)

be less than that between patient and inverted aërial image,
Figs. 32 and 105, R'; and as R' is in front of the myopic
eye the image will always be invisible if the observer go
close to the patient. Hence, if on going close to the
patient the observer cannot, either by relaxing or using
his accommodation, see any details of the fundus clearly,

FIG. 108.

Description of Fig. 108. This figure exhibits the effect on the size of the inverted image caused by withdrawing the objective lens from the eye, in the indirect ophthalmoscopic examination.

A shows that in emmetropia the image remains of the same size on withdrawal of the lens. *Ob* is the retina lying at the principal focus of the dioptric media of the eye, represented by L; *l* and *l'* show the objective lens at different distances from the eye; *Im* and *Im'* the oph-thalmoscopic images formed in each case. Rays from any point on *Ob* emerge from L parallel, and are united by *l* at the point *Im* (the prin-cipal focus of *l* for the rays indicated) on the secondary axis 1, which forms with the principal axis the angle *a*. If *l* be removed to *l'* it will still intercept some of the same bundle of parallel rays, and these will be united in *Im'*, at the same distance as before, on the secondary axis 2, which forms with the principal axis the angle $b =$ the angle *a*. The relative sizes of *Im* and *Im'* depend on (1) their respective distances, *d* and *d'*, from the lens, and (2) on the size of the angles *a* and *b*. As in the present case $d = d'$ and $a = b$, *Im* must $= Im'$.

B shows the diminution of the image in hypermetropia. The letter-ing is as before, but F is the principal focus of L, and v.f. the virtual focus of the retina *Ob*. The letters *d* and *d'* are omitted, but can easily be supplied. The angle *b* is now smaller than *a*, because the rays emerge from L divergent (as if from v.f.), and hence (*d* and *d'* being nearly equal) *Im'* must be smaller than *Im*.

C shows the increase of the image in myopia : the retina, *Ob*, is now beyond F; c.f. is the "far point" of the eye, conjugate to *Ob*. The angle *b* is now larger than *a* because the rays emerge from L conver-gent (toward c.f.), and hence (*d* and *d'* still being nearly equal) *Im'* must be larger than *Im*.

------

the patient is myopic, opacities of the media being, of course, excluded. This test is applicable to all degrees of M., accommodation being completely relaxed.

(4.) By *retinoscopy* with concave mirror (p. 82), the shadow obtained on rotating the mirror moves in the direc-tion of rotation. The tests (1), (2), and (4) are, on the whole, most generally useful for beginners.

In a large proportion of cases the elongation of the eye causes atrophy of the choroid on the side of the optic disc next to the y. s., the apparent inner side in indirect exami-nation. This atrophy gives rise to a crescentic patch, Fig.

107, of yellowish-white or grayish color, whose concavity
is formed by the border of the disc, whilst its convex side
curves towards the y. s.; it is known as a "myopic crescent,"
also as a "posterior staphyloma," because it indicates a
localized bulging of the sclerotic, Fig. 106.   It varies in
size from the narrowest rim to an area several times that
of the disc, and may form a zone entirely surrounding the
disc, Fig. 109, instead of a crescent; there may also be
several spots of atrophied or thinned choroid beyond the
bounds of the crescent, and these are apt to occur in horizontal lines near the y. s.   Extensive choroidal changes
are generally assumed to be the result of choroiditis, "myopic choroiditis."   As a rule, the higher the M. the more

FIG. 109.

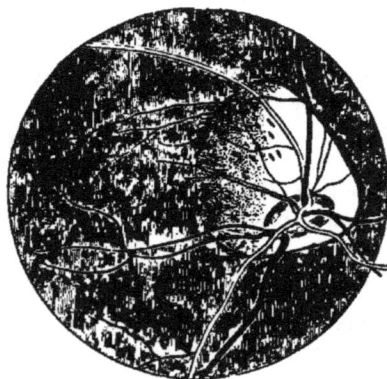

Large annular posterior staphyloma.   (Liebreich.)

extensive are the choroidal changes, but the relation is by
no means constant, and occasionally even in high degrees
we find no crescent.   Hemorrhages may occur from the
choroid in the same region, and leave some residual pigment.   Owing to the steepness of the bulging the disc is
often tilted and appears oval because seen at "three-quarter
face" instead of "full face," Fig. 109.   It is sometimes

very pale on the side next the y. s. when the staphyloma is large.

There is in M. a great liability to liquefaction of, and the formation of opacities in, the vitreous, and, still worse, to detachment of the retina. A large proportion of all retinal detachments occur in myopic eyes. A blow on the eye sometimes appears to have caused the detachment, though often not until after a considerable interval. In high degrees of M. the lens frequently becomes cataractous, the cataract generally being cortical and complicated with disease of the vitreous.

Thus we arrive at a sum total of serious difficulties and risks to which myopic persons are subject, especially when the myopia is of high degree. It is only when the degree is low (2 D. or less), and the condition stationary, that the popular idea of "short sight" being "strong sight" is at all borne out, or that the later onset of Pr. counterbalances the disadvantages of bad distant vision.

CAUSES.—M. is very rarely present at birth. The elongation of the globe which constitutes M. comes on gradually during the growing period of life, and especially between the ages of ten and twenty;[1] the eye begins to elongate during childhood. Though M. is strongly hereditary, it may also begin independently, especially from the prolonged use of the eyes for near work. The strain on the internal recti, counterbalanced, it may be, by a corresponding tension on the external recti, is believed to act by compressing the eyeball, and thus causing the unprotected posterior pole of the sclerotic to bulge. The concomitant tension of the ciliary muscle probably aids by bringing on congestion of the uveal tract (as it certainly appears to do of the disc), and thus predisposes to softening

[1] Recent examinations by Schleich and Germann upon several hundred infants show that the human eye is almost invariably hypermetropic at birth.

and yielding of the tunics; to this congestion the habit of stooping over the book or work contributes by retarding the return of blood. It is evident that if such causes are able to start the disease they must constantly tend to increase it. M. seldom increases after the age of twenty-five, unless under special circumstances; but general enfeeblement of health, as after severe illness or prolonged suckling, seriously increases the risk of its progress, even after middle life. Any condition in which during childhood better vision is gained by holding objects very close is likely to bring on M.; and so we find it disproportionately common amongst those who from childhood have suffered from corneal nebulæ, partial, especially lamellar, cataract, severe choroiditis, or a high degree of astigmatism. A bad supply, or bad management, of light, bad print, and seats or desks so proportioned as to encourage children to stoop over their lessons, are now generally believed to be largely answerable for the production of myopia. It is, however, to be noted that some of the very worst cases occur in persons who have never used their eyes for close observation of any kind.

TREATMENT.—The treatment is divisible into (1) prophylactic and (2) remediable. 1. Much may be done to prevent M., or to check its increase when it has begun, by regulating the light, books, and desks used by children, so as to remove the temptations to stooping. Children should not be allowed to read or work by flickering or dull light; and as we write and read from L. to R. it is best, whenever possible, to admit the light from the left, so that the shadow of the pen is thrown toward the right, away from the object looked at. A myopic child should not be allowed fully to indulge his bent, which is generally strong, for excessive reading. 2. By means of suitable glasses (*a*) distant objects may be seen clearly, *i. e.*, the eye be rendered emmetropic, (*b*) reading and working become possible at a

greater distance. The strain on the internal recti usually
ceases when the gaze is directed into the distance, whether
vision be distinct or not ; glasses for distant vision have,
therefore, no effect on the progress of the myopia, and are
of value only for educational purposes, that the patient may
see what is about him as clearly as other people; their use
is, therefore, to a great extent optional. But if we can
increase the distance of the natural far point (*r*) from the
eyes, we lessen the tension on the internal recti in near
vision, diminish the temptations to stooping and to reading
by bad light, and so help to check the progress of the disease; hence glasses for near work are very important in
the higher degrees of M. (3 D. and more) in early life.
When M. has been stationary for years, however, the decision even on this point may be left to the patient.

Before ordering glasses for either purpose we must
measure accurately the degree of M. In Fig. 110 let *r* be
the far point, and let it be 25 cm. in front of the patient's
eye, so that he can see nothing clearly at a greater distance
than 25 cm. (*a*) He is required to see distant objects
(objects seen under parallel rays) clearly. A concave lens
is interposed of strength sufficient to give to parallel rays a
degree of divergence, as if they came from *r*, Fig. 110. The
focal length of this lens will be the same as its distance
from *r*; and, as it is placed close to the eye, its focal
length will be very nearly the same as (a little shorter than)
the patient's far point. Therefore, if we measure the distance of *r* from the patient's eye, a lens of nearly the same
focal length will neutralize his M. He will choose a lens
rather higher than this test would lead us to expect, if the
M. be uncomplicated ;[1] whilst if, owing to complications,

---

[1] It is sometimes stated that the glass chosen for distance is rather
weaker than is indicated by the distance of *r* from the crystalline lens,
the accommodation causing an apparent increase of M. This is true
only in low degrees of M., and not always in them ; most patients

there be considerable defect of vision, he will often choose
a somewhat lower glass. Hence, it is a good rule to begin
the trial with a lens weaker than the one which, judging

FIG. 110.

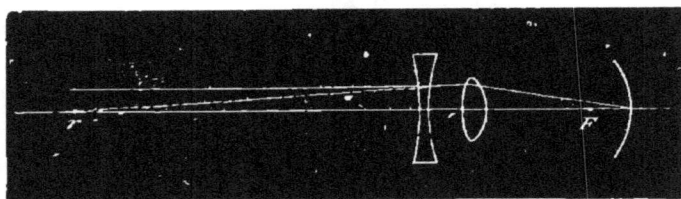

Myopia corrected by concave lens.

by the above test, we expect the patient to choose, and to
try successively stronger ones till the best result is reached.
The weakest concave glass which gives the best attainable
sight for the *distant* test types is the measure of the M.,
and this glass, *but not a stronger one,* may be safely worn
for distant vision. Beginners often test M. patients with
concave glasses for near types; neither + nor —glasses
give any information about the *refraction* when used for
near objects, since they merely either substitute, or call
into use, the *accommodation.*

(b) A glass is needed with which the patient will be able
to read or sew at a distance greater than his natural far
point. Theoretically the fully correcting glass (a) would
suit, since it gives to all rays a course which, in relation to
the myopic eye, is the same as that of the rays entering a
normal eye. But this glass can seldom safely be allowed
in the higher degrees of M. The lens which fully corrects
the myopia diminishes the size of the retinal images so
much that the patient is tempted to enlarge them again by

choose rather *stronger* lens than is indicated by *r—i. e.,* a lens whose
focus is shorter by the distance between its own central point and the
cornea.

bringing the object nearer; again, the accommodation is often defective in the higher degrees of M., and, as the fully correcting lens requires full accommodation, it will lead to over-straining if this function be weakened, and so cause discomfort, if nothing worse. For these two reasons the rule is to give, for near work, a glass which will diminish the myopia, but not fully correct it. Glasses for near work are seldom needed unless M. exceed 3 D.

Let M. be 7 D. then r will be at 14 cm. (p. 40) from the eye. If a glass be required with which the patient shall be able to read at 30 cm., or which shall remove r from 14 cm. to 30 cm., $i.\ e.$, shall leave the patient with M. 3 D., we must correct the difference between 7 D. and 3 D. (7 D.—3 D.=4 D.); a concave lens of 4 D. will make rays from 30 cm. diverge as if they came from 14 cm. But even this partial correction may diminish the images so much that, if vision be imperfect, from extensive choroidal changes, reading at the increased distance will be difficult, and the patient will prefer to bring the object nearer again at the expense of his accommodation, and will thus be inconvenienced instead of bettered; it is, therefore, often advisable, even for partial correction, to order a weaker lens than is optically correct.

Aching from preponderance of the external over the internal recti (insufficiency of the internal recti), if not cured by partially correcting glasses, is often best treated by division of the external rectus of one or both eyes. This operation may always be done when there is a marked divergent squint, even if the squint be variable. Prismatic spectacles (p. 35), the bases of the prisms being toward the nose, are very serviceable for reading in cases of slight muscular insufficiency. By deflecting the entering light toward their bases the prisms give to rays from a certain near point a direction as if they came from a greater dis-

tance, and thus lessen the need for convergence of the optic
axes. The prisms may be combined with concave lenses.

M. may also be caused by an increase of the curvature,
or of the refractive power of the media, *myopia of curvature*. Thus, in conical cornea the curvature of the central
part of the cornea is increased (*i. e.*, its focal length
shortened), and the principal focus of the lens system lies
in front of the retina, often very far in front, without any
change of place of the parts at the back of the eye. M.,
usually of low degree, often comes on in commencing senile
cataract from a shortening of the focal length of the crystalline lens, but whether this is due to increase of convexity
or of refractive index is uncertain. M. is sometimes simulated in H., and actual M. increased, by needless and uncontrollable action of the ciliary muscle.

HYPERMETROPIA (H).

H. is optically the reverse of M. It is one of the commonest conditions we have to treat. The eyeball is too
short, *axial hypermetropia*, so that when the accommodation is relaxed the retina lies within the principal focus of
the eye. As rays from an object within the principal focus of
a convex lens emerge from the lens divergent, so pencils of

FIG. 111.

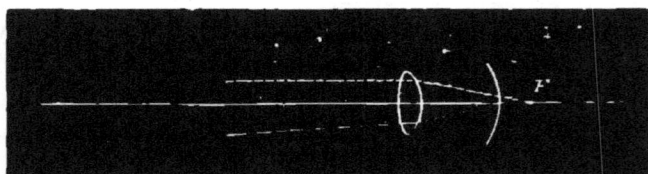

Hypermetropia. Parallel rays focussed behind retina. Rays already
convergent focussed on retina.

rays leaving a hypermetropic eye are divergent (Fig. 115);
and, conversely, only rays already convergent can be

focussed on the retina.   H. always dates from birth, and
does not afterwards increase, except slightly in old age. But
it may diminish and even give place to M. by elongation of
the eye. In Fig. 111 the curved line representing the retina
is in front of F.   Parallel rays will, after passing through
the lens, meet the retina before focussing and form a blurred
image, whilst divergent rays, meeting the retina still further
from their focus, will form an even worse image ; hence
neither distant nor near objects will be seen clearly.   But
by using accommodation the focal length can be shortened
until the focus falls upon the retina (Fig. 112), and distant

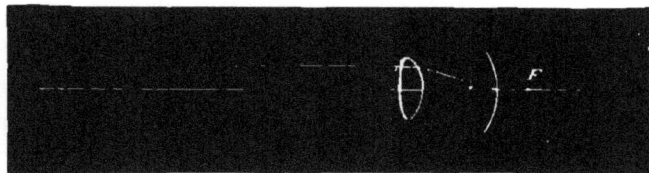

Fig. 112.

Hypermetropia corrected by accommodation.   Parallel rays focussed
on retina.

objects are then seen clearly ; and additional accommodation will give also distinct vision of near objects.   A little
consideration will show that the competence of the ciliary
muscle to give these results will depend in any given case :
(1) on the degree of advancement of the retina in front of
F, i. e., on the degree of shortening of the eye; and (2) on
the strength of Acc., i. e., on the extent to which the focal
length of the lens can be altered.

    The same result may be gained by placing a convex
lens in front of the eye, instead of using the accommodation.   In a given case, Acc. being relaxed, let the ray, Fig.
113, on leaving the eye diverge from the axis, as if it pro-
ceeded from a point v. F. 25 cm. behind the cornea.   If
the ray a', parallel with the axis, pass through a convex

lens, l, of 25 cm. focal length held close to the eye, it will be made to converge toward this same point, and, therefore,

FIG. 113.

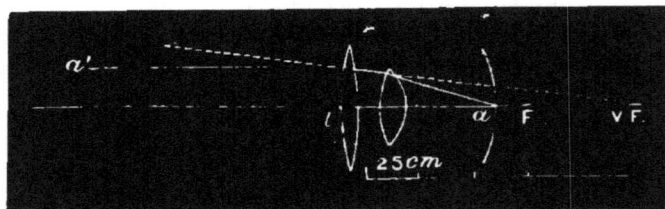

Hypermetropia corrected by a convex lens whose focus coincides with the virtual focus of the retina.

in accordance with § 12 (p. 31), will be focussed on the retina at a.

Fig. 114 may be taken for a section of a very highly hypermetropic eye, the rays emerging from which are

FIG. 114.

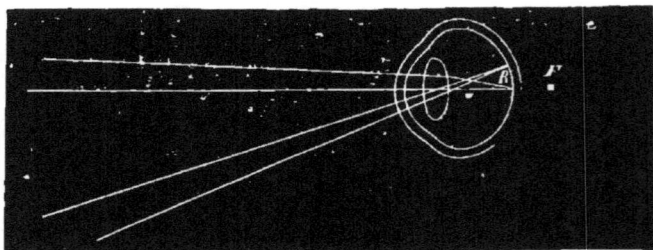

Course of the rays emerging from a hypermetropic eye.

divergent. The image formed on the retina of a hypermetropic eye is smaller than that of the same object placed at the same distance from a normal eye.

In old age the refractive power of the crystalline lens seems normally to diminish, and, therefore, an eye originally emmetropic becomes unable to focus parallel rays on the retina; this condition causes slight *acquired hyper-metropia*, and begins at the age of 65.

SYMPTOMS AND RESULTS OF H.—The *direct* symptoms are due to insufficiency of the accommodation; for distinct vision of any object, whether near or distant, requires Acc. proportionate to the degree of shortening of the eye, and the absolute power (amplitude) of Acc. is not increased in H., at any rate, not enough to meet the demand.

If H. is slight or moderate and Acc. vigorous, no inconvenience is felt either for near or distant vision. But if Acc. have been weakened by disease or ill-health, or have failed with age, the patient will complain that he can no longer see near objects clearly for long together; that the eyes ache or water, or that everything " swims" or becomes "dim" after reading or sewing for a short time, *accommodative asthenopia*. There is not usually much complaint of defect for distant objects. Many slight or moderately H. patients find no inconvenience till 25 or 30 years of age, when Acc. has naturally declined by nearly one-half.

Women are often first troubled after a long lactation, and other persons after prolonged study or deskwork, or when suffering from chronic exhausting diseases. Children often complain of watering, blinking, and headache, rather than of dimness.

In very high degrees of H., as a large part of Acc. is always needed from childhood upward for distant sight, even the strongest effort does not suffice to give clear images of near objects, which consequently such a person never sees well. Such patients often partly compensate for the dimness of near objects by bringing them still nearer, thus enlarging the visual angle and increasing the size of the retinal images. This symptom may be mistaken for M., but can be distinguished by the want of uniformity in the distance at which the patient places his book, and by his being often unable, at any distance whatever, to see the print easily or to read fluently.   In the highest degrees even distinct distant vision is not constantly maintained, the patient often being content to let his accommodation rest except when his attention is roused.

As age advances, a point is reached, even in moderate degrees of H., at which Acc. no longer suffices even for distant, and much less for near vision.   Such persons tell us that they early took to glasses for near work, but add that lately the glasses have not suited, and that they are now unable to see clearly either at long or short distances. Ophthalmoscopic examination shows no change except H., and suitable convex glasses at once raise distant vision to the normal.   Occasionally photophobia, conjunctival irritation, and redness are present in H., but the first-named symptom is less common than in M.

The most important *indirect result* of H. is *convergent strabismus.*   To understand this we must remember that there is a certain constant relation between the action of the ciliary muscles and of the internal recti,—that Acc. can be exerted only to a very limited degree without convergence of the optic axis, and that for every degree of Acc. there is, in the normal state, a constant amount of convergence.   In H. accurate near sight needs, as we have seen, an excess of Acc., thus e. g. with H. of 2 D., clear vision of an object at 50 cm. will require as much Acc. as vision at 25 cm. by a normal eye, and this Acc. cannot be exerted without converging for 25 cm., or nearly so. Such a person, therefore, has to do two things at once—to look at an object distant 50 cm., and to make his optic axes meet at 25 cm.   The former he does by directing one eye, e. g., the R., to the object 50 cm. off; the latter by converging the visual axes so that the L. meets the R. at 25 cm. instead of 50 cm.   In this case the L. eye will squint inwards, but *both* internal recti will act equally in bringing about the convergence, and both eyes will use as much Acc. as a pair of normal eyes would do at 25 cm.

This "concomitant" convergent strabismus generally comes on early in childhood, as soon as the child begins to look attentively and use Acc. vigorously in regarding near objects. In examining cases we shall be struck by finding that: (1) in some the squint is noticed only when Acc. is in full use—that it appears and disappears under observation, according as the child fixes its gaze on a near object or looks into space (*periodic squint*).

Periodic squint often occurs, chiefly when the child is nervous or tired; several patients have assured me that their occasional convergent squint scarcely ever came on except when eating.

(2) In others the squint is constant, but is more marked during strong Acc.; (3) it is constant, invariable, and of high degree; (4) in most cases the squint always affects the same eye, and this is generally accounted for by some original defect of the eye itself, such as a higher degree of H., or As., or a corneal opacity, which leads to its fellow being chosen for distinct sight; but patients who see equally well with each eye often squint with either indifferently, *alternating squint*. The squint causes diplopia, and to avoid this inconvenience patients for the most part soon learn to ignore, or "suppress," the image formed in the squinting eye, the result usually being that this eye becomes very defective. This power of suppressing the false image is learnt most easily in very early life. In alternating squint no permanent suppression occurs, and consequently both eyes remain good.

It will soon be noticed that squint is not present in every case of H. In very low degrees the necessary extra Acc. can often be used without any extra convergence. In very high degrees, on the other hand, the effort needed for distinct vision, even of distant, and *à fortiori* of near, objects,

15*

is so great that the child often sacrifices distinctness to comfort and binocular vision, using only so much Acc. as can be employed without over-convergence. The squint disappears sometimes spontaneously as the child grows up; this might be explained by an increased power of dissociating Acc. from convergence, or by a diminution of H. from elongation of the eye, or by a general tendency in all persons, and of this there is other evidence, to weakening of the internal recti with advancing age.

TREATMENT.—The treatment of H. consists in removing the necessity for overuse of Acc. by prescribing convex spectacles which, in proportion to their strength, supply the place of the increased convexity of the crystalline lens induced by Acc. In theory, the whole Acc. ought to be corrected by glasses in every case, and the eye be rendered emmetropic. But, in practice, we find it often better to give a weaker glass, at least for a time.

If Acc. in a H. eye be in abeyance, paralyzed by atropia, vision for distant objects will be distinct only if the rays pass through a convex lens, held in front of the eye, whose focus coincides with the virtual focus of the retina. The strength of this lens is the measure of the H.; thus the patient has H. 2 D. if a convex lens of 50 cm. focal length is necessary for this purpose.

But if Acc. be intact, then, as it has constantly to be used for distant sight, the patient is often unable to relax it fully, when a corresponding convex lens is placed in the front of the eye; he will relax only a part, and this part will be measured by the strongest convex lens with which he can see the distant types clearly. That part of the H. which can be detected by this test is called "manifest" (m. H.). The part remaining undetected, because corrected by the involuntary use of Acc , is latent (l. H). The sum of the m. H. and l. H. is the total H.

Now, most H. people can habitually use some Acc. for

distance (and a corresponding excess for near vision) without inconvenience, and hence the full correction of H. is by no means always needful, or even agreeable to the patient. In many cases correction of the m. H. is enough to relieve the asthenopic symptoms, at any rate for a considerable time; but we often find that after wearing these glasses for some weeks or months, the symptoms return, and a fresh trial will show a larger amount of m. H., which must then again be corrected by a corresponding increase in the strength of the glasses. This process may have to be repeated several times until after a few months the total H. becomes manifest and may be corrected. This method is most suitable for adults in whom the use of atropine to paralyze Acc., and allow the immediate estimation of the total H., is inconvenient or impossible ; or for whom the glasses which correct the total H., as estimated by the ophthalmoscope, without atropinization, are found, if ordered at once, to be inconveniently strong. But for children there is seldom any gain, and often no little inconvenience, from following this gradual plan ; with them the better way is to estimate the total H., and to order glasses slightly (about 1 D.) weaker than that amount.

To EXAMINE FOR H.—(1.) For m. H. Note the patient's vision for distant types at 6 m., then hold in front of his eyes a very weak convex lens (+ 0.5 D.), and if he sees as well, or better, with it, go to the next stronger lens, and so on until the strongest has been found which allows the best attainable distant vision ; this lens is the measure of the m. H.

(2.) For H. (total).—The easiest and most certain plan is to direct the patient to use strong atropine drops (F. 31) three times a day for at least two days, and then to test his distant vision with convex glasses. As in (1), the strongest lens which gives the best attainable sight is the measure of the H.

OPHTHALMOSCOPIC TESTS.—(3.) The image of the disc seen by the indirect method becomes smaller when the lens is withdrawn from the eye.

(4.) The retinoscopic test is described at p. 82

(5.) By direct examination an erect image is seen at whatever distance the observer be from the patient. The observer may learn to estimate H. with almost as great accuracy with a refraction ophthalmoscope as by trial lenses, and this plan, like retinoscopy, is extremely valuable with children who are too young or too backward to give good answers. The total, or nearly the total, H. may often be found in this way without atropine if the examination be made in a dark room, for then Acc. is generally quite relaxed, however persistently it may have acted when the patient was able to look attentively at objects in the light. The objective estimates (4 and 5), however, are more easily made after the use of atropine.

The next question is, whether the glasses are to be worn always, or only when Acc. is specially strained, *i. e.*, in near work. They are to be worn constantly (1) whenever we are attempting to cure a squint by their means; (2) in all cases of high H. in children, whether with or without strabismus. But patients who come under care for the first time as young adults, in whom the H. is, as a rule, of moderate or low degree, may generally be allowed to wear them only for near work. Elderly persons require two pairs—one for distance, neutralizing the m. H., the other stronger, neutralizing the presbyopia also, for near work; the use of the former may, however, be left to the patient's choice.

Treatment of Convergent Hypermetropic Squint.

(1.) If the squint be periodic, it can be cured by the constant use of spectacles which nearly correct total H.

(2.) The same is true in some cases where the squint,

though constant, varies in degree, being greater during Acc. for near than for distant objects.

(3.) If the squint be constant in amount and of some years' standing, operation is usually necessary. As the squinting eye is then usually very defective, the removal of the deformity is the chief object of the operation, binocular vision being comparatively seldom restored. Hence, in view of the tendency to spontaneous cure already mentioned, I think it better, as a rule, not to operate on children below the age of six, especially as in younger children we cannot always tell whether or not the squint be still periodic. The most rational treatment for children under four (when glasses may often be begun), is to cover the eyes alternately with a blind, for some hours daily, to insure each eye alternately used; but this plan can seldom be carried out.

When operation is decided upon, it is a safe rule to divide only one internal rectus at a sitting. At the end of a few weeks, if the squint still be considerable, the operation is performed on the other eye.[1]

Muscular asthenopia is very likely to come on some years later, if both tendons are needlessly divided. It is safer to leave slight convergence than to run this risk. (See also Divergent Strabismus.)

ASTIGMATISM (As.).

In the preceding cases (M. and H.) the refracting surfaces of the eye (the front of the cornea and the two surfaces of the lens) have been regarded as segments of spheres.

All the rays of a cone of light which issue from a

---

[1] Regulations for operating in convergent strabismus in relation to its degree have been laid down by various authors; recently by Hirschberg, Centralbl. f. A., 1886, p. 5.

round spot and pass through such a system are, neglecting "spherical aberration," equally refracted, and meet one another at a single point—the *focus* of the system.   For if such a cone of incident light be looked upon as composed of a number of different planes of rays, situated radially around the axis of the cone, the rays situated in any plane, say the vertical, will, after passing through the lens-system, meet behind it at its focus, whilst those forming any other plane, as the horizontal, will meet at the same point; and the same will be true of all the intermediate planes.

But let the curvature, and, therefore, the refractive power, of one of the media, for instance, the cornea, be greater in one meridian, say the vertical, than in the horizontal, then the vertical-plane rays will meet at their focus, whilst the horizontal-plane rays at the same distance, not having yet met, will, if received on a screen, form a horizontal line of light.   If the intermediate meridians had regularly intermediate focal lengths, they would form, at the same place, lines of intermediate lengths, and the image of the round spot of light, if caught on a screen at this distance, would form a horizontal oval.   To a retina receiving such an image, the round point of light would appear drawn out horizontally.   Such an eye is called astigmatic, because unable to see a point as such, all round points appearing drawn out more or less into lines.

A little reflection will show that in the same case, at the focal point of the horizontal-plane rays, the rays of the vertical plane will already have met and crossed, and that the image at this point will form a vertical oval.

If the screen be placed midway between these two extreme points, the image will be circular, but blurred, because the vertical-plane rays will have crossed, and begun to separate, while the horizontal ones will not yet have met, and each set will be equally distant from its focus.   The meridians of the astigmatic medium which refract most,

shortest focus, and least, longest focus, are the *principal
meridians.* The distance between their foci is the *focal
interval,* and represents the degree of astigmatism.

The astigmatism of the eye may be *regular* or *irregular.*
In *regular astigmatism,* the meridians of greatest and least
refractive power, "principal meridians," are always at
right angles to each other; and every meridian is nearly a
segment of a circle. Of the principal meridians the most
refractive, the one with shortest focal length, is, as a rule,
vertical, or nearly so, and the least refractive, therefore,
horizontal, or nearly so. The cornea is the principal seat
of this asymmetry. The crystalline lens, however, is also
astigmatic, to a less degree, and its meridians of greatest
and least curvature are usually so arranged as in some degree to neutralize those of the cornea; it thus partially
corrects the corneal error. Corneal astigmatism is often
caused by operations for cataract or iridectomy.

FIG. 115.

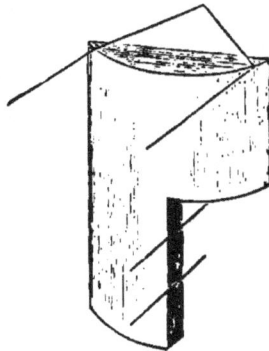

Course of rays passing through the two "principal meridians" of
a cylindrical lens.

Regular astigmatism is corrected by a lens which equal-
izes the refraction in the two principal meridians. Such a
lens, Fig. 115, must be a segment of a cylinder, instead of,

like an ordinary lens, a segment of a sphere. Rays traversing a cylindrical lens in the plane of the axis of the cylinder are not refracted, since the surfaces of lens in this direction are parallel; but rays traversing it in all other planes are refracted more or less, and most in the plane or meridian at a right angle with the axis.

Irregular astigmatism may be caused either by irregularities of the cornea, arising from ulceration, inflammation, or conicity ;[1] or by various conditions of the crystalline lens, such as differences of refraction in its various sectors, tilting or lateral dislocation of the lens, so that its axis no longer corresponds, as it should nearly do, with the centre of the cornea. Irregular astigmatism causes much distortion of the ophthalmoscopic image, especially when the object lens is moved from side to side. It is seldom much benefited by glasses.

Returning to *Regular Astigmatism*, it will be seen that the optical condition of the eye depends upon the position

Fig. 116.

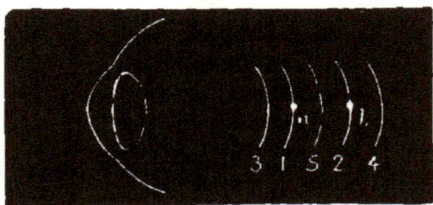

of the retina in respect to focal interval. In the above diagram, Fig. 116, let the most refractive meridian be vertical and its focus be called *a*, the least refracting meridian horizontal and its focus *b*. The astigmatism is here

[1] There can be little doubt from clinical observation with a refraction ophthalmoscope, that corneal As. is often complicated by the curvature of each meridian being naturally more or less elliptical instead of circular, and this without any tendency toward "conical cornea," as commonly understood.

represented as caused by altered *position of the retina* in
different planes instead of by altered *curvature of the cornea*
in different planes, the diagram being, of course, only intended to aid the comprehension of the principle. (1) Let
a fall on the retina, 1, Fig. 116, and *b*, therefore, behind
it. There is E. in the vertical meridian, and therefore H.
in the horizontal meridian ; this is simple H. As. (2) Let
b fall on the retina, 2, Fig. 116, and *a* in front of it. The
horizontal meridian is, therefore, E., and the vertical meridian M.; simple M. As. (3) Let *a* and *b* both lie behind
the retina, 3, Fig. 116. There is H in both meridians,
but more in the horizontal than the vertical meridian ;
compound H. As. (4) *a* and *b* are both in front of the
retina, 4, Fig. 116. There is M. in both meridians, but
more in the vertical than the horizontal : compound M. As.
(5) *a* as in front of the retina, and *b* behind it, 5, Fig. 116.
There is M. in the vertical and H. in the horizontal meridian ; mixed As.

The general symptoms of As. resemble those caused by
the simpler defects of refraction ; but attention to the patient's complaints and to the manner in which he uses his
eyes, will, in the higher degrees, often give the clue to its
presence. Low degrees, especially of simple H. As., often
give rise to no inconvenience till rather late in life. As. is
most commonly met with in connection with H., because
H. is so much commoner than M. But it is said to occur
with greater *relative* frequency in M., when, if complications be present, it may, if not of high degree, be readily
overlooked, unless specially sought for. The higher grades
of As. cause much inconvenience, no objects being seen
clearly ; and spherical glasses, though of use if the As. be
compound, are nearly useless if it be simple. As. is always
to be suspected if, with the best attainable spherical glasses,
distant vision is less improved than it ought to be, supposing, of course, that no other changes are present to

account for the defect. No definite rule can be laid down
as to the degree of defect which should raise the suspicion
of As.; indeed, in the higher degrees of even simple M.
and H, acuteness of vision is often below normal. There
seems no doubt that in young persons with vigorous accommodation the astigmatism of the cornea is often partly
corrected by the ciliary muscle acting unequally on the
different meridians of the lens; and that the seemingly
greater frequency of astigmatism in the presbyopic is due
to the impairment of this power.

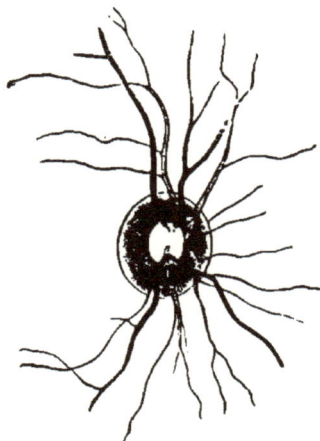

Fig. 117.

Erect image of disc in Astigmatism
with meridian of greatest refraction
nearly vertical. (Wecker and Jaeger.)

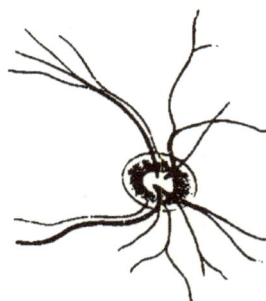

Fig. 118.

The same disc, seen by the
indirect method. (Wecker
and Jaeger.)

As. may be measured either by trial with glasses, by
retinoscopy, or by ophthalmoscopic estimation of the refraction of the retinal vessels in the two chief meridians. A
comparatively easy qualitative test is found in the apparent
shape of the disc, which, instead of being round, is more
or less oval. In the erect image the long axis of the oval
corresponds to the meridian of greatest refraction, and is,
therefore, as a rule, nearly vertical. Fig. 117.

In the inverted image, Fig. 118, the direction of the
oval is at right angles to the above, provided that the
object lens be nearer than its own focal length to the eye.
As. is suspected when, in the erect image, an undulating
retinal vessel appears clear in some parts and indistinct in
others, an appearance which may be taken for retinitis if
the examination be confined to the erect image. It may
be imitated by looking at a wavy line through a cylindrical lens.

In the indirect examination the shape of the disc changes
on withdrawing the lens from the patient's eye. It will be
remembered that in M. the image increases as the lens is
withdrawn; that in E. its size remains the same, whilst in
H. it diminishes, Fig. 108. Thus, in a case of simple M.
As. in the vertical meridian, that dimension of the disc
which is seen through the vertical meridian will enlarge
on distancing the lens; from being oval horizontally when
the lens is close to the eye, it becomes first round and then
oval vertically on withdrawing the lens. In the other
forms of As. the same holds true; the image enlarges
either absolutely, as in M. As., or relatively, as in H. As.,
in the direction of the most refracting meridian.

The subjective tests for As. are very numerous, but all
depend on the fact, that if an astigmatic eye look at a
number of lines drawn in different directions, some will be
seen more clearly than others. The form of this test is not
a matter of great consequence, provided that the lines are
clear, not too fine, and are easily visible with about half the
normal V. at from 3 m. to 6 m. The forms resembling a
clock-face with bold Roman figures at the ends of the radii
are very convenient, and I prefer the pattern recommended
by Mr. Brudenell Carter (see Appendix) to any other that
I have used. On this face are three parallel black lines
separated by equally wide white spaces, and which collec-

tively form a "hand" that can be turned round into the positions of best and worst vision.

The easiest case for estimation is one of simple H. As., in which the eye is under atropine. Many cases of simple M. As. are almost as easy to test. In a given case let the eye be E. in the vertical meridian, and H. in the horizontal. With Acc. paralyzed, rays refracted by the vertical meridian will be accurately focussed on the retina, whilst the focus of those refracted by the horizontal meridian will be behind the retina, Fig. 116, 1, and consequently form on it a blurred image. Now, the rays which strike in the plane of the vertical meridian are those which come from the borders of horizontal lines; hence the patient under consideration will see the lines at a distance of 3 m. to 6 m. quite clearly when the "hand" is horizontal, except their ends, which will be blurred. The rays which strike in the plane of the horizontal meridian are those which proceed from the sides of vertical lines, and as this meridian is hypermetropic, the lines in the "hand," when placed vertically, will be indistinct, except their ends, which will be sharply defined. We now leave the "hand" vertical, and test the refraction for the lines in this position, i. e., for the horizontal meridian, in the ordinary way, and find, e. g., that with $+ 2$ D. they are seen most clearly, though not perfectly. On substituting for the spherical glass, $+ 2$ D. cylinder with its curvature horizontal, i. e., its axis vertical, the lines of the hand and all the figures on the clock will be seen perfectly; the vertical lines and figures will be seen through the horizontal meridian, corrected by the cylinder lens, and the horizontal figures through the unaided vertical meridian, the rays which pass through the cylinder in this meridian not being refracted.

In a case of simple M. As. in the vertical meridian the lines of the "hand" will be dull or invisible when horizontal, whilst when vertical they will be clear On trial a

concave cylinder will be found, which, with its curvature
vertical, axis horizontal, makes the lines of the hand quite
clear when horizontal, and all the figures quite plain.

The cases of compound and mixed As. are less easily
dealt with by this test. It is generally best to find, in the
usual way, the spherical glass which gives the best result
for the distant types, and then, arming the eye with this
glass, to test for As., with the clock-face and cylindrical
lenses, as in the simple cases described above.

We may use, instead of a cylindrical glass, a narrow slit
in a round plate of metal, which can be placed in the direction of either of the chief meridians, the spherical glass
being then found with which, in each meridian, the patient
sees best. One chief meridian may be ascertained by finding
the direction of the slit which gives the best sight with the
spherical glass chosen in the preliminary examination, and
the other meridian by finding the glass which gives the best
result with the slit at a right angle to the former direction.

Another method, that of Javal, consists in making the
patient highly myopic for the time being, by means of a
convex lens (unless he be myopic already); then accurately
finding his far point for the least myopic meridian, and,
lastly, finding the concave cylinder which is needed to
reduce the opposite meridian to the same refraction. A
special apparatus is needed.

Ophthalmoscopic estimation and retinoscopy, however,
save much time, especially in mixed As. If As. be measured by direct ophthalmoscopic examination, we may remember that the axis of the correcting cylinder will be
parallel to the vessel used as a guide to either of the chief
meridians; and that in retinoscopy the same axis is parallel
to the *edge* of the shadow. Thus, if a vertical vessel be
clearly seen with + 2 D., the horizontal vessels being best
seen with no lens, retinoscopy will also show H. 2 D. for
the shadow moving horizontally, *i.e.*, with a vertical edge,

and the patient will choose a cylinder of + 2 D. with the axis vertical, i. e., its curvature horizontal because the horizontal meridian of his eye has H. 2 D., the vertical meridian being E.

Whatever means be employed the degree of As. is expressed by the difference between the glasses chosen for the two chief meridians; or by the cylindrical lens which, added to the chosen spherical, gives the best result for the lines or the distant types. When cylindrical glasses are ordered the whole of the astigmatism should be corrected. It is not usually necessary to correct astigmatism of less than 1 D. ; but exceptions to this rule are not uncommon, some patients deriving marked relief from the correction of lower grades.

Vision is often defective in As., and in the high degrees we are often obliged to be content with a very moderate improvement at the time of examination. This may sometimes be explained by the retina never having received clear images, i. e., never having been accurately practised ; V. in such cases often improves after proper glasses have been worn for some months. In other cases regular As. is the cause of the defect. Much also depends on the intelligence of the patient ; some persons are far more appreciative of slight changes in the power, or in the direction of the axis, of the cylinder than others, and this apart from the absolute acuteness of sight.

Unequal refraction in the two eyes (An-iso-metropia.) —It is common to find that one eye has more H., more M., or more As than its fellow ; or that one is normal, while the other is ametropic. When the difference is not more than is represented by 1.5 D., and V. is good in both, the refraction may with advantage be equalized by giving the glasses which correct each eye, and the development of divergent squint may sometimes be prevented by the increased stimulus to binocular vision thus given. But equalization is seldom possible if the difference be greater, though, especially in myopic cases, advantage is sometimes gained by partial equalization. On the other hand, some patients, probably those who do not possess binocular vision, will not permit even a partial equalization. When no attempt is made to harmonize the eyes, the spectacles ordered should suit the *less* ametropic eye. Often, when one eye is E. and the other M., each is used separately for different distances, and both remain perfect; but if one be As. or very H. it is generally defective from want of use.

Contrary to what might be expected, anisometropia is seldom, if ever, corrected by unequal action of the two ciliary muscles.

PRESBYOPIA (PR.).

Presbyopia, old sight, often called "long sight," is the result of the gradual recession of p, which takes place as life advances, and which causes curtailment of the range or amplitude of Acc. From the age of ten, or earlier, onward, p is constantly receding from the eye. When it has reached 9″ (22 cm.), *i. e.*, when clear vision is no longer possible at a shorter distance than 22 cm., Pr. is said to have begun. The standard is arbitrary, 22 cm. having been fixed by general agreement as the point beyond which p cannot be removed without some inconvenience, the point where age begins to tell on the practical efficiency of the eyes unless glasses are worn. In the normal eye this point is reached soon after forty, and the rate of diminution is so uniform that the glasses required to bring p to 22 cm. may often, if necessary, be determined merely from the patient's age. But, as there are exceptions to this rule, even for normal eyes, and as allowance has to be made for any error of refraction (H. or M.), it is unsafe in practice to rely upon age except as a general guide.

The slow failure of Acc., causing Pr., depends upon

senile changes in the lens, which render it firmer and less elastic, and therefore less responsive to the action of the ciliary muscle. There can be little doubt, however, that failure of the ciliary muscle itself, or of its motor nerves, also forms an important factor in those cases (and they are well known) where Pr. comes on earlier or more quickly than usual ; but it is a curious fact that in these cases of premature Pr. the mobility of the iris is not affected.

As Pr. depends on a natural recession of the near point, it occurs in all eyes, whether their refraction be E., M., or H. In M., however, Pr. sets in later than in a normal eye, because for the same *range* of Acc. the *region* is always nearer than in the normal eye. In H., on the contrary, Pr. is reached sooner than is normal, because for the same *range* of Acc. the *region* is always further than in the normal eye. Thus, in an E. eye a power of Acc. $= 4.5$ D. gives a *range* from $r =$ infinity to $p = 22$ cm., the focal length of 4.5 D., *i e.*, Pr. is just about to begin ; at æt. 50, Acc. $= 2.5$ D., and $p = 40$ cm. (the focal length of 2.5 D.). In a case of M. 3 D., æt. 50, the *range* being $= 2.5$ D., the *region* of Acc. lies between 33 cm. (the r for this eye) and 18 cm. ($=$ focal length of $3 + 2.5$ or 5.5 D.) ; Pr. has not yet begun. In a case of H. 3 D. with 4.5 D. of Acc., 3 D. of it are used in correcting the H., *i. e.*, in bringing r to infinity, and only 1.5 D. remains; p is therefore at 66 cm. ($=$ focal length of $4.5 - 3$, or 1.5 D.), and a $+$ lens of 3 D. is needed to bring p to 22 cm. ; there is Pr. $= 3$ D. The only cases in which Pr. cannot occur are in M. of more than 4.5 D. Thus if M. $= 7$ D., r is at 14 cm., and though, with advancing years, p will recede to 14 cm., it cannot go further, cannot reach 22 cm. ; the patient, who never could see at a greater distance than 14 cm., has simply lost the power to see at a shorter distance. Fig. 119 shows these facts in a graphic manner.

TREATMENT.—Convex spectacles are found, by the aid of the Table at p. 362, with which the patient can read at 22 cm.

In practice it is always proper to examine for H. or M., by taking the distant vision, and trying the patient for

FIG. 119.

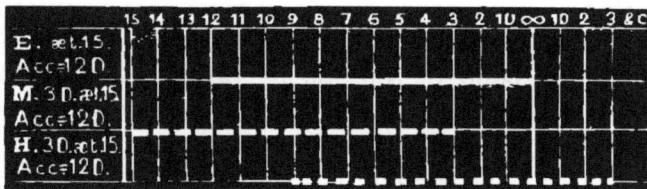

Region and range of Acc. in E., M., and H.

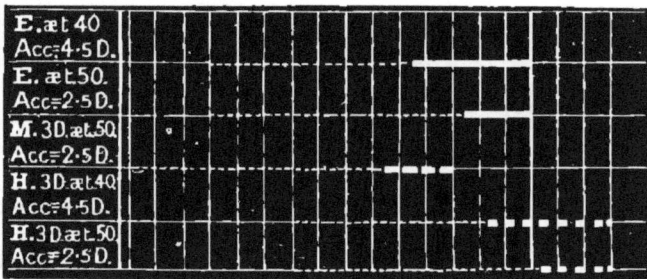

Range of Acc. diminishes with age.

The numbers along the top show the range of Acc. in Dioptres from infinity (∞) (or beyond it in H.) to 15 D. The numbers beyond ∞ represent Dioptres of Acc. necessary to correct H. Observe that the *range* of Acc. is always the same at the same age, though its *region* varies with the refraction of the eye.

m. H. and M. If m. H. be found, arm the patient with the glass which neutralizes it and makes him E., and then add the convex glass that should, by the Table, be required

16

to bring p to 22 cm. If M. be found, subtract its amount from the corresponding convex glass.

In prescribing for Pr. we must often order rather less than the full correction. For instance, if Acc. be almost entirely lost, p is practically removed to r, and the glass which will bring p to 22 cm. will also bring r to the same, or nearly the same point, and the patient will be able to see clearly only just there. Now, 22 cm. is too near for sustained vision, and such patients often prefer a glass which gives them a near point of from 30 to 40 cm. (12″ to 16″), though in choosing it they sacrifice the power of easily reading very small print. The difficulty experienced by these patients in reading with glasses which give $p = 22$ cm. depends on the unaccustomed strain thereby thrown on the internal recti; and it may be removed or lessened by adding to the convex glasses, prisms, with their bases toward the nose; or by decentering the ordinary convex lenses inward.

Presbyopia Table for Emmetropic Eyes.

Age.	Distance of p.		Pr. expressed by the lens necessary to bring p to 22 cm. or 9″.	
	Cm.	Inches.	Dioptres.	Paris inch scale.
40	22	9	0	0
45	28	11	$+1$	$+\frac{1}{38}$
50	43	17	2	$\frac{1}{18}$
55	67	27	3	$\frac{1}{12}$
60	200	72	4	$\frac{1}{9}$
65	infinity		4.5	$\frac{1}{8}$
70	acquired H. $= 1$ D.		5.5	$\frac{1}{6}\frac{1}{2}$
75	" " 1.5 D.		6	$\frac{1}{6}$
80	" " 2.5 D.		7	$\frac{1}{5}$

CHAPTER XXI.

STRABISMUS AND OCULAR PARALYSIS.

STRABISMUS exists whenever the two eyes are not, as they ought to be, directed toward the same object. The eye is "directed toward" an object when the image is formed on the most sensitive part of the retina, the yellow spot; the straight line joining the centre of this image with the centre of the object is the "visual axis." The action of the ocular muscles is normally such as to keep both visual lines always directed to the object under regard, binocular but single vision being the result. Although each eye receives its own image, only one object is perceived by the sensorium, because the images are formed on parts of the retinæ which "correspond" or are "identical" in function, *i. e.*, which are so placed that they always receive identical and simultaneous stimuli.

But if, owing to the faulty action of one or more of the muscles, one eye deviate, and the visual lines cease to be directed toward the same object, the image will no longer be formed on the y. s. in both eyes. In one of them it must fall on some other and non-identical part of the retina, and the result is that two images of the same object are seen. In Fig. 120, *y* is the y. s. in each eye, and the visual line of the R. eye (the thick-dotted line) deviates inward; hence the image of the object (*ob*) which is formed at *y* in the L. eye, will in the R. eye fall on a non-identical part to the inner side of *y*. *Ob* will be seen in its true position by the L. eye; to the R. eye, however, it will appear to be at *F. ob*, because the part of the R. retina which now

receives the image of *ob* was accustomed, when the eye was
normally directed, to receive images from objects in the
position of *F. ob;* and in consequence of this early habit

Fig. 120.

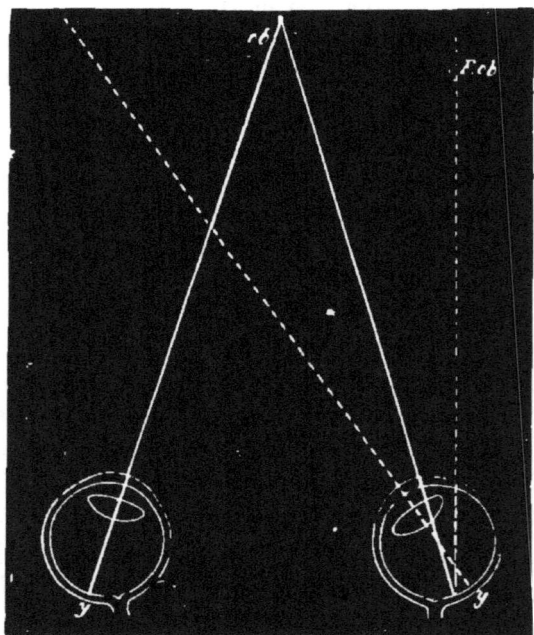

Shows the position of the double images in diplopia from convergent or crossed strabismus. The images are homonymous, or correspond in position to the eyes.

F. ob is the position to which every image formed on this
part of the retina is referred.

Hence, if the eye deviate toward its fellow, convergent
squint, as in Fig. 120, the false image will seem to the
squinting eye to be in the opposite direction; the image
(*F. ob*) for the R. eye being referred to the patient's R.,
and that for the L. eye (*ob*) to his L.; in convergent or
crossed strabismus the double images correspond in position

to the eyes, or are *homonymous.* Similar reasoning will show that if the eye deviate away from its fellow (Fig. 121, divergent squint), the position of the double images must

FIG. 121.

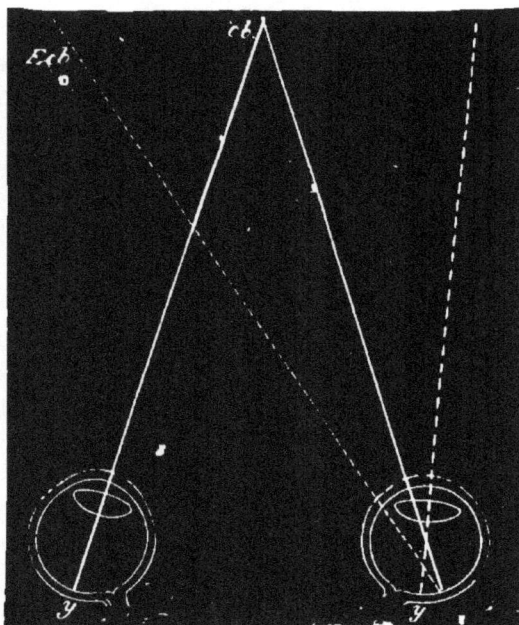

Position of double images in divergent strabismus. The images are crossed.

be reversed, and the image belonging to the R. eye appear to be to the left of the other; hence, in divergent squint, the double images are *crossed.*

Since the image of *ob* in the squinting (R.) eye is formed on a portion of the retina more or less distant from the most perfect part (the y. s.), it will not appear so clear or so bright as the image formed at the y. s. of the sound (or "working") eye; it is called the "false" image, that formed in the working eye being the "true" one. The greater the deviation of the visual line (*i. e.*, the greater the squint), the wider apart will the two images appear, and the less distinct will the "false" image be.

[The v. s. (*y*) of the squinting (R.) eye will receive an image of some different object lying in its visual line (shown by the thick-dotted line); this image, if sufficiently marked to attract attention, will be seen, and will appear to lie upon the image of *ob* seen by the "working" (L.) eye, two equally clear objects will be seen superimposed. But, as a rule, only one of these images is attended to, the perception of the other being habitually suppressed, even sooner than that of the "false image"; the suppressed image always belonging to the squinting eye.]

Squinting is not always accompanied by double vision, because—(1) if the deviation be extreme, the false image is formed on a very peripheral part of the retina, and is so dim as not to be noticed; conversely, the less the squint the more troublesome is the diplopia, when present; (2) after a time the "false image" is suppressed; or the eye may have been very defective before the squint came on.

For the method of examining for strabismus and diplopia, see pp. 57 and 60.

Strabismus may arise from any one of the following muscular conditions : (1) over-action ; (2) weakness following over-use ; (3) disuse of an eye whose sight is imperfect ; (4) stretching and weakening of a tendon after tenotomy ; (5) paralysis of one or more of the muscles.

Fuchs[1] has lately shown that considerable variations occur in the attachments of the recti and obliqui to the sclerotic. Such variations in the attachment and power of the muscles probably operate as predisposing causes of the squint in groups 1, 2, and 3.

---

[1] Fuchs, Graefe's Arch., xxx., abstracted in Ophth. Review, vol. iv. 143, 1885.

(1.) Over-action of the internal recti gives rise to the convergent squint of hypermetropia (p. 344). Occasionally convergent squint occurs in myopia. Both forms are concomitant (p. 58), but in cases of long standing the range of movement of the squinting eye is often deficient.

(2.) Strabismus from weakness is always divergent, depending upon relaxation, or absolute weakening, of the internal recti. It is commonest in M., but is not infrequent in H., and even in E. This form of squint sets in gradually, with difficulty in using the eyes for long together for reading, etc., the internal recti not being able to keep up convergence; in this stage it may often be detected by covering one eye whilst the patient looks attentively at some near object, for the covered eye will diverge when thus excluded, *latent divergent squint*, though in the interest of binocular vision convergence may be maintained for a short time when both eyes are open. Latent divergent strabismus is sometimes a temporary condition due to overuse of the eyes, or want of general vigor, in young adults. Anything which lessens the importance of binocular vision predisposes to divergent squint, *e. g.*, defective sight of one eye from anisometropia Latent divergence is extremely apt to pass gradually into manifest permanent divergent squint. In this form of strabismus the eye can be moved into the inner canthus, even in extreme cases, by making the patient look sideways, though not by efforts at convergence, and it is thus but rarely that the cases simulate paralysis. Tenotomy of the external rectus, and even "advancement" of the weakened muscle, are often needed. In slight cases the symptoms are sometimes quite cured by wearing prisms with their bases toward the nose; but, as far as I know, one can seldom predict success with any certainty from their use. One of the most troublesome features in muscular asthenopia is its great variability with the patient's state of health; the symptoms sometimes disappear entirely in a bracing climate, returning as soon as the patient comes back to his less invigorating home air.

(3.) Strabismus from disuse is also nearly always divergent, depending, as it does, on relaxation of the internal rectus. It occurs in cases where convergence is no longer of service, as when one eye is blind from opacity of the cornea, or other cause, or where the refraction of the two eyes is very different. Tenotomy of the external, with or without advancement of the internal, rectus may be performed.

(4.) Stretching and weakening of the internal rectus after division of its tendon for convergent squint may give rise to divergence simulating that caused by paralysis of the internal rectus. The caruncle in these cases, however, is generally much retracted, and this, together with the history of a former operation, will prevent any mistake in diagnosis. Such a squint can always be lessened, and often quite removed, by an operation for readjustment or advancement of the defective muscle.

(3.) **Paralytic squint.**—The deviation is caused by the unopposed action of the sound muscles. When the palsied muscle tries to act, the eye fails, in proportion to the weakness, to move in the required direction. In many cases there is only slight paresis, and the resulting deviation is too little to be objectively noticeable; but in such cases the diplopia, as mentioned already, is very troublesome, and it is for this symptom that the patient comes under care. Further, in these slight cases, the symptoms often vary with the effort made by the patient. In paralysis of the third nerve, the several branches are often affected in different degrees, and the strabismus and diplopia are then complex. When paralysis of any ocular muscle is of long standing, secondary contraction of the opponent seems sometimes to occur, and complicates the symptoms. Further difficulty in diagnosis is occasionally caused by the sound yokefellow[1] of the paralyzed muscle acting too much, in obedience to efforts made by the latter; when this happens the squint will sometimes, even when both eyes are uncovered, affect the sound instead of the paralyzed eye, *i. e.*, it will alternate.

The commonest forms of paralytic squint are due to affection, separately, of the external rectus (sixth nerve), superior oblique (fourth nerve), or of one or all of the muscles supplied by the third nerve (internal, superior, and inferior recti, inferior oblique, levator palpebræ).[2]

Paralysis of the external rectus (*sixth nerve*) causes a convergent squint, from preponderance of the internal rectus, which, except in the slightest cases, is usually very noticeable. Movement straight outward is impaired, and if the paralysis be complete the eye cannot be moved outward beyond the middle line of the palpebral fissure. There is homonymous diplopia; the two images, when in the horizontal plane, are upright and on the same level; the distance between them increases as the object is moved toward the paralyzed side, but it diminishes, or the images even coalesce, in the opposite direction. Thus in paralysis of the left external rectus, Fig. 122, uppermost figure, the images separate more as the object is moved to the patient's left, but approach one another, and finally coalesce, as it is moved over to his right. In slight cases the diplopia ceases when the patient looks at an object a few inches off, but reappears when he gazes straight forward at a distant object. In the upper part of the field the false image is sometimes lower, and in the lower part of the field higher,

---

[1] Yoked or conjugate muscles are the muscles of opposite eyes which act together in producing lateral and vertical movements; *e. g.*, the internal rectus of one eye acts with the external rectus of the other in movement of the eyes to the R. or L.

[2] In 77 cases of paralysis of a single oculo-motor nerve I found the third nerve affected in 31 cases, the fourth in 9, and the sixth in 37.

than the true one. I have many times noticed that the
pupil is larger in the affected eye than in the other, a condition which we should not expect.

In **paralysis of the superior oblique** (*fourth nerve*) there
is either no visible squint, or only a slight deviation upward
and inward. But when the eyes are directed below the
horizontal, very troublesome diplopia arises from the defective downward and outward movement, and loss of rotation
of the vertical meridian inward, to which the lesion gives
rise. In downward movements, especially downward and
toward the paralyzed side, the eye remains a little higher
than its fellow ; in trying to look straight down, inferior
rectus and superior oblique, the unopposed action of the
inferior rectus carries the cornea somewhat inward, convergent squint, and at the same time rotates the vertical
axis outward, whilst the cornea remains on a rather higher
level than its fellow ; in following an object from the horizontal middle line down-outward, it will be seen that the
vertical meridian of the cornea does not, as it should, become inclined inward.

In many cases, however, the slight defects of movement
caused by paralysis of the superior oblique are not clearly
marked, and the diagnosis has to be based on the characters
of the diplopia. In all positions below the horizontal line
the false image is below the true one, and displaced toward
the paralyzed side (homonymous); thus, if the R. muscle
be at fault, the false image will be below and to the
patient's R., Fig. 122, arrow-head figure; further, it is not
upright, but leans toward the true image. The difference
in height between the images is greatest in movements
toward the sound side ; the lateral separation is greater the
further the object is moved downward ; the leaning of the
false image is greatest in movements toward the paralyzed
side. When the patient looks on the floor, *i. e.*, projects
the images on to a horizontal surface, the false image seems

nearer to him than the true one. The images are always near enough together to cause inconvenience, and as the diplopia is confined to, or is worst in, the lower half of the field, the half most used in daily life, paralysis of the superior oblique is very annoying, especially in going up or down stairs, in looking at the floor, counting money, eating, etc.

FIG. 122.

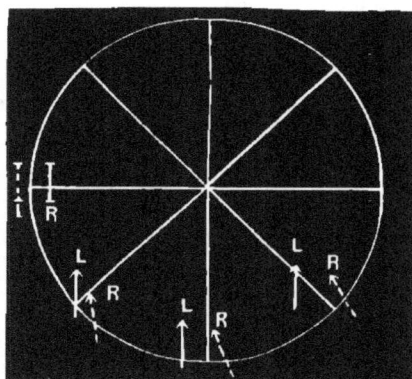

Chart showing position of double images, as seen by the patient in paralysis of L. external rectus and R. superior oblique.

Paralysis of the third nerve, when complete, causes ptosis, loss of inward, upward, and downward movements, loss of accommodation, and partial mydriasis, well-marked divergent strabismus from unopposed action of the external rectus and crossed diplopia. The downward and outward movement, with rotation of the vertical meridian inward effected by the superior oblique, remains. The mydriasis is much less than that produced by atropine. In many cases the paralysis is incomplete, affecting some branches (and muscles) more than others, and the symptoms are then less typical. Isolated paralysis of a single third-nerve muscle is rare.

Peculiarities of paralytic strabismus.—(1.) If a patient suffering, *e. g.*, from paresis of one external rectus, look at an object distant about two feet, and the sound eye be then covered by holding a card or piece of ground-glass before it, the paralyzed eye will make an attempt, more or less successful according to the degree of palsy, to look at the object. The movement effected will call for a greater effort than if the sixth nerve were healthy, and as the eye muscles always work in pairs, the same effort will be transmitted to the internal rectus of the healthy eye. The latter will, in consequence, describe a larger movement than the paralyzed eye, *i. e.*, the secondary squint will be greater than the primary. This test is sometimes of use in distinguishing which is the faulty eye in cases where the squint is slight and the patient unable to distinguish between the false and true images. (2) Giddiness is often present when the patient walks with the sound eye closed. This symptom depends on an erroneous judgment of the position of surrounding objects, which is caused by the weakened muscle not being able to achieve a movement of the eye corresponding in magnitude to the effort made. It is absent when both eyes are open, and when the paralyzed eye is covered. It often helps us more than does the former symptom in determining which is the faulty eye; but it varies much in severity in different cases, and may be quite absent. Patients with ocular palsy often keep one eye closed, *nearly always the paralyzed one*, to avoid diplopia.

Paralysis of the ocular muscles is seldom symmetrical; in the rare cases where it is so, the disease is usually intracranial In uncomplicated symmetrical "ophthalmoplegia externa," paralysis of all the external muscles, the iris and ciliary muscles escaping, the disease is usually nuclear, whilst in cases of symmetrical disease of oculo-motor nerve trunks, both external and internal muscles are paralyzed; but even in nuclear ophthalmoplegia the disease may spread forward and attack the centres for the iris and ciliary muscle, and the differential diagnosis may then be exceedingly difficult to make. In the later stages of nuclear ophthalmoplegia, other cranial nerves, especially the optic and fifth, may be involved, and symptoms of spinal or bulbar disease be present.

It is believed, as the result chiefly of experiments by Hensen and Völckers, that there are separate centres for different parts of the third (and fourth) nerve in the floor of the aqueduct of Sylvius; most anteriorly is the centre for accommodation, next that for the sphincter of the pupil, next for the internal recti (convergence), and further back those for the other ocular muscles. It has also been made out that there is a direct connection between the nucleus of the sixth nerve on one side, and part of the fibres of the third and fourth on the opposite side, an arrangement which may explain the association of the external rectus of one eye with the internal of the other in looking sideways. Mauther suggests that the limitation of nuclear ocular palsies to the external muscles in some cases, and to the internal muscles in others, may be explained by vascular supply ; the centres for accommodation and pupil being fed by the posterior communicating artery, the centres for the external muscles by the posterior cerebral.

AFFECTIONS OF THE INTERNAL MUSCLES OF THE EYEBALL.

Physiological outline.—The nerves of the iris are : *a*, The third for contraction of the pupil ; *b*, the cervical sympathetic for its dilatation ; and *c*, the fifth supplying sensory fibres. The sympathetic fibres (*b*) come from the cord probably through the anterior root of the second dorsal nerve and reach the eye —(1) through the Gasserian ganglion from the carotid plexus ; (2) through the lenticular ganglion from the cavernous plexus ; (3) it is stated that sympathetic (dilator) fibres accompany the fifth nerve directly from its origin. The ciliary muscle has not hitherto been thought to contain any nerve-fibres corresponding to the dilator nerves of the iris, but it is now thought, by Jessop, that such fibres, capable of causing complete relaxation, are present in the long ciliary nerves. The filaments of the fifth (c), form—(1) the long root of the lenticular ganglion (which gives off the short ciliary nerves) ; (2) the long ciliaries, two or three in number, independent of the ganglion. The human iris contains a circular (sphincter) unstriped muscle close to the pupil ; but there seems to be no dilator muscle, the thin layer of radiating fibrous structure with staff-shaped nuclei, which lies immediately beneath (i. e., in front of) the uveal layer, being probably only elastic.[1]

If the third nerve be divided or paralyzed, the pupil dilates moderately (never extremely) and becomes motionless to light and accommodation, and accommodation is lost. Of contraction of pupil and spasm of accommodation from irritation of the nerve, we have little clinical knowledge ; but experimental stimulation of the nerve produces those effects. Section, or paralysis of the cervical sympathetic causes some contraction of pupil and destroys its power of dilating when shaded ; stimulation of it, or of the anterior root of the second dorsal (in monkeys, Ferrier), causes well-marked dilatation, which, however, is less than that due to atropine ; irritation of the skin, stimulating the dilator nerve, causes slight, momentary dilatation.

All the drugs which act upon the iris act upon the ciliary muscle too, but the iris is affected sooner, for a longer time, and by weaker solutions, than the ciliary muscle.

Atropine[2] dilates the pupil and paralyzes the accommodation; the effect on the pupil in old people is often, and in children sometimes, lessened ; the mydriasis of atropine is greater than that due to paralysis of a third nerve, but is somewhat increased if the third nerve be cut. It acts in old-standing paralysis of iris (third nerve) and of cervical sympathetic, but in both conditions the mydriasis is apt to be rather less than full ; the

---

[1] The different views that have been held by various anatomists as to the nature of this layer (Henle's layer) show that the question is exceedingly difficult to decide on microscopical evidence alone.

[2] And all the mydriatics except cocaine.

mydriasis is said to be rather increased by stimulating the long ciliary nerves, and diminished by cutting the fifth.[1] Atropine dilates the pupil of a freshly excised (rabbit's) eye, and of the eye of an animal bled to death, and it acts a little if put on to the human eye very soon after death. From the above it is inferred that atropine acts directly upon the muscular fibres, paralyzing them, and not upon the nerve fibres. Atropine does not act upon the iris of birds (containing striped muscle).

Eserine[2] contracts the pupil and causes spasm of accommodation ; it has the same action in long-standing paralysis of iris (third nerve), and after section of the third nerve and of the sympathetic ; it has very little effect if atropine have been used, but it immediately overcomes the mydriasis of cocaine. Eserine therefore probably acts directly on the muscular fibres, stimulating them.

Cocaine dilates the pupil, but does not prevent its action to light and accommodation, and has but little action on the ciliary muscle ; hence it does not act by paralyzing either the third nerve fibres or the muscular fibres. It causes further dilatation of a pupil dilated by atropine or by section of third nerve ; whilst it does not dilate the pupil if the cervical sympathetic have been cut or paralyzed for some little time. It also causes retraction of the eyelids and contraction of the superficial blood-vessels of the eye. Hence, cocaine probably acts by stimulating the sympathetic nerve fibres. (Consult Michael Foster's *Physiology;* Ferrier, *Functions of Brain* (2d ed.), and *Proc. of Roy. Soc.*, 1883 ; Gowers, *Diseases of Nervous System*, vol. i.; Jessop, *Proc. of Roy. Soc.*, 1885–6 ; Marshall, *Lancet*, 1885, ii. 286 ; Author's own cases.)

The following forms of paralysis, or altered innervation, of iris and ciliary muscle agree tolerably with the above physiological facts:

A. **Pupil alone.**—(1) Paralysis of dilatation : Pupil in good light, equal to or smaller than the other; but when

---

[1] The relation of the fifth nerve to the iris is evidently not yet fully understood.

[2] And pilocarpine.

shaded, dilates little, if at all, so that in dull light it is much the smaller, *paralytic miosis;* accommodation not affected. This uncommon condition is, when well marked, generally one-sided, and due to paralysis of cervical sympathetic by pressure, *e. g.*, by aneurism or tumor at the root of the neck, or injury to the brachial plexus; it should therefore always lead to careful examination. A degree of miosis and non-dilatability of pupils is common in old age. (2.) The opposite state, *spasmodic mydriasis,* is very rare as a permanent symptom, though temporary, varying dilatation of one pupil is sometimes seen in young or neurotic persons. Persistent spasmodic mydriasis is said to occur in the early irritative stage of lesions which afterward produce paralytic miosis ;[1] in this state we should expect the pupil, though dilated, to act both to light and to accommodation, as after cocaine. (3.) Of paralytic mydriasis[2] paralysis of third-nerve fibres of the sphincter muscle without paralysis of accommodation, we know but little, except in a slight degree as a residue after recovery from the double condition, paralysis of the sphincter iridis and ciliary muscle, the pupil often not recovering so well, or so soon, as the accommodation ; compare the action of the drugs above given. (4.) Paralysis of iris, *iridoplegia*, without defect of accommodation, usually affects only the action to light, *reflex iridoplegia*, the associated action remaining. It occurs as a very early symptom in locomotor ataxy, and sometimes without any other symptoms of that disease, and should always lead to full investigation. It is probably due to degeneration in that part of the nucleus of the third which presides over the reflex action of the pupil.

[1] Gowers, Dis. of Nervous Sys., i. 152. I can hear very little of this symptom from physicians, and I have only once seen anything of the kind.
[2] See several cases reported by the author in Ophth. Hosp. Reports, vol. xi., iii., pp. 260-264.

B. **Paralysis of accommodation alone** (*cycloplegia*) is often seen after diphtheria. It is often incomplete, and the pupils are usually unaffected; but if the cycloplegia be complete there is sometimes mydriasis. In ataxy there is occasionally cycloplegia with a pupil active to light. Accommodation is sometimes quite lost without any alteration of pupil in what is spoken of as premature presbyopia, but this is not called cycloplegia, not being supposed to be paralytic.

C. **Ciliary muscle and iris affected.**—(1) *Cycloplegia with mydriasis;* loss of accommodation and pupil dilated to about 5 mm. and motionless; the ordinary condition in complete paralysis of third nerve. It is now and then seen without failure of any other part of the third nerve, and the pupil may then be quite widely dilated. When an old person gets paralysis of the third, the pupil is often very little dilated. (2) Total iridoplegia, with cycloplegia, *ophthalmoplegia interna;* accommodation lost; pupil motionless to reflex and associated stimuli, and of medium size; this is sometimes a later stage of (A. 4), but it may be primary; the paralysis, both of iris and ciliary muscle, is often incomplete. In paralysis of sixth nerve, the pupil of the paralyzed eye is often rather larger than that of the other.

Causes of ocular paralysis.—It is convenient to separate the external and mixed forms from those in which only the internal muscles are involved, since the local lesions are, as a rule, different in the two groups.

Paralysis of the third, fourth, or sixth nerve, may be the result of tumors or other growths in the orbit, but in such cases, as a rule, the paralysis forms only one amongst other well-marked local symptoms. In the vast majority of uncomplicated ocular palsies we are quite unable to decide, either from the state of the eye, or the orbital parts, whether the lesion be in the orbit or within the cranium. Menin-

gitis, morbid growths, and syphilitic periostitis at the base
of the skull, or involving the sphenoidal fissure, often cause
ocular palsy, seldom confined to one nerve, and aneurism
of the internal carotid in the cavernous sinus occasionally
does so. Syphilitic gumma of the nerve-trunk is probably
the commonest cause of single paralysis; the intracranial
portion of the nerves is known to be often the seat of such
growths, but small neural gummata probably occur also
on the orbital part of the nerves. Injuries to the head
often cause ocular paralysis; the paralysis is usually noticed
very soon after the accident, and is probably always a sign
of fracture of the base involving the middle fossa, or of
some part of the walls of the orbit. Direct damage to, or
thickening subsequent to fracture near the pulley, seems to
account for some cases of traumatic paralysis of the superior
oblique. Pain in the temple or front of the head is very
common in ocular palsies due to periostitis and gummata.
In certain cases neither the symptoms nor history enable
us to locate the seat or prove the cause of the paralysis; the
term "rheumatic" is often applied to such cases, on the
assumption that the palsy is peripheral and caused by cold,
that it is, in fact, to be compared to peripheral paralysis of
the facial nerve; no doubt some of these are in reality
syphilitic. Paralysis, usually of short duration and affecting only one nerve, is not uncommon at any early stage of
locomotor ataxy. Ophthalmoplegia externa generally sets
in slowly, is bilaterally symmetrical and permanent; it
usually indicates sclerotic disease of the nerve centres,
often caused by syphilis; but it is sometimes caused by
tumor centrally placed, or by symmetrical gummata on
nerve-trunks. Occasionally ocular palsies are "functional," or occur in company with symptoms apparently
of hysterical nature, and pass off. Paralysis of oculo-
motor muscles is in rare cases congenital, and occurring
in several members of the same family. These cases are

perhaps of the same nature as those of congenital ptosis, absence or imperfect development of muscles. Occasionally paralysis of oculo-motor nerves from birth has been attributed to instrumental labor.

In respect to the causation of the purely internal paralyses we have but little positive knowledge Mydriasis with cycloplegia and no other paralysis, would be accounted for by disease of the short (third-nerve) root of the lenticular ganglion. Iridoplegia and ophthalmoplegia interna are probably the result of chronic, very strictly localized, disease of the centres for the pupil and accommodation (Gowers), which have been shown to form separate parts of the nucleus of the third nerve. Complete ophthalmoplegia interna would also be expected if the lenticular ganglion (Hutchinson), or the intra-ocular ganglionic cells of the choroid (Hulke), were disorganized; but such changes have not yet been proved *post mortem*. Paralysis from blows on the eye is referred to at p. 180. (See also Diphtheria, Chap. XXIII.)

TREATMENT OF OCULAR PARALYSES.—In estimating the results of treatment it is well to remember that some cases recover spontaneously, that in many the defect is a paresis rather than paralysis, and that in the latter cases the symptoms often vary in severity from day to day, or even whilst under observation at a single visit, according to the attention given and effort made by the patient. The questions of syphilis and of injury to the head must always be carefully inquired into, especially when only one nerve is paralyzed. When several nerves are involved, tumor, aneurism, or syphilis, either gummatous inflammation at the base, or sclerotic nuclear disease, is to be suspected. Iodide of potassium and mercury are the only internal remedies likely to be beneficial, and unless syphilis be quite out of the question they should have a full trial; many cases recover quickly under moderate doses of iodide.

Faradization of the paralyzed muscles is sometimes used. Operation for paralytic squint of old standing may sometimes be undertaken.[1]

Nystagmus (involuntary oscillating movement of the eyes) is generally associated with serious defect of sight dating-from very early life, such as opacity of the cornea after ophthalmia neonatorum, congenital cataract, choroido-retinitis, or disease of the optic nerve. It is, however, also seen in cases of infantile amblyopia without apparent cause, and constantly in albinoes. Nystagmus is often developed during adult life in coal-miners; it has been attributed to the insufficiency of light furnished by the safety lamps, and with more probability to the necessity which the miner is under of constantly looking in an unnatural direction, upward or sideways, for example. It is often present only when the collier takes up his mining posture. Nystagmus also occurs as a symptom in some cases of disseminated sclerosis, and in other forms of central nervous disease.

Usually both eyes oscillate, but when only one eye is defective, it alone may oscillate. The movements in nystagmus, whatever the cause of the condition, vary much in rapidity, amplitude and direction in different cases, and even in the same case at different times; they are generally worse when the patient is nervous, and often there is a particular position of the eyes in which the oscillation is least. Nystagmus often becomes much less marked as life advances. Treatment is useless.

[1] Rules for operations for paralytic squint have been laid down by Alfred Graefe, Arch. f. Oph., xxxiii. 3, 179.

CHAPTER XXII.

OPERATIONS.

A. Operations on the Eyelids.

1. **Epilation of eyelashes.**—Position: Patient seated; surgeon standing behind. The forceps to be broadened, with smooth, or very finely roughened, blades which meet accurately in their whole width. Stretch the lid tightly by a finger placed over each end. Pull out the lashes at first quickly in bundles, and finish by carefully picking out the separate ones that are left.

2. **Eversion of upper lid.**—Position as for 1, or the surgeon may stand in front. The patient looks down, a probe is laid along the lid above the upper edge of the "cartilage;" the lashes, or the edge of the lid, are then seized by a finger and thumb of the other hand, and turned up over the probe, which is simultaneously pushed down. After a little practice the probe can be dispensed with, and the lid everted by the forefinger and thumb of one hand alone, one serving to fix and depress the lid, the other to turn it upward.

Fig. 123.

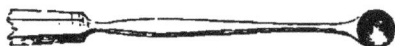

Meibomian scoop.

3. **Removal of Meibomian cyst.**—Position as for 1. Instruments: A small scalpel or Beer's knife, Fig. 159, and a curette, or small scoop; Figs. 123 and 155. (1) Evert the

lid ; (2) make a free crucial incision into the tumor from
the conjunctival surface ; (3) remove the growth, either
by squeezing the lid between finger- and thumb-nail, or by
means of the scoop. The cavity fills with blood, and may
thus for a few days be larger than before. These tumors
have no distinct cyst-wall.

4. **Inspection of cornea** in purulent ophthalmia, etc.
Position : If the patient be a baby or child, the back of its
head is to be held between the surgeon's knees, its body
and legs being on the nurse's lap ; if an adult, the same as
for 1. If the lids cannot be easily separated by a finger
of each hand, enough to allow a view of the cornea, re-
tractors should be used—a convenient pattern is shown in
Fig. 124—by which one lid, or both, can be raised and held

FIG. 124.

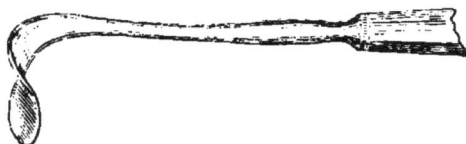

Desmarres' lid elevator.

away from the globe. If this instrument be gently used
we avoid all risk of causing perforation of the cornea
should a deep ulcer be present ; an accident which may
happen in cases attended by much swelling or spasm of the
lids if the fingers be used.

5. **Entropion.**—*Spasmodic entropion of the lower lid*,
with relaxed skin, in old people. Position as for 1. Instruments: T-forceps, Fig. 125, scissors, Fig. 140, toothed
forceps. With the T-forceps pinch up a fold of skin as close
as possible to the edge of the lid, and of width proportionate to the degree of inversion, and cut it off close to the
forceps ; now pinch up and cut out a portion of the exposed
orbicularis muscle ; sutures need not be used. Another

good plan is to enter a threaded needle close to the edge of the lid, bring it out half an inch vertically below, tie the intervening skin and muscle tightly and allow the thread to cut its way out; two or three such stitches will be

FIG. 125.

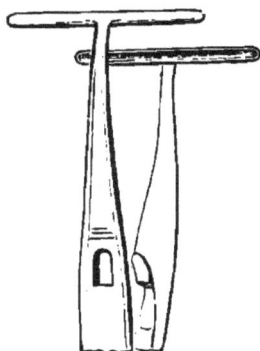

Entropion forceps.

wanted at equal distances apart; the resulting scars being vertical are rather conspicuous.

6. **Organic entropion and trichiasis.**—When the whole row of lashes is turned inward, and the inner surface of the lid much shortened by scarring, the radical extirpation of all the lashes is the quickest and most certain means of giving permanent relief, but it leaves an unsightly baldness and exposes the cornea to unnatural risk from dust, etc. Position: Recumbent; the surgeon stands behind the patient. Anæsthesia seldom necessary. Instruments: A horn or bone lid-spatula, Fig. 127, s, or a lid clamp, Fig. 126, a Beer's knife, Fig. 159, and forceps. Make an incision from end to end, beginning just outside the punctum, between the hair-follicles and Meibomian ducts, as if to split the lid into two layers. Make a second incision through the skin and tissues, about a twelfth of an inch above the border

of the lid, parallel with, but in a plane at right angles to, the first. The strip of skin and tissues included between these two cuts will now be almost free, except at its ends, which are to be united by a cross-cut, and the strip dissected off; it should include the hair-follicles in their whole

FIG. 126.

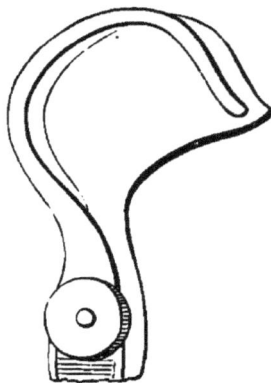

Snellen's lid clamp (for the R. upper lid).

depth. Examine the white edge of the "cartilage," now exposed, for any hair-follicles accidentally left behind; they will appear as black dots, and are to be carefully removed.

In the same or slighter cases, the inversion of the border of the lid may be much lessened by complete division of the "cartilage" from the conjunctival surface along a line parallel with, and 3 mm. from the free border (Burow's operation), Fig. 128, Bu. The wound gapes and the inverted border of the lid falls forward and is kept in its natural place by the cornea. The only instruments needed are a scalpel and scissors. Position as for 1, or recumbent. The lid is kept well everted while the incision is being made. A puncture is made with the knife parallel to the edge of the lid, close to the inner or outer end, one blade of the scissors passed through this puncture and made to run along the outer surface of the "cartilage" between it and the orbicularis muscle, and then the "cartilage" divided by closing the blades parallel to the border. The wound should be at right angles to the surface. A bluish

FIG. 127.

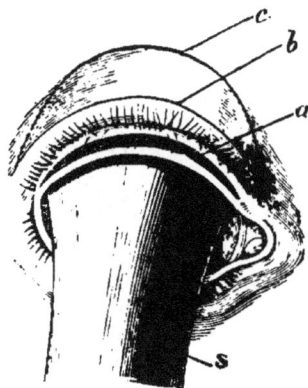

Arlt's operation for trichiasis. (After Schweigger.)

line should be seen through the skin on replacing the lid. This operation gives complete relief for the time, but may need repetition in a few months.

Various operations are performed for transplantation of the displaced lashes forward and upward, so as to restore their natural direction. *Arlt's operation:* The free border of the lid is split from end to end, leaving the punctum as for extirpation of the lashes, but more deeply, Fig. 127, *a*. A second incision (*b*), extending beyond the ends of the first, is now made through the skin parallel to, and about two lines from, the border of the lid, and down to, but not through the "cartilage;" thirdly, a curved incision (*c*) is made, joining *b* at each end and including a semilunar flap of skin, of greater or less width according to the effect

17

desired ; fourthly, this flap is dissected off without injury to the orbicularis, and the wound, bounded by the lines *b* and *c*, closed by sutures. The anterior layer of the lid border, which contains the lashes, is thus tilted forward and drawn upward.

FIG. 128.

FIG. 129.

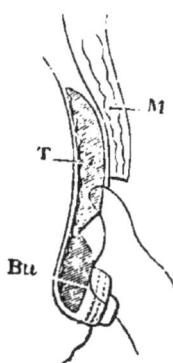

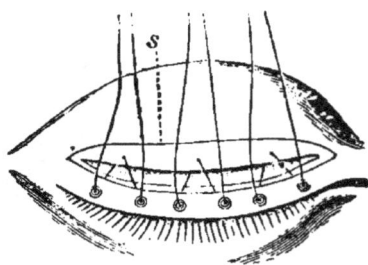

Snellen's operation for trichiasis. (After Wecker.) *s.* Edge of retracted skin and muscle.

Diagrammatic section of upper lid; showing Snellen's operation, and line of section in Burow's operation (Bu). (Altered from Wecker.)

A third operation (Streatfeild's) consists in the simple removal of a wedge-shaped strip of the "cartilage," with its superjacent skin and muscle, from the whole length of the lid, at a distance of a line or two from its border, *b*, Fig. 127. No sutures are used.

Snellen operates as follows: The incision, *b*, Fig. 127, is carried down to the tarsus, the muscle and skin separated from it and pushed upward, and a wedge, shown by the groove in Fig. 128, cut from the exposed tarsus, as in Streatfeild's operation. The border of the lid is now everted, and kept in its new position by passing two or three threads, as shown in Figs. 128 and 129, and tying them over beads. The skin wound need not be sutured.

All these operations (except 1) are apt to need repetition sooner or later.

The above operations are most suitable when the whole length of the upper lid is affected ; in most hands Arlt's proceeding probably gives better average results than any other.   In cases of partial trichiasis, where only a part of the border is affected, these operations sometimes only transfer the seat of the affection, by causing displacement of the adjacent healthy lashes.   In such cases, transplantation of a strip of mucous membrane from the patient's lip, into the gap made by splitting the diseased part of the lid, Fig. 130, is the best operation.   This may be done as follows (van Millingen) : (1) Split the affected part of the

FIG. 130.

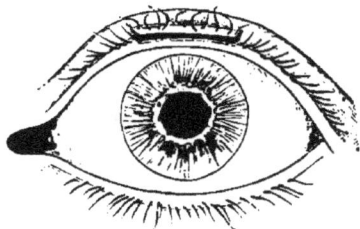

Van Millingen's operation.—1st stage ; the portion of lid containing misdirected lashes split parallel to its surfaces, leaving the lashes in the anterior layer.   The incision at each end is carried a short distance into the skin at a right angle with the split.

lid as in Arlt's operation, but turn the cut forward, into the skin a little at each end, as in Fig. 130.   (2) Separate a strip of mucous membrane from the lower lip, parallel to its length, leaving its ends attached ; the strip should be longer and wider than the gap it is to fill.   (3) Take two needles, each with a long thread attached, and pass one through each end of the lid incision from the skin surface into the angle of the wound, draw the needles through,

carry them down to the lip, and pass each one through the
corresponding end of the bridge of mucous membrane from
the deep to the free surface.   (4) Cut the attached ends of
the bridge, turn the strip over on the thumb-nail, and clean
its under surface with scissors, taking care not to cut the
thread at each end.   (5) Draw the strip up into its new
position by pulling on the upper ends of the threads, and
tie the threads.   A very fine stitch may be inserted at the
centre of the flap, if thought necessary, but this can be
dispensed with.   The split in the lid should be cleaned
from clot before the strip is brought into position.   The
strip usually lives and adheres well under an antiseptic
dressing ; the stitches may be left to come out.

   · 7. **Ectropion.**— Ectropion from thickening of the conjunctiva, aided by relaxation of the tissues of the lower
lid, seen chiefly in old people, may be treated by the removal of a V-shaped piece of the whole thickness of the lid,
the edges being brought together with a harelip-pin ; or
the everted mucous membrane may be drawn back into the
sulcus between lid and globe by a suture, entered into the
conjunctiva at two points $\frac{1}{3}$ inch apart, passed deeply,
brought out on the cheek, and tied over a bit of India-
rubber tube ; the thread is tightened from day to day until
it has nearly cut through (Snellen).   An operation of
which the principle is nearly the same, but the execution
more complicated, is described by Argyll Robertson.[1]
Slighter cases may be satisfactorily treated by the excision,
or destruction by burning deeply with a fine galvanic cautery, of a strip of the palpebral conjunctiva parallel to the
border of the lid ; the contraction of the scar draws the
margin of the lid into place.

   For ectropion from cicatricial changes in the skin a
plastic operation is generally needed.   At the same time

---

[1] A. Robertson, Edin. Clin. and Path. Journ., Dec. 1883.

the eyelids should be united by fine sutures, after paring a
narrow strip from the border of each lid just within the
line of the lashes (blepharoplasty), a proceeding which at
once assists the restitution of the displaced lid, and gives
protection to the cornea ; the lids may be separated a few
weeks later.   The operation for the cure of the ectropion
will naturally vary with the seat, extent, and cause of the
deformity, but we may conveniently distinguish three varieties of organic ectropion, according as the condition has
followed—(1) a wound of the eyelid with faulty union ;
(2) a deeply adherent scar from abscess, disease of bone, or
deep ulceration of the lid ; or (3) extensive scarring of the
face from burns, lupus, etc.   When the cause is quite
localized, and there is not much loss of tissue (groups 1 and
2), the scar may be included in a V-shaped incision, the
flap separated and pushed up till the lid is in position, and
the lower part of the wound then brought together by a pin
or sutures, so that what was a v now becomes a y, the
edges of the flap being attacked by sutures to the limbs of
the y, Fig. 131.   As the lid has generally become too long,

FIG. 131.

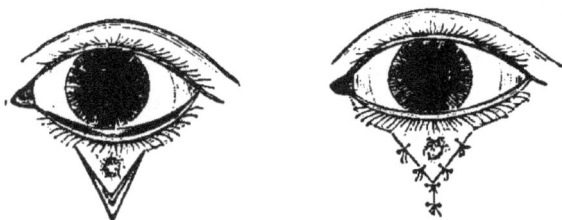

V Y operation.   (From Ritterich.)

from prolonged eversion, we have often, at the same time,
to shorten it by removing a small triangle from its outer
end, and uniting the edges of the gap.   When the position
of the deformity prevents the above operation it is necessary
to introduce new skin into the gap, made by dissecting out

the cicatricial tissue and putting the everted lid into position. This may be done by bringing a flap with a broad
pedicle, either by sliding or twisting, into the gap; or by
the method (introduced into our country by Dr. Wolfe) of
transplanting from a distant part a single graft of skin without a pedicle, large enough to fill the gap; or, again, by fill-
ing the gap with several small pieces of skin (dermic grafts).
Where there is extensive destruction of skin (group 3)
these grafting methods seem particularly valuable. If a
single large graft be used the important points are to make
it considerably larger than the deficiency it is to supply, to
free the under surface of the graft very thoroughly of all
subcutaneous tissue, to unite it by numerous fine sutures,
and to apply warm dressings. The single-graft operation
has now been tried many times, and with a good proportion
of successes.

8. Paralytic and congenital **ptosis** have often been treated
by the removal of an oval of skin from the upper lid,
parallel to its length, the orbicularis muscle not being
touched. This simple method, however, has but little
effect, unless the piece removed be so large as to shorten
the lid materially, and thus endanger the power of complete closure. More complicated operations, intended to
raise the lid by producing contraction of the subcutaneous
tissues, or adhesion between these parts and the tendon of
the occipito-frontalis at the eyebrow without the removal
of any skin, have been recommended by Pagenstecher,
Dransart, Meyer, and Panas. I have had, and have seen
in the hands of others, satisfactory results from Panas'
operation in several cases.

9. **Canthoplasty**, for lengthening the palpebral fissure at
the outer canthus. The canthus is divided by scissors or a
knife as far as may seem necessary. The contiguous ocular
conjunctiva is then slightly dissected up and attached by
sutures to the cut edges of the skin, so as to prevent re-

union, one suture being placed in the angle of the wound, one above and one below, Fig. 132.

FIG. 132.

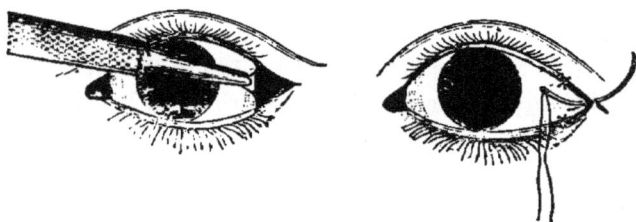

Canthoplasty. (From Ritterich.)

10. **Peritomy** for obstinate cases of partial pannus. Anæsthesia is necessary. Instruments: Speculum, Fig. 139, fixation forceps, Fig. 141, scissors, and Beer's knife, Fig. 159. With the knife a circular incision is carried through the conjunctiva, round the cornea, at 5 mm. ($\frac{1}{5}''$), or less, from its border. The zone of conjunctiva so included, together with the whole of its subconjunctival tissue down to the sclerotic, is now carefully removed by the scissors. The bare surface thus left granulates, and finally contracts to a narrow band of white scar-tissue, by which the vessels running to the cornea should be obliterated. The subconjunctival fascia is often found much thickened in these cases. Care must be taken not to make the incision too far from the cornea, lest the insertions of the recti be damaged. The strip removed should extend completely round the cornea; removal of only a part of the zone is not satisfactory. The symptoms are generally made worse for a time, and the final result is not reached for several months. In some cases the operation has, in my experience, been very successful, whilst in others, without apparent reason, it has quite failed of its purpose.

Symblepharon, adhesion of lid to globe after destruction of conjunctiva, unless very extensive, can be greatly improved by operation. In slight cases we have merely to separate the adhesion from the globe and bring together the edges of the ocular conjunctiva to cover the surface thus exposed and thus prevent reunion. But when the surface exposed by the dissection is large, flaps of conjunctiva with broad pedicles must be brought down to cover the deficiency in the manner first proposed by Mr. Teale;[1] or mucous membrane may be transferred from the lip of the patient or even from the conjunctiva of a rabbit. Snellen has lately used a flap of neighboring skin with a pedicle, pushing it through a sort of buttonhole in the lid and attaching it in the gap made by separating the adhesions.

B. OPERATIONS ON THE LACHRYMAL APPARATUS.

1. **Lachrymal abscess.** (See p. 101.)
2. **Slitting up the lower canaliculus.**—This is best done by means of a knife with a blunt or probe point, and a blade narrow enough to enter the punctum. The best forms of these knives are Weber's knife, with a probe end, Fig. 134; Bowman's, with nearly parallel borders and a rounded end, Fig. 135, and Liebreich's, Fig. 136. Position as for 1. (1) The lower lid is drawn tightly outward and downward by the thumb. (2) The canaliculus knife is passed *vertically* into the punctum, then turned horizontally and passed on through the neck of the canaliculus till it reaches the bony (inner) wall of the lachrymal sac. It is then raised up from heel toward point, and thus made to divide the canaliculus, care being taken that the neck is freely divided. Liebreich's knife cuts its own way without being raised. The lower canaliculus may also be divided with a Beer's knife, Fig. 159, which is run along a

---

[1] Teale, Ophth. Hosp. Reports, iii. p. 253, 1861.

fine grooved director, Fig. 133, previously introduced. In cases of mucocele, it is good practice to divide the wall of the sac freely, and some surgeons open the upper as well as the lower canaliculus. The canaliculus requires to be kept open every three or four days till its cut edges are healed, or they will unite again.

3. **Probing the nasal duct.**—After dividing the canaliculus pass a good-sized lachrymal probe

FIG. 134.

Weber's canaliculus knife.

FIG. 135.

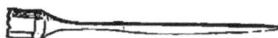

Bowman's canaliculus knife.

FIG. 136.

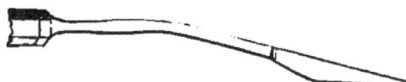

Liebreich's knife for canaliculus and nasal duct.

horizontally along its floor till it strikes the inner, bony, wall of the sac. Then raise it to the vertical position and push it steadily down the duct (downward and a very little outward and backward) till the floor of the nose is reached. Bowman's earlier probes were in six sizes, of which the largest was $\frac{1}{20}$ inch in diameter. Bowman afterward adopted much larger probes with bulbous ends, and several such patterns are now in use. The probe used should be the largest that will pass easily.

4. **A stricture of the duct** may be incised with any of the canaliculus knives, although Weber's and Bowman's are

too slender to be used with safety. Liebreich's is intended to be so used, and a special knife for the purpose had previously been introduced by Stilling. The knife is used as a probe, being pushed quite down the duct, then partly withdrawn, turned in another direction, and pushed down again. There is generally bleeding from the nose.

In all these procedures we must be certain that the probe or knife rests against the bony (nasal) wall of the lachrymal sac before it is raised into the vertical direction. If the probe be stopped at the entrance of the canaliculus into the sac, as may easily happen if the canal be not thoroughly slit in its whole length, the lid will be pulled upon and puckered whenever the instrument is pushed toward the nose; but if the probe have reached the sac, backward and forward movements will not usually cause puckering of the lid. If in the former case the instrument be turned up and an attempt made to pass it down the duct, a false passage will probably be made.

The direction of the two nasal ducts is either parallel or such that if prolonged upward they would converge slightly; they very seldom diverge. The probe when in the duct should, even if, as usual, its lower end be curved forward, rest against and indent the eyebrow; if it stand forward from the brow it is usually in a false passage.

Lachrymal syringes are of two kinds: (1) Anel's syringe with a nozzle fine enough to pass into the unopened punctum, Fig. 137. By injecting a little water into the duct through the canaliculus we can sometimes clear out slight, apparently mucous, obstruction and relieve epiphora without cutting or probing; and by the same method we can often decide whether or not there is an obstruction needing the severer treatment. (2) Hollow probes attached to syringes of various patterns are used for passing down the duct and syringing at the same time. Fig. 138 shows a simple form sold as Bowman's.

Fig. 137.   Fig. 138.

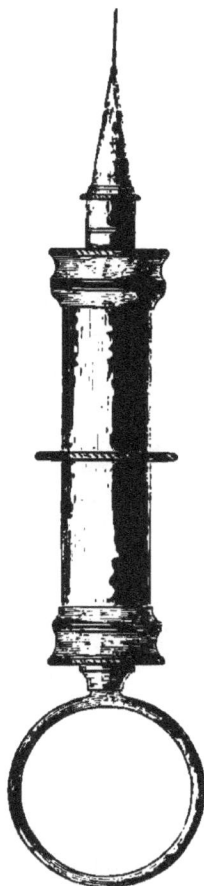

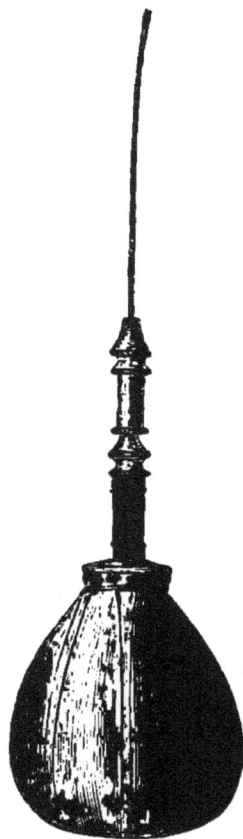

Anel's syringe, full size.   Bowman's syringe, about half
                               full size.

C. Operations for Strabismus.

Tenotomy.—The object is to divide the tendon close to its insertion into the sclerotic.   In this country Critchett's subconjunctival operation is commonly used; abroad the operation of Von Graefe, in which the tendon is more or less exposed, is more often employed. The internal and external recti are the only tendons commonly divided, the internal far the more frequently. Anæsthesia is seldom necessary except for young children. Instruments: Stop speculum, Fig. 139, straight scissors, with blunted points, Fig.140, toothed fixation forceps, Fig.141, strabismus hook, Fig. 142. There are several forms of hook, differing in the length and sharpness of the curve and the shape of the tip.

FIG. 139.

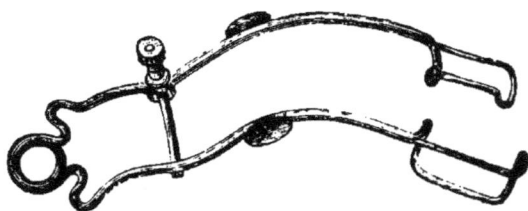

Stop spring speculum.

Operations. *Graefe's.*—An incision is made transversely over the insertion of the tendon, and, the conjunctiva being pushed aside, Tenon's capsule is opened below the tendon ; the hook is then passed under the tendon, and the latter divided with the scissors. The whole width of the tendon is exposed. The conjunctival wound may be closed by a single stitch. Snellen makes the conjunctival wound parallel to the muscle to avoid gaping. The effect in this and all operations may be considerably increased if the various facial or indirect connections of the muscle be divided as well as its tendon. This is done (1) by separating the conjunctiva from the fascia and its muscle by a burrowing dissection with the scissors before the tendon is cut ; (2) by freely dividing the fascia above and below the tendon, by cutting with the scissors upward and downward after having divided the tendon itself; (3) by tying the eye out with a

FIG. 140.

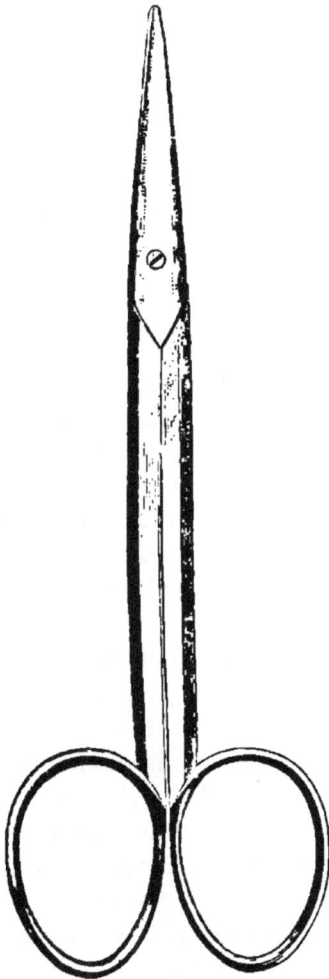

Strabismus scissors (drawn too thick in the blades).

FIG. 141.

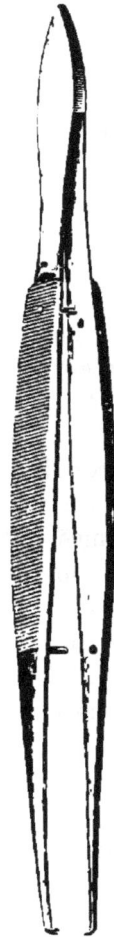

Fixation forceps.

silk suture passed through the conjunctiva and surface
fibres of the sclerotic, close to the outer border of the
cornea, and attaching it to the temple for two days by
strapping.

FIG. 142.

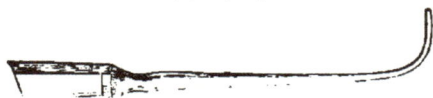

Strabismus hook (the bent part is represented too thin).

Critchett's operation.—(1.) Introduce the speculum, and
with the fixation forceps in the left hand, pinch up a fold
of conjunctiva over the lower border of the tendon (say of
the right internal rectus) at its insertion ; with the scissors
in the right hand make a small opening close to the end of
the forceps, and parallel with the border of the tendon.
The exposed fascia, capsule of Tenon, is now easily recognized ; it is to be pinched up, and an opening made in it
corresponding to the conjunctival wound.   By taking deep
hold with the forceps, both conjunctiva and fascia may
sometimes be divided at one stroke.   As a rule, both conjunctiva and Tenon's capsule are thicker in children than
adults.

(2.) Take the hook in the right hand, holding the wound
open with the forceps in the left, and pass it, concavity
downward and point backward, through the opening in the
fascia as far as its elbow, keeping its end always flat against
the sclerotic.   Next turn the end of the hook upward, still
guided by the sclerotic, between the tendon and the globe,
until its end is seen projecting beneath the conjunctiva
above the upper border of the tendon.   On now attempting to draw the hook toward the cornea it will be stopped
by the tendon.   If Tenon's capsule have not been well
opened, the hook cannot be passed beneath the tendon nor
swept round the sclerotic.

(3.) Lay down the forceps, transfer the hook to the
left hand, holding its handle parallel with the side of the
nose and tightening the tendon by traction forward and
outward ; pass the scissors, with the blades slightly opened,

into the wound, and push them straight up *between the hook and the eye;* the tendon is divided at two or three snips with a crisp sound and feeling. When the whole breadth of the tendon is divided the hook slips forward beneath the conjunctiva up to the edge of the cornea. It is well, by reintroducing the hook, to make sure that no small strands of the tendon have escaped, for the operation does not succeed unless the division be complete.

No after-treatment is needed, but the patient is more comfortable if the eye be tied up for a few hours.

The difficulties for beginners are: (1) to be sure of opening the fascia; (2) to avoid pushing the tendon in front of the scissors, especially when only the upper part remains undivided.

Simple division of one internal rectus without separation and division of fascia diminishes the squint by about two lines (4 mm.). The effect, however, is often much less if the patient be adult or nearly so.

Liebreich's operation is Critchett's with the addition of the separation of the conjunctiva from the fascia and division of the fascia beyond the edges of the tendon described at p. 398. These additions to simple tenotomy can be more easily and thoroughly applied to Graefe's operation when the incision is over the tendon, and after a considerable trial I have ceased to use Liebreich's method. In any case of considerable convergent squint or squint operated on in an adolescent or adult I prefer Graefe's method, which admits of the maximum effect being easily obtained.

The immediate effect of the tenotomy of a rectus muscle is lessened after a few days by the reunion of the tendon with the sclerotic, but after a few weeks or months it is sometimes again increased by the stretching of this new tissue.

Readjustment or *Advancement* consists in bringing for-

ward to a new attachment the tendon of a rectus, generally
the internal, which has become attached too far back after
a previous tenotomy, or is acting inefficiently, as in various
cases of primary divergent squint; advancement of the
external rectus is also used in simultaneous conjunction
with tenotomy of the internal in high degrees of convergent squint, especially when the squint is of many years'
duration. Indeed, whether performed for divergent or
convergent strabismus, tenotomy of the opponent muscle is
generally needed. There are several different operations,
but in all of them the tendon is held in its new position by
sutures. The operation is tedious, but may often be done
under cocaine. Instruments are the same as for tenotomy.

I now generally perform the operation as follows (essentially the method described by Tweedy[1]): (1) A stitch of
fine silk is first put through conjunctiva and surface fibres
of sclerotic, close to the inner edge of cornea, and exactly
on the horizontal line; this is to serve as a guide in case
the eyeball rotates afterward. (2) The tendon is exposed
by a vertical wound in the conjunctiva about 5 mm. from
the corneal border, the fascia opened above and below, and
a hook passed under the tendon. (3) A stitch is passed
through the upper part of the muscle alone, not including
conjunctiva, some way from its attachment, and tied round
the included part of the muscle, and the needle then passed
beneath conjunctiva and fascia and brought out above the
upper edge of the cornea; the lower part of the muscle is
treated in the same way, and the tendon then divided from
the sclerotic with scissors, and, if thought necessary, shortened by cutting off the portion in front of the sutures. The
needle carrying the central (guide) thread is now passed
from behind forward through the muscle between the other
two sutures and overlying conjunctiva, and tied. The upper

[1] Tweedy, Lancet, March 22, 1884.

and lower stitches are then tied slightly. The conjunctiva is a good deal dragged upon above and below, but soon stretches, or the sutures partly cut through. The opponent rectus is divided before the sutures are tied. The eyes should both usually be kept quietly tied up for several days, and the stitches be left in for a week, or until they come away, if silk.

De Wecker's method of advancement by folding the tendon on itself, so-called advancement of Tenon's capsule, does not seem to have gained general acceptance, and need not be described here. I have had very good success with it once or twice.

D. Excision of the Eye.

Instruments as for squint, but the scissors curved on the flat. The operator may stand either behind or in front. (1) Divide the ocular conjunctiva all round, close to the cornea. (2) Open Tenon's capsule, and divide each rectus tendon and the neighboring fascia on the hook; the two obliques are seldom divided on the hook. (3) Make the eye start forward by pressing the speculum back behind the equator of the globe. (4) Pass the scissors backward along the sclerotic until their open blades can be felt to embrace the optic nerve, recognized by its toughness and thickness, and divide it by a single cut, while steadying the globe with a finger of the other hand. Finish by dividing the oblique muscles and remaining soft parts, close to the globe. Apply pressure for a minute or two, and then tie up tightly for six or eight hours with an elastic pad of small sponges overlaid by cotton wool. There is scarcely ever serious bleeding. The artificial eye may be fitted in from three to four weeks.[1]

---

[1] The glass eye must be renewed as often as it gets rough, generally at least once a year. Some persons have much difficulty in tolerating

After some weeks or months a button of granulation tissue occasionally grows from a scar at the bottom of the conjunctival sac, and should be snipped off.

The operation is more difficult when the eye is ruptured or shrunken, or the surrounding parts much inflamed and adherent. The order of division of the muscles is immaterial. The important points are to leave as much conjunctiva as possible, so as to form a deep bed for the glass eye, and by keeping the scissors close to the globe during the whole operation, to avoid unnecessary laceration of the tissues.

When, as in some cases of intra-ocular tumor, it is desired to remove another piece of the optic nerve, the nerve should be felt for with the finger, seized and drawn forward with the forceps, and cut off further back with the scissors.

Substitutes for excision of the eyeball.—*Abscission* is the removal of a staphylomatous cornea with the front part of the sclerotic, leaving the hinder part of the globe, with the muscles attached, to serve as a movable stump for carrying the artificial eye. Four or five semicircular needles carrying sutures are made to puncture and counter-puncture the sclerotic, just in front of the attachments of the recti; the part of the globe in front of the needles is cut off, the needles drawn through, and the sutures tied. The operation is admissible only when the ciliary region is free from disease, and has therefore a very limited application; even in the most favorable cases the stump is not entirely free from the risk of setting up sympathetic inflammation, and I therefore never perform it. It is said that if the sutures are passed only through the conjunctiva or the muscles, the risk is less than when they are passed through the sclerotic.

The operation of *optico-ciliary neurotomy*, in which the optic nerve and all the ciliary nerves are divided without removal of the globe, with the view of preventing sympathetic disease, appears to me to be bad surgery. The sensibility of the cornea,

it, and they must be content to wear it for only a part of the day. It is always to be removed at bedtime.

abolished by the operation, often returns, proving that the ciliary nerves have reunited. The cut ends of the optic nerve have also been found reunited, and though union may be prevented by exsection of a considerable piece of the optic nerve, the same cannot be done with the ciliary nerves. The operation, therefore, cannot be relied upon to destroy these, nor, it may be added, any of the other possible paths along which sympathetic irritation and inflammation may travel; indeed, sympathetic inflammation has been observed to follow the operation in at least one case.

Evisceration of the eye, long ago performed in certain cases by sundry operators, has been systematically practised and advocated lately by Mr. Mules,[1] of Manchester, and Professor Graefe, of Halle. The front of the eye is removed at the sclero-corneal junction, and the whole contents of the globe emptied out with any convenient instrument, very great care being taken to remove every trace of choroid and ciliary body. Mr. Mules then, after enlarging the scleral opening by a vertical slit, introduces into its cavity a hermetically closed, hollow glass ball, and stitches the sclerotic carefully over it with fine catgut, the conjunctiva being separately sewn afterward. The parts should be irrigated or sprayed during the whole operation. There is more reaction than after excision, and if the sclerotic be much inflamed, or if suppuration occur, the stitches may give way. The introduction of the glass globe is not an essential part of the proceeding, its object being merely to improve the stump. Graefe advocates evisceration as less likely than excision to be followed by meningitis—a terrible accident, which every now and then occurs.[2] Mules defends it as likely to be, equally with excision, a safeguard against sympathetic disease whilst allowing a better stump for the artificial eye.

Mr. Frost,[3] wishing, in common with many others in the present imperfect state of our knowledge of sympathetic in-

---

[1] Mules, Trans. Ophth. Soc., v. 200, 1885.

[2] The known cases of meningitis after excision, about thirty-five in number, are collected in a paper by the author in vol. vi. of the Ophth. Soc. Transactions, 1886.

[3] Frost, Brit. Med. Assoc., Brighton Meeting, 1886.

flammation, to get rid of all properly ocular tissue, proposes the introduction of Mules's glass globe into the cavity of Tenon's capsule, uniting the muscles and conjunctiva over it.

The operation of stretching the infra-trochlear, or external nasal nerve, has been introduced by Dr. Badal, as an alternative to excision for the relief of pain, *e.g.*, in absolute glaucoma. The nerve—or nerves, for there are two or three twigs—is found by making a nearly vertical incision through skin and orbicularis muscle, rather below and external to the inner end of the eyebrow.

E. Operations on the Cornea.

1. **Removal of foreign bodies.**—Instruments: A steel spud, Fig. 143, or a broad needle with double cutting edge, Fig. 144. A 2 per cent. solution of cocaine is to be dropped

FIG. 143.	FIG. 144.
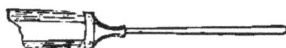	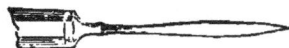
Corneal spud.	Broad needle.

in two or three times within five minutes. The operator stands behind the patient, and, keeping the lids apart with his index and ring fingers, steadies the eyeball by placing his middle finger against its outer or inner side. The chip is gently picked or tilted off by placing the edge of the spud beneath it, or, if firmly embedded, a certain amount of scraping may be necessary. If the foreign body be barely embedded in the epithelium, a touch with a little roll of blotting-paper will often detach it. When a fragment of iron has been present for more than a couple of days its corneal bed is usually stained by rust, and a little plate or ring of brown corneal slough can often be picked off after the removal of the chip; but, as a rule, this minute slough may be left to separate spontaneously.

[1] Badal, Bull. de la Soc. de Chir., Dec. 1882; Lagrange, Arch. d'Ophthal., vi. 43, 1886.

AFTER-TREATMENT.—Tie the eye up, so as to protect the corneal surface from friction and irritation. Atropine is to be used if there be marked congestion and photophobia.

When a splinter is deeply and firmly embedded, especially if it have penetrated the cornea and is projecting into the anterior chamber, its removal is often very difficult.

Unless great care be taken the splinter in such a case may be pushed on into the chamber, and the iris or lens be wounded. This may sometimes be prevented by passing a broad needle through the cornea at another part, and laying it against the inner surface of the wound, so as to form a guard or foil to the foreign body, the latter being removed by spud or forceps from the front.

A foreign body in the anterior chamber should, in recent cases, always be removed, and the piece of iris on which it lies must generally be excised. In cases of old standing we may judge by the symptoms whether to operate or not.

2. **Paracentesis of the anterior chamber.**—Position as for 1, or recumbent; general anæsthesia not necessary. Instruments: A paracentesis needle, Fig. 145, with a very small, short, triangular blade, bent at an obtuse angle, like a minute bent keratome; or a broad needle, Fig. 144. The former is more safe, as the blade is too short to reach the iris or lens, even if the patient should jerk his head. If the contents of the chamber do not follow the needle on its withdrawal, a small probe, Fig. 145, is passed into the

FIG. 145.

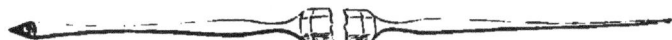

Paracentesis needle and probe mounted on same handle.

wound. In cases where the operation needs repeating every day or two, the original wound can generally be

reopened with a probe.   Speculum and fixation forceps
should be used, unless the patient has good self-control.

3. **Corneal section for hypopyon ulcer.**—Position recumbent; general anæsthesia seldom needed.   Instruments: A
Graefe's or Beer's cataract knife, Figs. 153 and 159, speculum, and fixation forceps.   The incision is carried through
the whole thickness of the cornea from one side of the
ulcer to the other, being both begun and finished in sound
tissue.   Or it may be placed entirely in sound cornea, or
at the sclero-corneal junction, leaving the ulcer untouched;
the last position avoids all risk of wounding the lens.

The knife is entered at an angle with the plane of the
iris, its edge straight forward; when its point is seen, or
judged to have perforated the cornea, the handle is depressed until the back of the knife lies parallel with the
iris, and the blade then pushed straight across the ulcer to
the point chosen for counter-puncture; often in practice it
is simply pushed on till it cuts out.   The aqueous ought
not to escape until the point of the knife is engaged in its
counter-puncture, but an earlier escape cannot always be
avoided.   If it be desired to keep the wound open, its
edges are to be separated by a probe every second or third
day.   The wound closes quickly at first, unless kept open,
but after having been opened a few times, it sometimes remains patent for longer.

4. **Cauterization** of the cornea is best performed with a
very fine galvano-caustic terminal, which should be very
intensely hot—yellow or almost white heat.   The finest
terminal of Paquelin's instrument may be used, but its
action cannot be so well localized, owing to the greater
bulk of the heated metal.   If the eye be much congested
I generally apply solid cocaine hydrochlorate to the part
to be burnt, and to the part where the fixation forceps will
be applied.

Operations for conical cornea.—The object is to produce a scar at the apex of the cone, which by contracting shall reduce the curvature, and so diminish the high degree of irregular myopic astigmatism to which the condition gives rise.

There are several methods. (1.) Graefe's treatment consisted in first carefully shaving off the apex of the cone, without entering the anterior chamber, and then producing an ulcer by touching the raw surface with solid mitigated nitrate of silver (F. 1), and so obtaining a scar. This method is more painful and less safe than others, and is now seldom used. (2.) In another operation the apex of the cone is cut off with a cataract knife, the anterior chamber being entered, and the wound either left to close or united by sutures; there are several different modes of removing the little piece. (3.) Sir William Bowman removes the outer layers of the cone by means of a very delicate cutting trephine, and leaves the surface to heal and contract. (4.) The galvanic cautery is now being a good deal used instead of the knife or trephine; I have found that the opacity left by the cautery is apt to engage a larger area than that caused by cutting operations, but more experience is needed before deciding on the relative merits of Nos. 2 and 4.

AFTER-TREATMENT.—Atropine and compressive bandage until the wound has closed; antiphlogistic treatment, and heat locally, if inflammatory symptoms arise.

All operations for conical cornea are difficult to perform and somewhat uncertain in result, but in many cases vision improves, from barely seeing very large letters before operation to reading small print afterward. The final result is never gained for several months. An artificial pupil may be necessary if a large corneal opacity finally remain.

F. Operations on the Iris.

A portion of the iris is very often removed by operation
(iridectomy), and with various objects. The principal of
these are: (1) the direct improvement of sight by altering
the position and size of the pupil (artificial pupil); (2) to
influence the course of an active disease—glaucoma, iritis,
ulcer of cornea with hypopyon; (3) to remove the risks
attending "exclusion" and "occlusion" of the pupil, by
restoring communication between the anterior and posterior
chambers; (4) as a stage in the extraction of cataract.

Iridectomy often causes astigmatism by giving rise to flattening of that meridian of the cornea which forms a right angle
with the operation wound, and by bringing the edge of the
cornea and lens into use permits the spherical aberration (Fig.
9) which the iris naturally prevents; striæ, if present in the
lens, add to these difficulties, all of which are, *cæteris paribus*,
greater if the artificial pupil be large and uncovered by the
upper lid. Thus it is evident that an artificial pupil should
seldom be made for the optical improvement of sight unless
the opacity in or over the natural pupil be such as to interfere
seriously with visual acuteness.

Artificial pupil.—The object is to remove the portion of
iris in the position best adapted to sight; thus, in cases of
leucoma the iridectomy is made opposite the clearest part
of the cornea. When the state of the cornea allows it, the
new pupil should be made down-inward or straight downward; the next best place is outward or out-upward; and
straight upward is, of course, least useful, because the new
pupil will be covered by the lid. The coloboma should
generally be small, and often only 'the inner (pupillary)
part of the chosen portion is to be removed, the outer (ciliary) part being left, Fig. 146, so as to prevent the light
passing through the margin of the lens. After such an
operation the pupil will be oval or pear-shaped, and widest

towards the centre. The incision should lie in the corneal
tissue, if only the pupillary part of the iris is to be removed;
but if only a narrow zone of cornea remain clear the incision must lie a little outside the sclero-corneal junction,

Fig. 146.

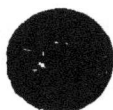

Iridectomy downward and inward for artificial pupil.

lest its scar should interfere with the transparency of the
remaining clear cornea. The loop of iris should be cut off
with a single snip.

In iridectomy for glaucoma the coloboma is to be large,
the iris to be removed quite up to its ciliary attachment,
and the incision to lie as far back in the sclerotic as possible, 1 to 2 mm. from the border of the cornea is not too
far. The coloboma should be wider towards the wound
than towards the pupil, so as to form a "keyhole pupil,"
Fig. 147. The loop of iris, when drawn out, is usually

Fig. 147.

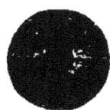

Iridectomy for glaucoma. (De Wecker.)

cut first in one angle of the wound, then torn from its ciliary attachment by carefully drawing it over to the other
angle of the wound, and its other end cut there.

The difficulty of making an artificial pupil, for optical
purposes, of the best shape, i. e., broad towards the natural
pupil and narrow towards the circumference, is, owing to

18

the small size of the parts, much greater than would be at
first supposed, and several methods are in use. In Mr.

FIG. 148.

Critchett's *iridodesis* a loop of iris is
drawn out, and strangulated by a fine
ligature tied round it over the incision;
the little loop soon drops off, and the
result is a pear-shaped pupil, with its
broad end towards the centre. Irritation, and even destructive irido-cyclitis, sometimes follow, and the operation
has therefore been abandoned. Another plan is to draw out a small loop
of iris with a blunt hook (Tyrrell's
hook), and to cut off only the pupillary
portion; this method is uncertain, but,
on the whole, it gives good results.

Iridotomy (*iritomy*).—In this operation an artificial pupil is formed by
the natural gaping of a simple incision
in the iris. It is only applicable when
the lens is absent. Through a small
incision in the cornea, between the
centre and margin, the scissors (shears)
shown at Fig. 148 are passed; the more
pointed blade is passed behind the iris
as far as is deemed necessary, and the
iris and false membrane divided by a
single closure of the blades. It is sometimes necessary to make a second cut
at an angle with the first, so as to in-

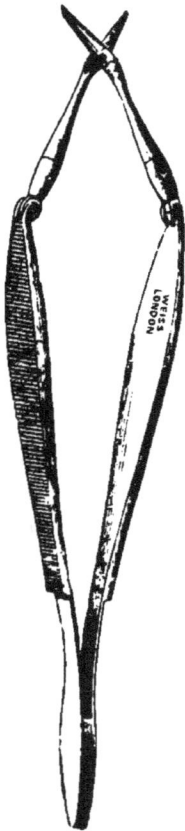

Iridotomy scissors.

clude a V-shaped tongue of iris which
will shrink and allow a larger pupil.

Iridotomy is most useful when the iris has become tightly
drawn towards the operation scar by iritis occurring after
cataract extraction, Fig. 160. The line of the cut in the

iris should lie, as nearly as may be, *across* the direction of
its fibres, and should always be as long as possible. In
cases of this sort, or when, even without such dragging of
the iris towards the scar, the pupil is filled with iritic or
cyclitic membrane after cataract extraction, iridotomy
yields a better pupil than iridectomy, and with less disturbance of, and no dragging upon, the ciliary body.

THE OPERATION OF IRIDECTOMY.—Position recumbent;
the operator usually stands behind. Anæsthesia is often
advisable, but many operators prefer cocaine; I myself
prefer general anæsthesia whenever the operation is critical
or likely to be difficult. Instruments: stop speculum, Fig.
139, fixation forceps, bent keratome, Fig. 149, iris forceps,
bent at various angles according to the position of the iridectomy, Fig. 151, iris scissors with elbow bend, Fig. 151,
of which some patterns have one or both blades probe-
pointed, a curette, Fig. 155, or small vulcanite or tortoise-shell spatula for replacing the cut ends of the iris,
and preventing their incarceration in the angles of the
wound. The iridotomy scissors, Fig. 148, are very convenient, especially for downward and inward operations,

FIG. 149.

Bent triangular keratome.

and for the left hand. Some operators prefer Graefe's
cataract knife, Fig. 153, to the triangular keratome, in
iridectomy for glaucoma.

The conjunctiva is held by the fixation forceps near the
cornea, at a point opposite to the place selected for puncture. (1) The keratome is to be entered slowly, steadily
pushed on across the anterior chamber till the wound is of
the desired size, then slowly withdrawn, and, in withdrawal,

its blade carefully turned to one side, so as to lengthen the internal wound. Two points need attention: as soon as the point of the knife is visible in the anterior chamber, it

FIG. 150.   FIG. 151.

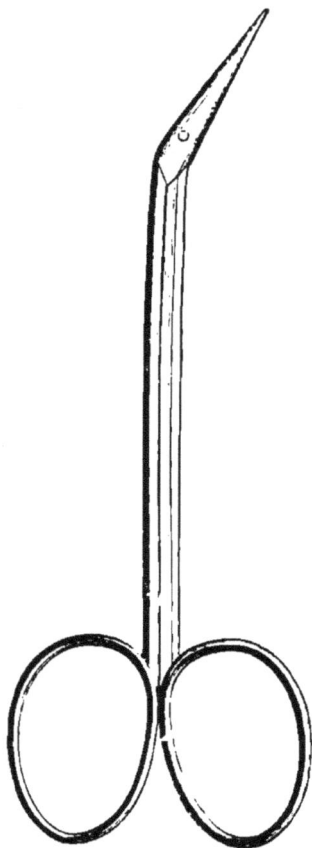

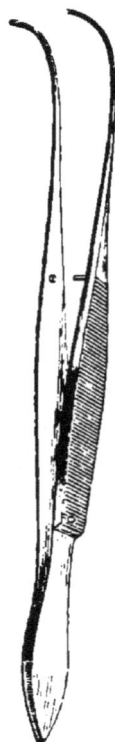

Iridectomy scissors.   Iris forceps.

must be tilted slightly forward to avoid wounding the iris and lens; and care must be taken not to tilt it sideways, for if this be done the wound, instead of lying paral-

lel with the border of the cornea, will lie more or less across
that line. The incision is made almost as much by lifting
the eye against the knife with the fixation forceps, as by
pushing the knife against the eye. The forceps are now
laid down, or, if fixation be still necessary, they are given
to an assistant, who is gently to draw the eye into the position required for the next step ; in so doing he is to draw
away from the eye, not to push the ends of the forceps
against the sclerotic. (2) The iris forceps are introduced,
closed, into the wound, and passed very nearly to the pupillary border of the iris, before being opened and made to
grasp it. By seizing the pupillary part of the iris its inner
circle is certain to be brought outside the wound, when the
forceps are now withdrawn ; if the iris be seized in the
middle of its breadth, a buttonhole may be cut out, and
the pupillary part left standing. Often the iris is carried
into the wound by the gush of aqueous as the keratome is
withdrawn, and it is then seized without passing the forceps
so far into the chamber. (3) The loop of iris having been
cut off, either at a single snip, or by cutting first one end
and then the other, as in glaucoma, the tip of the curette
or spatula is passed into each angle of the wound to free
the iris, should it be entangled ; it is important to make
sure that no iris is left incarcerated in the track of the
wound. The speculum is now removed, and the eye, or
both eyes, bandaged over a pad of cotton-wool, either with
a four-tailed bandage of knitted cotton, or two or three
turns of a soft cotton or flannel roller.

The anterior chamber is refilled in twenty-four hours,
except in cases of glaucoma, when the wound frequently
leaks more or less for several days. It is as well in all
cases to keep the eye bandaged for a week, the wound being
but feebly united and likely to give way from any slight
blow or other accident. When the incision lies in or
partly in the sclerotic, some bleeding generally occurs ;

when the eye is much congested this hemorrhage is considerable, and the blood may run into the anterior chamber either during or after the excision of the iris; it can be drawn out by depressing the lip of the wound with the curette, but if the chamber again fills no prolonged efforts need be made, since the blood is usually absorbed without trouble in a few days. In diseased, especially glaucomatous eyes, however, its absorption is often slow. Secondary hemorrhage sometimes occurs from a diseased iris several days after the operation.

Sclerotomy is an operation for dividing the sclerotic near to the margin of the cornea. It is employed in glaucoma instead of iridectomy, or after iridectomy has failed. The pupil is to be contracted as much as possible by eserine before the operation. It is often performed subconjunctivally, a Graefe's cataract knife, Fig. 153, being entered through the sclerotic near the margin of the cornea,[1] passed in front of the iris, and brought out at a corresponding point on the other side, so as to include nearly one-third of the circumference; the puncture and counter-puncture are then enlarged by slow sawing movements; the central quarter of the sclerotic flap and the whole of the conjunctiva, except at the punctures, are left undivided. The knife is then slowly withdrawn. The whole operation is to be done very slowly, that the aqueous humor may escape gradually; any rush of fluid is likely to carry the iris into the wound and cause a permanent prolapse, a result to be carefully avoided. If prolapse occur the iris should be excised, and the operation then becomes a very peripheral iridectomy. A moderate degree of bulging and separation of the lips of the two scleral wounds takes place for a week or two, when the scar flattens down and finally

---

[1] De Wecker makes it 1 mm. from the clear cornea. In my own operations the distance is generally about 2 mm.

a mere bluish line is left. Sclerotomy is also performed with a triangular keratome, Fig. 149, the incision being just as for a very peripheral iridectomy, but no iris being

FIG. 152.

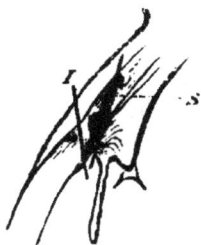

Diagrammatic section of ciliary region. showing path of wound in iridectomy for glaucoma (*I*) and in sclerotomy (*S*).
(Compare Fig. 100, 1 and 2.)

removed or allowed to prolapse. Sclerotomy is difficult to perform well, is not free from risk, and on the whole has not answered early expectations; it is, however, valuable as a reserve for certain cases. In Fig. 152, *I* shows the line of incision in iridectomy for glaucoma, and *S* the line in sclerotomy; comparison with Fig. 100, however, will show that even in iridectomies for glaucoma the position of the wound may vary a good deal.

G. Operations for Cataract.

1. *Extraction of cataract* has been systematically practised for nearly a century and a half. The operation has passed through several important changes, and procedures differing more or less from each other are still in use. All the operations are difficult to perform well, and much practice is needed to insure the best prospect of success. The sources of possible failure are many, and as in avoiding one we are apt to fall into another, it cannot be expected that any one operation will, in all its details, ever be uni-

versally adopted. At present the majority of surgeons adhere more or less closely to the operation known as the "modified linear" method of von Graefe, in which iridectomy forms a step in the proceeding. There is, however, a strong tendency, especially amongst operators of large experience, to dispense with iridectomy on account of the cosmetic and optical advantages of a round pupil. For the last twelve months I have operated, as a rule, without iri-

FIG. 153.

Graefe's cataract knife.

FIG. 154.

Cataract spoon.

dectomy. That many cataracts can be easily and safely extracted without iridectomy admits of no doubt; and it appears equally certain that some cases, especially where the lens is very hard, cannot be dealt with properly in this way. Any operator of experience is fully justified in leaving the iris intact unless there be difficulty in delivering the lens through the pupil, or difficulty in perfectly replacing the iris afterward, or the patient be very restless; in either of these events iridectomy should be performed at the moment when required. Eserine used just before and a few times after the operation appears to assist in preventing prolapse of the iris afterward. If prolapse occurs, as it may, several days after operation, it is best to remove it carefully as in a case of accidental wound.

FIG. 155.

Cystitome (upper end) and curette (lower end).

All operations for extraction of hard cataract agree in the following points: (1) An incision is made in the cornea, at the junction of the cornea and sclerotic, or even slightly in the sclerotic, large enough to give exit to the crystalline lens unbroken and unaltered in shape. The knife now almost universally employed is the narrow, thin, straight knife of von Graefe, Fig. 153. (2) The capsule is freely opened with a small, sharp-pointed instrument, cystitome or pricker, Fig. 155. (3) The lens is removed through the rent in the capsule (the latter structure remaining behind), either by pressure and manipulation outside the eye, or by means of a traction instrument, scoop or spoon, Fig. 154, passed into the eye just behind the lens. Few operators, however, use the scoop, except for certain emergencies and special cases. (4) Iridectomy is very often performed as the second stage. This part of the operation was originally introduced less with the object of facilitating the exit of the lens, than of preventing prolapse of the iris and lessening the after-risks of iritis. But these untoward results do not occur so often, with cocaine and antiseptics, as formerly; and, as already stated, many now omit iridectomy. A few of the many surgeons who adhere to iridectomy prefer to perform it some weeks or months before the extraction of the lens, *preliminary iridectomy;* the theory being that iritis is less likely to follow if the cut edges of the iris are soundly healed before the lens rubs against them on its way out. Patients, however, will not, or cannot, always submit to this subdivision of the operation for cataract, and for this and other reasons of expediency preliminary iridectomy cannot be employed so largely as may, perhaps, on theoretical grounds, be desirable. In my own practice I keep it for cases where special risks or difficulties are present, as, *e. g.*, where the patient has only one eye.

The following are the chief varieties of operation for cataract at present practised:—

18*

(*a*) *Simple linear extraction*, best described here, though not applicable to hard cataract. A small incision (4 to 6 mm.) is made by a keratome, Fig. 149, well within the margin of the cornea, with a small iridectomy, if necessary. After opening the capsule the lens is squeezed out piecemeal, or coaxed out by depressing the outer lip of the wound with the curette, Fig. 155. Only quite soft cataracts, or those in which the nucleus, though firm, is very small, can be so dealt with.

The wish to extend the principle of a straight wound to full-sized hard cataracts, led von Graefe, in 1865, to introduce (*b*) the *modified linear* or *peripheral linear* extraction, in which the incision lies slightly beyond the sclerocorneal junction, Fig. 157, 2, and consequently involves the conjunctiva, of which a flap is made. The incision is intended to form an arc of the largest possible circle, *i. e.*, of the scleral, not of the corneal, curve; its plane, therefore, must lie as nearly as may be in a radius of the scleral curve, and at a considerable angle with that of the iris, Fig. 158, 2. A large iridectomy is performed as the second stage. The incision is made with the Graefe knife, Fig. 153, which is at first directed toward the centre of the pupil and then brought up to the seat of counter-puncture. The edge is turned somewhat forward during the greater part of the proceeding, and the cut completed by sawing movements, if needful. The disadvantages of the peripheral linear extraction are: the frequency of bleeding from the conjunctiva into the anterior chamber, the parts being thus obscured; a considerable risk of loss of vitreous, owing to the peripheral position of the wound and sometimes a difficulty in making the lens present well; a small but appreciable risk that the operated eye will set up sympathetic inflammation, the wound lying in the " dangerous region ;" lastly, there is a tendency to make the wound rather too short in order to avoid some of these risks, and thus difficulties are introduced in the clean removal of the lens. Its great advantage lies in the very small attendant risk of suppurative inflammation.

A variety of this operation consists in placing the incision rather further down, and at the same time giving it a somewhat sharper curve, so that it forms an arc of a smaller circle than before, but is still not concentric with the cornea, Fig. 157, 3, upper section. The puncture is directed somewhat downward (as at the right-hand end of the figure), and its plane, which at the puncture and counter-puncture is almost parallel with the iris, alters to nearly a right angle at the summit of the flap. The track of the wound, if shaded, would appear as in the figure.

(c) *Short flap* (De Wecker).—The incision, made with the same knife, lies exactly at the sclero-corneal junction, and is of such an extent that it has a height of about 3 mm. ($\frac{1}{4}$ of the diameter of the cornea), Fig. 156. A narrow

FIG. 156.

Short flap.

rim of conjunctiva remains attached to the flap. The iridectomy, if made, is small, as in Fig. 148. For very bulky cataracts this incision is not quite large enough.

(d) The incision has nearly the same curve and plane as in b, but the greater part of it lies considerably within the margin of the cornea, *corneal section*, and iridectomy is usually dispensed with. Liebreich and Bader made the section downward, its plane forming an angle of about 45° with that of the iris, Fig. 158, 3, lower section. In Lebrun's corneal operation an almost identical section is

made upward; the upper section of 3, Fig. 157, if placed
further in the cornea, would nearly represent it. The corneal operations, without iridectomy, are easy to perform,

FIG. 157.

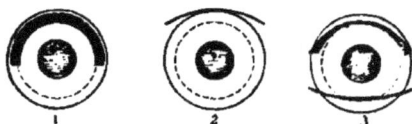

Paths of incision for extraction of cataract. 1, old flap; 2, peripheral
linear; 3 (upper Fig.), a variety of the peripheral linear; (lower Fig.)
corneal section. The wound appears as a narrow slit (2) or a broad
tract (1), when seen from the front, according to the inclination of its
plane. The dotted circle shows the average outline of the lens.
Compare Fig. 158.

compared with those in which the section lies further back;
the wound, however, does not, on the whole, heal so quickly,
and is more likely to reopen about the fourth or fifth day.

FIG 158.

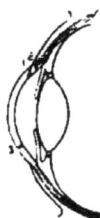

The same sections seen
in profile, showing the
plane of the incision in
1, 2, and the lower sec-
tion of 3.

(e) *Old flap extraction* (Daviel,
Beer, now very little used).—The
incision was slightly within the visible margin of the cornea, concentric
with it, and equal to at least half
its circumference, 1, Fig. 157, thus

FIG. 159.

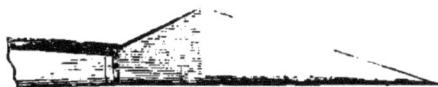

Beer's cataract knife.

forming a large arc of a small circle; the plane of the incision being parallel with that of the iris, 1, Fig. 158; no
iridectomy was made. The incision was made with the
triangular knife of Beer, Fig. 159, in which the blade near
its heel is somewhat wider than the height of the flap, the

section being completed by simply pushing the knife across the anterior chamber flat with the iris, its back corresponding to the base of the intended flap.   The inner length of the wound is less than the outer by the thickness of the obliquely cut cornea at each end. 1, Fig 157.

The flap operation was usually done without either anæsthesia, speculum, or fixation forceps.   The after-treatment was troublesome.   But the great height of the flap, in proportion to its width, renders it very liable to gape or even to fall forward, and this, with the fact that the whole wound lies in corneal tissue, considerably increases the risks of large and dangerous prolapse of the iris and of rapid suppurative inflammation of the cornea.   For these reasons the old flap extraction has been almost abandoned in favor of the peripheral linear, corneal section, and short flap operations, which yield a much larger average of useful eyes.

Historically, the flap operation was the earliest; then came the linear operation ; thirdly, the modified or peripheral linear operation, with iridectomy ; then the modern corneal operations and short flap, the aim of which is to gain the substantial advantages both of the old flap and the modified linear methods, without the great risks of the former or the imperfections of the latter; lastly, iridectomy has, as stated above, been again abandoned, more or less completely, by many operators.

Of other operations the most important is Pagenstecher's, in which the lens is removed by a scoop in its unbroken capsule.   It is most applicable to cataracts which are over-ripe or are complicated with old iritis, and to Morgagnian cataract.

(For methods of dealing with unripe senile cataract see p. 202.)

The chief *complications* which may arise *during extraction of cataract* are: (1) too short an incision ; this is best remedied by enlarging with a small bent "secondary knife." (2) Escape of vitreous before expulsion of the lens; this is a signal for the prompt removal of the lens with a scoop, Fig. 154, the vitreous being afterwards cut off level with the wound by scissors. (3) Portions of the lens remaining behind after the chief bulk has been expelled; they should be coaxed out by gentle manipulation after removal of the speculum.

AFTER-TREATMENT OF EXTRACTION.—The patient is best in bed for from four to seven days. The dressing consists of a piece of soft linen overlaid by a pad of cotton-wool or alembroth tissue, and kept in place by a four-tailed bandage of knitted cotton, or narrow flannel or open tissue roller. Both eyes are to be bandaged. The room is usually kept partly dark for about a week, all dressings and examinations being made by the light of a candle.

Some operators keep their cataract patient from the first in daylight, and with no other dressing than some strips of isinglass plaster to maintain closure of the lids. Others bandage only the operated eye. Old people occasionally get delirious if kept in bed and in the dark after extraction of cataract or iridectomy, and for such, at any rate, the ordinary rules as to bandaging, darkness, and confinement to bed must be relaxed. In my experience the subjects of this delirium have usually been alcoholics; but I believe that imprudent use of strong mydriatics may produce it in some old persons who have not been habitual drinkers.

During the first few hours there will be some soreness and smarting, and at the first dressing, from twelve to twenty-four hours after operation, a little blood-stained fluid, but after this there should be no material discomfort, and nothing more than a little mucous discharge, such as old people often have. The dressings are removed, and the lids gently cleansed with warm water once or twice a day, their edges being separated by gently drawing down the lower

lid, so as to allow any retained tears to escape ; this cleansing is very grateful to the patient. Some surgeons open
the lids and look at the eye the day after the operation ;
but many prefer to leave them closed for several days
unless there are signs that the case is doing badly. It is a
good practice to use one drop of atropine daily after the
third day, to prevent adhesions should iritis set in ; but if
no iridectomy have been made, I prefer not to use atropine
till about the fifth day, because if the wound should reopen
whilst the pupil is dilated prolapse of iris is more likely to
occur than if the pupil be small. When first examined
from two to seven days after operation, the eye is always
rather congested from having been tied up; but there
should be no chemosis, the wound should be united so as
to retain the aqueous, and its edges clear. The pupil is
expected to be black, unless it is known that portions of
lens matter have been left behind. If all be well, the
bandage may be left off during the daytime at the end of
a week or ten days, a shade being worn ; but it should be
reapplied at night for the first two or three weeks to prevent accidents from movements during sleep. At the end
of a fortnight, if the weather be fine, the patient may
begin to go out, the eyes being carefully protected from
light and wind by dark goggles, and he may be out of the
surgeon's hands in from three to four weeks.

AFTER-OPERATIONS.—When iritis occurs the pupil becomes more or less occluded by false membrane, and the
subsequent contraction of this membrane may draw the iris
toward the scar, so that the pupil is at once blocked and
displaced, Fig. 160. In slight cases, where the pupil is not
dragged out of place, sight is greatly improved by simply
tearing across the membrane and capsule with a fine needle,
and treating the case as after discission of soft cataract.
In doing this the needle should be passed deeply enough to
tear the posterior capsule also, so that the vitreous by bulg-

ing forward may keep the opening in the capsule patent
(compare Discission of Soft Cataract), in which care is
taken *not* to go so deeply. But in severer cases an artificial
pupil must be made, either by iridectomy or iridotomy.

FIG. 160.

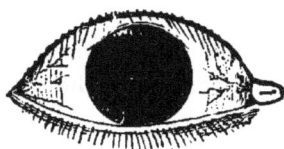

Diagram of occlusion and displacement of pupil from iritis, after
upward extraction of cataract.

2. **Solution (Discission) operations.**—In these the lens
is gradually absorbed by the action of the aqueous humor
admitted through a wound in the capsule. (1) The pupil
is fully dilated by atropine; (2) the lids are held open by
the fingers, or a stop speculum and fixation forceps used;
(3) a fine cataract needle, Fig. 162, is directed to a point
a little within the border of the cornea (usually the outer
border), and when close to its surface is plunged quickly
and rather obliquely into the anterior chamber. Its point

FIG. 161.   FIG. 162.

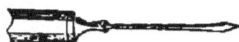

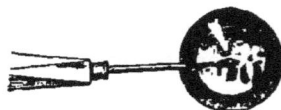

Cataract needle.   Discission of cataract.

is then carried to the centre of the pupil, Fig. 162, dipped
back through the lens-capsule, and a few gentle movements
made so as to break up the centre of the anterior layers
of the lens; (4) the needle is then steadily withdrawn.
Special care is taken not to wound, nor even touch, the iris,

either on entering or withdrawing the needle, not to stir up the lens too freely, nor to go so deeply as to perforate the posterior capsule and so engage the vitreous. A general anæsthetic is necessary only for young children or excessively nervous patients; but it should always be in readiness, and the patient prepared.

AFTER-TREATMENT.—The pupil is kept widely dilated with atropine (F. 31), a drop being applied after the operation, and at least six times a day afterward, or much oftener if there be threatening of iritis. Ice or iced water is usually to be applied constantly for twenty-four to forty-eight hours after the operation,[1] as for threatened traumatic iritis (p. 160), and the patient to remain in bed in a darkened room for a few days. A little ciliary congestion for two or three days need cause no uneasiness, but the occurrence of pain, increase of congestion, and alteration in the color of the iris (commencing iritis) are indications for the application of leeches near the eye, and the more frequent use of atropine.

If the cataract was complete, no marked change will be seen for some weeks; if partial (e. g., lamellar), in a day or two the part of the lens near the needle wound, and in a few days the whole lens, will become opaque. In from six to eight weeks the lens will have become notably smaller, flattened, or hollowed on the front surface. If the eye be perfectly quiet, but not unless, the operation may now be repeated in exactly the same way, and with the same after-treatment and precautions, but the needle may be used more freely. The bulk of the lens will generally disappear after the second operation, but the needle may have to be used a third or a fourth time for the disintegration of small residual pieces, or in order to tear the capsule if it

---

[1] I have to thank my colleague, Mr. Gunn, for this valuable suggestion.

have not retracted enough to leave a clear central pupil. A small whitish dot remains in the cornea at the seat of each needle puncture.

3. **Extraction by suction.**—This operation, like *simple linear extraction*, is applicable to completely soft cataracts. The pupil is to be dilated by atropine. The lens-capsule is opened as in discission, but more freely. Then an incision is made obliquely through the cornea, between its centre and margin, with a keratome, Fig. 149, or broad needle, Fig. 144, and the nose of the syringe passed through the wound and gently dipped into the lacerated lens-substance. By very gentle suction the semi-fluid lens-matter is then drawn gradually into the syringe. The instrument is not to be passed behind the iris in search of fragments. Nearly the whole of the lens can thus be removed. The after-treatment is the same as for needle operations. Two forms of syringe are in use: Teale's, in which the suction is made by the mouth applied to a piece of flexible India-rubber tubing; Bowman's, in which the suction is obtained by a sliding piston worked by the thumb moving along the syringe. It is often better, and in lamellar cataract necessary, to break up the lens freely with a fine needle a few days before using the syringe, and thus allow it to be thoroughly macerated and softened in the aqueous humor; atropine and ice must be used freely in the interval between this needle operation and the suction; and the surgeon must be prepared to interfere before the day appointed for the suction, should severe pain or increase of tension occur from the rapid swelling of the lens (p. 207). Suction is more difficult to perform, and perhaps less safe, than simple linear extraction, but I have myself no objection to make against it.

Anæsthesia in Ophthalmic Surgery.—Before the introduction of cocaine (October, 1884) there was much diversity of practice in respect to anæsthesia, many surgeons pre-

ferring to perform extraction of cataract, tenotomy for
squint, and simple iridectomy, without anæsthesia, whilst
others preferred ether or chloroform for nearly all operations. Cocaine has immensely facilitated operating without
general anæsthesia, but of course some will continue to use
ether or chloroform, where others feel able to rely solely on
the local anæsthetic. In using cocaine for the eye we have to
remember that it does not affect the sensibility of the borders
of the lids, nor in any constant manner that of the iris,
unless used many times for at least half an hour, nor that
of the muscles and deeper parts, unless injected under the
conjunctiva. Hence the introduction and pressure of the
speculum are always more or less felt, there is usually some
little pain when the iris is seized and drawn out, and decided pain when, in tenotomy, the tendon is stretched on
the hook, unless subconjunctival injection have been resorted
to. It must further be remembered that the patient is conscious and knows that something critical is being done, and
that his good behavior depends almost as much on absence
of fear as on absence of feeling ; and, again, that the pain-
lessness of one step of an operation, e. g., the section in
extraction of cataract, contrasts strongly with the sensation of pain felt in another stage, e. g., the iridectomy, and
that the patient will be likely to start or jump, unless
warned, at such a stage. My own experience leads me to
use cocaine in all cataract extractions and discissions, unless
for some peculiar reason ether or chloroform be needed, for
nearly all tenotomies and operations for corneal ulcer and
conical cornea, and for some simple iridectomies; and to
avoid it usually in iridectomy for glaucoma and for synechiæ
whether anterior or posterior. I have not myself used it
much for lachrymal cases ; nor have I excised the eyeball
under its influence ; but it may be used for both purposes
with fair success. For small lid tumors, subcutaneous
injection is very successful. For granular lids or lupus of

conjunctiva, a strong solution, 10 to 20 per cent., may be painted on before touching with actual cautery or caustics; but it is better for such cases, and also whenever the eyeball is congested and painful, to use the solid cocaine salt, powdered and rubbed over the surface with a brush or the finger. For cataract, a solution of 2 per cent., or a single disc containing $\frac{1}{200}$ grain, repeated three times within five minutes of the operation, is generally quite enough. Solutions should be freshly made.

PART III.

DISEASES OF THE EYE IN RELATION TO GENERAL DISEASES.

CHAPTER XXIII.

In stating very shortly the most important facts bearing on the connection between diseases of the eye and of other parts of the body, it is convenient to make the following subdivisions: (**A**) the eye-changes occur as part of a general disease; (**B**) the ocular disease is symptomatic of some local malady at a distance; (**C**) the eye shares in a local process, affecting the neighboring parts.

(For the clinical details of the various eye diseases referred to in this chapter, see Part II.)

A. General diseases, in which the eye is liable to suffer.

Syphilis is, directly or indirectly, the cause of a large proportion of the more serious diseases of the eye.

1. Acquired syphilis.—Primary stage: Hard chancres are occasionally seen on the eyelid, and even far back on the conjunctiva.

Secondary stage: Sore-throat, shedding of hair, eruption, and condylomata. *Iritis* is common between two and eight or nine months, and does not occur later than about eighteen months, after the contagion; in from two-thirds to three-fourths of the cases both eyes suffer; there is a marked tendency to exudation of lymph, plastic iritis, shown by keratitis punctata, haze of cornea, and less commonly by

lymph-nodules on the iris. In some cases there are symptoms of severe cyclitis, leading to detachment of retina and
secondary cataract, and but little iritis ; but the cyclitis of
acquired syphilis does not give rise to ciliary staphyloma.
Syphilitic iritis, though sometimes protracted, rarely relapses after complete subsidence. *Choroiditis* and *retinitis*
generally set in rather later, from six months to about two
years after the chancre ; seldom as late as four years.[1] The
two conditions are most often seen together, but either may
occur singly ; and in each the vitreous generally becomes
inflamed. These conditions are essentially chronic, the
retinitis being often, and the choroiditis sometimes, liable
to repeated exacerbations or recurrences ; whilst in some
cases the secondary atrophic changes progress slowly for
years, almost to blindness, often with pigmentation of the
retina. Syphilitic choroiditis and retinitis usually affect
both eyes, but often in an unequal degree, and even when
severe the disease is occasionally limited to one eye. *Keratitis*, indistinguishable from that of inherited syphilis, is
amongst the rarest events in the acquired disease ; when it
occurs it is usually in the secondary stage of the disease.

Later periods : Ulceration of the skin and conjunctiva
of the lids, gummatous infiltration of the lids and sclerotic,
and nodes in the orbit, whether cellular or periosteal, occur
but rarely. *Oculo-motor paralysis* is one of the frequent
ocular results of syphilis. It may depend upon gumma,
syphilitic neuroma, of the affected nerve or nerves in the
orbit or in the skull, or upon gummatous inflammation of
the dura mater at the base of the skull, matting the nerves
together, or on disease of nerve-centres. The gummatous
nerve-lesions seldom occur very late in tertiary syphilis.

The optic disc is often inflamed or atrophied as an indi-

---

[1] A few cases are on record in which it appeared not to have begun
till about ten years after infection.

rect result of syphilitic disease of the eye or of the nervous
system; but the terms "syphilitic optic neuritis" or
"syphilitic optic atrophy" are not often applicable in any
more direct sense. The retinitis of the secondary stage
affects the disc, and, when atrophy of the retina and choroid occurs, the disc becomes wasted in proportion; whilst
in rare cases the retinitis of secondary syphilis is replaced
by well-marked papillitis. Such cases must not be confused
with others, still more rare, in which double papillitis, passing into atrophy, occurs with all the symptoms of severe
meningitis, in secondary syphilis. Tertiary syphilitic disease, anywhere within the cranium, commonly causes optic
neuritis, in the same way as do other coarse intracranial
lesions; but neuritis may also be caused more directly by
gummatous inflammation of the trunk of the optic nerve,
cr of the chiasma. Primary progressive atrophy of the
discs occurs in association with locomotor ataxy and ophthalmoplegia externa of syphilitic origin; probably in a
few instances the optic atrophy occurs alone, or for a time
precedes the other changes in syphilitic, as it is known to
do in non-syphilitic, ataxy.

Sight is liable to be rapidly damaged from severe acute
loss of blood, especially from the stomach; usually both
eyes suffer, but often unequally. When seen quite early
papillitis has been found, but the cases are often not seen
till the appearances of atrophy have come on.

2. **Inherited syphilis.**—In the secondary stage: *Iritis*
corresponding to that in the acquired disease is seen in a
small number of cases, and occurs between the ages of
about two and fifteen months. • It often gives rise to much
exudation, leading to occlusion of the pupil, and is frequently accompanied by deeper changes, cyclitis and disease of vitreous. It is very often symmetrical, and is much
commoner in girls than boys. *Choroiditis* and *retinitis*, of
precisely the same forms as in acquired syphilis, occur at

the corresponding period of the disease, *i. e.*, between six months and about three years of age; and they show as much (some observers think more) tendency to the degenerative and atrophic results already described; in severe cases there are not uncommonly signs of cerebral degeneration. In the later stages, *keratitis*, which is the commonest eye disease caused by inherited syphilis, occurs. It is commonest between six and fifteen years old, but is sometimes seen as early as two or three years, and is occasionally deferred till after thirty. The disease is frequently complicated with iritis and cyclitis, and, though tending to recovery, shows a considerable liability to relapse. It almost always attacks both eyes, though sometimes at an interval of many months. When the patient is unusually young, the disease as a rule runs a mild and short course. The *oculo-motor palsies* occur but rarely in inherited syphilis, but a few well-authenticated cases are on record.

Smallpox causes inflammation and ulceration of the cornea, leading, in the worst cases, to its total destruction, but in a large number to nothing worse than a chronic vascular ulcer. The corneal disease comes on some days after the eruption (tenth to fourteenth day from its commencement), and after the onset of the secondary fever. Iritis, uncomplicated and showing nothing characteristic of its cause, sometimes occurs some weeks after an attack of smallpox. Only in very rare cases do variolous pustules form on the eye, and even then they are always on the conjunctiva, not on the cornea.

Scarlet fever, typhus, and some other exanthemata may be followed by rapid and complete loss of sight, lasting a day or two, showing no ophthalmoscopic changes, and ending in recovery. Such attacks are believed to be uræmic, or at any rate dependent on some toxic condition of the blood. A peculiarity of these cases is the preservation of the action of the pupils to light. Very severe purulent or

diphtheritic ophthalmia sometimes occurs during scarlet
fever.

Diphtheria.—By far the commonest result is paralysis,
often incomplete, of both the ciliary muscles, *cycloplegia;*
the pupils are not affected except in severe cases, when
they may be rather large and sluggish.[1] The symptoms
generally come on from four to six weeks after the commencement of the illness, last about a month, and disappear completely. Diphtheritic cycloplegia is usually, but
not invariably, accompanied by paralysis of the soft palate.
In most of the cases seen by ophthalmic surgeons the attack
of diphtheria has been mild, sometimes extremely so, the
case often being described as "ulcerated throat;" but inquiry often yields a history of other and severer cases in
the family, and of general depression and weakness in the
patient out of proportion to his throat symptoms. We
find that most of the patients who apply with diphtheritic
cycloplegia are hypermetropic, doubtless because those with
normal, and, *à fortiori,* with myopic, refraction are much
less troubled by paresis of accommodation, and often do
not find it necessary to seek advice. Concomitant convergent squint sometimes develops in hypermetropic children
during diphtheritic paresis, owing to the increased efforts
at accommodation. Paralysis of the external muscles is
occasionally seen; I have never myself seen any except
the external rectus affected, and recovery has been rapid.

Diphtheritic and membranous ophthalmia are occasionally caused by direct inoculation of the conjunctiva of the
attendant by diptheritic material from the patient's throat;
or in the patient himself by extension up the nasal duct
to the conjunctiva. But in many cases of "diphtheritic"
and "membranous" ophthalmia the disease seems to be
local, the inflammation taking on this special form without

[1] Further observations are wanted.

19

ascertainable relation to any infectious disease. No doubt
there is often something peculiar in the patient's health or
in the state of his eye-tissues which gives a proclivity to
this kind of inflammation.   Thus, diphtheritic ophthalmia
of all degrees is more common in young children than in
adults; the worst cases generally occur after measles, or
during or after scarlet fever, broncho-pneumonia, or severe
infantile diarrhœa ; old granular disease of the conjunctiva
also confers a liability to a diphtheritic type of inflammation, and the same tendency is sometimes seen in ophthalmia neonatorum and in gonorrhœal ophthalmia.   As there
seems but seldom any reason to look upon diphtheritic
ophthalmia as the local manifestation of a specific blood
disease, the term "diphtheria of the conjunctiva" should,
I think, seldom be used.

Measles is a prolific source of ophthalmia tarsi in all its
forms, and of corneal ulcers, particularly of the phlyctenular forms.   It also gives rise to a troublesome muco-
purulent ophthalmia, and under bad hygienic conditions
this may be aggravated, by cultivation and transmission,
into destructive disease of purulent, membranous, or diphtheritic type.   Double optic neuritis has been seen in several patients after measles.

Mumps.—Dr. Swan M. Burnett[1] has lately called attention to haze of disc with venous engorgement of retina
and failure of sight during mumps.   Œdema of lids and
conjunctiva, and in one case paresis of third nerve, point
to effusion in the orbit.   The symptoms, as a rule, quickly
subsided.

Chicken-pox is sometimes followed by a transient attack
of mild conjunctivitis.

Whooping-cough often, like measles, leaves a proneness
to corneal ulcers.   In a few rare cases the condition known

---

[1] Burnett, Amer. Journ. of Med. Sci., Jan. 1886, p. 86.

as *ischæmia retinæ* (sudden, temporary, arterial bloodless-
ness) has occurred.

Malarial fevers, especially the severe forms met with in
hot countries, are sometimes the cause of retinal and other
intra-ocular hemorrhages, and even of considerable neuro-
retinitis; when there is much pigment in the blood the
swollen disc may have a peculiar gray color. When renal
albuminuria is caused by malarial disease, albuminuric
retinitis may occur. Simple optic neuritis with failure of
sight, followed by recovery, seems to occur sometimes, and
amblyopia of more than one form is said to be produced
by malarial poisoning; some cases have recovered under
quinine. Loss of sight from malarial fever must not be
confused with blindness due to the quinine administered
for its cure (p. 439).

Relapsing fever is sometimes followed, during convales-
cence, by inflammatory symptoms with opacities in the
vitreous, cyclitis, with or without iritis; recovery takes
place. These cases are commoner in some epidemics than
in others. In a large outbreak Lubinski saw no eye cases
in patients under twenty years of age, and none in females.

Epidemic cerebro-spinal meningitis also, in a few cases,
gives rise to acute choroiditis, with pain, chemosis, and
great tendency to rapid exudation of lymph into the vitreous and anterior chambers, and often leading to disorganization of the eye and blindness.[1] It is believed that
the inflammation may extend to the eye along the optic
nerve, or it may occur independently in the brain and the
eye. Deafness from disease of the internal ear is even
commoner than the eye disease.

Purpura has been observed in a few cases to be accompanied by retinal or subretinal hemorrhages; they are

---

[1] Possibly a few of the cases in which similar eye conditions are seen
without apparent cause may be the accompaniments of slight and un-
recognized meningitis.

sometimes perivascular and linear, and in other cases form
large blotches. They have also, but rarely, been found in
Scurvy. Ecchymosis may also be seen in and around the
eyelids in scurvy. In that form of scurvy which occurs
in infants, especially rickety infants, extravasation may
also occur, as Dr. Barlow has shown,[1] into the orbit, and
probably between the roof of the orbit and its very loosely.
attached periosteum, thus causing proptosis and swelling
of the lids, as well as discoloration.

In **Pyæmia** one or both eyes may be lost by septic emboli
lodging in the vessels of the choroid or retina, and setting
up suppurative panophthalmitis. The symptoms are swelling of the lids, loss of sight, congestion, especially of the
perforating ciliary vessels, Fig. 27, chemosis, discoloration,
and dulness of aqueous and iris. There may or may not
be some protrusion and loss of mobility, and conjunctival
discharge. Pain, sometimes very severe, may be almost
absent; probably its presence indicates rise of tension. A
yellow reflex is often seen from the vitreous. The eyeball
generally suppurates if the patient live long enough. Sometimes both eyes are affected, together or with an interval.
In cases of *Septicæmia* abundant retinal hemorrhages of
large size may occur in both eyes; they come on a few
days before death, and are thus of grave significance. As
they are not present in typhoid and other fevers of corresponding severity, their presence is sometimes an aid in
differential diagnosis.[2]

Lead poisoning is an occasional cause of optic neuro-
retinitis leading to atrophy, of atrophy ensuing upon
chronic amblyopia, and of rapid, usually transient, amblyopia. The two former are the most common; the atrophy,

[1] Med.-Chir. Trans., vol. lxvi., and Keating's Encyclopædia of Diseases of Children, article " Scurvy."
[2] Gowers, Medical Ophthalmoscopy, 2d ed., p. 255.

whether primary or consecutive to papillitis, is generally
accompanied by very marked shrinking of retinal arteries,
and great defect of sight or complete blindness; it is generally symmetrical, but one eye may precede the other.
Other symptoms of lead poisoning, usually chronic, but
occasionally acute, are nearly always present. Care must
be taken not to confuse albuminuric retinitis from kidney
disease induced by lead with the changes here alluded to,
which are due in some more direct manner to the influence
of the metal.

The deposition of lead upon corneal ulcers has been referred to at p. 150.

Alcohol.—Some observers still hold that alcohol, especially in the form of distilled spirits, may cause a particular
form of symmetrical amblyopia, the so-called *amblyopia
potatorum*. Optic neuritis and paralyses of various single
oculo-motor nerves are described by Thomsen as occurring
in cases of alcoholic paralysis. The difficulty of arriving
at the truth depends chiefly upon the fact that most drinkers are also smokers, and that tobacco, whether smoked or
chewed, is allowed by all authorities to be one of the causes,
or, as most now hold, the sole cause, of a similar disease.
The question whether alcohol directly causes disease of the
optic nerves will not be settled until observers are much
more careful than they have hitherto been to record as
typical cases of alcoholic amblyopia only those in which
the patient does not use even the smallest quantity of tobacco in any shape.

Tobacco.—Whatever may be the truth, and it is confess-
edly difficult to arrive at, as to the direct influence of
alcohol, and of the various substances often combined with
it, there is no doubt whatever that tobacco, whether smoked
or chewed, does act directly on the optic nerves, and in
such a manner as to give rise to definite, and usually very
characteristic symptoms. The amblyopia seldom comes on

until tobacco has been used for many years. The quantity needed to cause symptoms is, *cæteris paribus*, a matter of idiosyncrasy, and very small doses may produce the disease in men who in other respects, also, are unable to tolerate large quantities of the drug. Predisposing causes exert a very important influence; amongst these are to be specially noted increasing age; nervous exhaustion from overwork, anxiety, or loss of sleep; chronic dyspepsia, whether from drinking or other causes; and probably sexual excesses and exposure to tropical heat, or light. A large proportion of the patients drink to excess, and thus make themselves more susceptible to tobacco, both by injuring the nervous system and the stomach. But some remarkable cases are seen in men who have for long been total abstainers, in others who have lately become abstainers without lessening their tobacco, and in yet others who are strictly moderate in alcohol, are in robust health, and in whom increasing age is the only recognizable predisposing cause. The strong tobaccos produce the disease far more readily than the weaker sorts, and chewing is more dangerous than smoking. Probably alcohol in very moderate doses counteracts, rather than increases, the injurious effect of tobacco upon the nervous system and optic nerves (Hutchinson).

The vapor of *Bisulphide of Carbon*, if inhaled in a concentrated form and for long periods, produces at first excitement, then general and severe loss of nerve power, with extreme mental and muscular debility and impotence. In some of the cases the sight fails chiefly in the centre of the field, central scotoma, with haze and pallor of the discs, chronic neuritis. The cases are met with either in India-rubber works or oil-mills, in both of which the bisulphide is largely used.[1]

[1] For full particulars, see Trans. Ophth. Soc., vol. v. pp. 149–175 (1885). Another case is reported by Gunn, ibid., vi. 372 (1886).

Quinine, taken in very large doses, at short intervals, has in a few cases caused serious visual symptoms. Sight in both eyes may be totally lost for a time, but recovery, more or less perfect, takes place eventually, sometimes in a few days, sometimes not for months. There is a great contraction of the visual field even after perfect recovery of central vision ; the discs are pale and the retinal arteries extremely diminished. The symptoms are therefore those of almost arrested supply of arterial blood to the retina.

Kidney disease.—The common and well-known retinoneuritis associatied with renal albuminuria, and of which several clinical types are found, has been already described. It need only be noted that the disease is commonest with chronic granular kidneys and in the kidney disease of pregnancy, but that it is also seen in the chronic forms following acute nephritis and in lardaceous disease, and that children suffering from chronic renal disease seem as liable to it as adults. Retinitis with renal albuminuria is usually a sign that the kidney disease is far advanced, and the prospect of life very bad. According to Miley, hospital patients seldom live more than six months after the onset of the retinitis (*Ophth. Soc. Trans.*, viii. 132). C. S. Bull finds that the average duration of life is somewhat longer, according to returns from patients of all classes. There is no doubt that the prospect of life for patients who are able to live carefully is considerably better than for others. It seems likely that there is also a group of cases in which the retinal change precedes the signs of kidney disease, these signs appearing later. Detachment of the retina is an occasional result in extreme cases. The prognosis as regards vision is best in the cases depending on albuminuria of pregnancy The retinal œdema and exudation are probably caused by the blood state ; but the disease of the small bloodvessels and the cardiac hypertrophy, no doubt, add to and complicate the changes. Indeed, the different types of retinal disease which are met probably depend in great measure on the varying parts played by the three factors alluded to. The failure of the sight caused by albuminuric retinitis has often led to the correct diagnosis of cases which had been treated for dyspepsia, headache, or "biliousness."

Diabetes sometimes causes cataract. In young or middle-aged patients the cataract usually forms quickly, and is of course soft. As it is always symmetrical, the rapid formation of double, complete cataract, at a comparatively early age, should always lead to the suspicion of diabetes. In old persons the progress of diabetic cataract is much slower, and often shows no peculiarities. The relation of the lenticular opacity to the diabetes has not been satisfactorily explained; the presence of sugar in the lens, the action of sugar or its derivatives dissolved in the aqueous and vitreous, the abstraction of water from the lens owing to the increased density of the blood; and, lastly, degeneration of the lens from the general cachexia attending the disease, have all been offered in explanation. It is important to know that diabetic cataract sometimes disappears entirely if the health improves, the lens completely clearing up.[1] In a few cases retinitis occurs; sometimes with great œdema and copious, probably capillary, hemorrhages into the retina and vitreous, in other cases with numerous white patches, but no œdema. Plastic iritis sometimes occurs in diabetes both with and without previous operation; Schirmer draws attention to the importance of examining the urine for sugar in cases of intractable iritis. Central amblyopia from disease of the optic nerves has also been observed, even, it is said, in patients who were not smokers.[2]

---

[1] See cases reported in the Trans. Ophthalmological Soc., vol. v. p. 107 (1885).

[2] See a paper by Dr. Edmunds and the author, Trans. Ophth. Soc., vol. iii., 1883. A doubtful case in a woman is recorded in the same

Leucocythæmia is often accompanied by retinal hemorrhages, less commonly by whitish spots bordered by blood, and consisting of white corpuscles; these spots may be thick enough to project forward. Occasionally there is general haziness of the retina. In severe cases the whole fundus is remarkably pale, whether there be other changes or not.[1] The changes are usually symmetrical.

Progressive pernicious anæmia is marked by a strong tendency to retinal hemorrhages; these are usually grouped chiefly near the disc, and are striated (Gowers). White patches are also common, and occasionally well-marked neuritis occurs. I have seen hemorrhages of different dates, and in one case, shown to me by Dr. Sharkey, there had evidently been a large extravasation from the choroid at an earlier period. The disc and fundus participate in the general pallor.

Heart disease is variously related to changes in the eyes and alterations of sight. Aortic incompetence often produces visible pulsation of the retinal arteries. This pulsation often differs from that seen in glaucoma in extending far beyond the disc, and in not being so marked as to cause complete emptying of the larger vessels during the diastole. In glaucoma the pulsation is confined to the disc. The difference is explained by the different mode of production in the two cases: in the one, incomplete closure of the aortic orifice lowers the pressure in the whole blood-column during the diastole, and allows a reflux of blood from the eye; in the other heightened intra-ocular tension, telling chiefly on

paper; and another, also not completely satisfactory, by Samuel, in Hirschberg's Centralblatt, 1882, p. 202. Paper by Moore, New York Med. Journ., 1858.

[1] For a full account of the changes see Gowers' Medical Ophthalmoscopy. Dr. Sharkey has shown me a case with diffuse retinitis, very numerous punctiform hemorrhages, chiefly peripheral, and dilatation, with extreme tortuosity of the veins.

the comparatively yielding tissues of the optic disc, increases the resistance to the entrance of arterial blood.
Valvular disease of the heart is generally present in the
case of sudden lasting blindness of one eye, clinically diagnosed as embolism of the arteria centralis retinæ; but in
some of these thrombosis of the artery or of its companion
vein, or blocking of the internal carotid[1] and ophthalmic
arteries, has been found *post-mortem*. Brief temporary
failure, or even loss, of sight may occur in the subjects of
valvular heart disease, and in some persons who are liable
to recurring headache (see Megrim). Repeated attacks of
this kind sometimes lead to permanent blindness of one eye,
and atrophy of the disc comes on; possibly repeated temporary failures of retinal circulation at length give rise to
thrombosis. In another group of cases which needs investigation, sight fails during successive pregnancies or lacta-
tions, recovering between times; some of these may be
cases of renal retinitis; others may be mere accommodative
asthenopia. It is probable that high arterial tension predisposes to intra-ocular hemorrhage in cases where the small
vessels are unsound, and that the frequent association of
retinal hemorrhage with cardiac disease is thus explained.

Tuberculosis is sometimes accompanied by the formation
of tubercles in the choroid. These may occur in acute
miliary tuberculosis, whether the meninges be involved or
not, but owing to the difficulty of thorough ophthalmoscopic examination in such patients, and the frequently
very small size of the choroidal growths, they are much
more often seen after, than before death. Chronic tubercular tumors of the brain may be accompanied by tubercles
of slow growth and larger size in the choroid, and occasionally these attain such dimensions, and cause such active

---

[1] Gowers' Medical Ophthalmoscopy, p. 29.

symptoms, as to simulate malignant tumors.[1] It is also probable that certain cases of localized choroidal exudation, not accompanied by serious general symptoms or by inflammatory symptoms in the eye, may be of tubercular nature.

Barlow[2] has seen tubercles in the choroid *post-mortem*, in 16 cases; in 13 with, 3 without, tubercular meningitis. Sometimes they took the form of extremely minute dots, "tubercular dust." In 44 children who died of tubercular disease, 42 showing miliary tubercles in the meninges, Dr. Money[3] found tubercles in the choroid of one or both eyes in 14.

Rheumatism.—In acute rheumatism Dr. Barlow informs me that he has more than once seen well-marked congestion of the eyes and photophobia; but neither iritis nor other inflammatory changes occur. The subjects of chronic rheumatism are, however, subject to relapsing inflammation of the eye, usually taking the form of iritis, but sometimes falling entirely on the scleral or episcleral tissues, whilst in others, less common, the changes are apparently confined to the conjunctiva—rheumatic conjunctivitis. But however superficial the inflammation, or congestion, may be, there is no muco-purulent discharge. Some of these patients give a history of acute articular rheumatism as the starting-point of their chronic troubles, others of a prolonged subacute attack, lasting for many months, whilst in others, again, the articular symptoms have never been severe. In yet another series a liability to fascial or muscular rheumatism, or to recurrent neuralgia from exposure to cold or damp, are the only "rheumatic" symptoms of which

---

[1] For interesting cases of and remarks on choroidal tuberculosis in its various forms and relations, see communications by Mackenzie, Barlow, Coupland, and others in Trans. Ophth. Soc., vol. iii. p. 119 *et seq.* (Oct. 1882).

[2] Barlow, Ibid., p. 132.   [3] Money, Lancet, 1883, ii. 813.

a history is given; in some of these the neuralgia is probably gouty. It is to be remembered that the eye is now and then the first part to be attacked by an inflammation which later events show to be clearly related to rheumatism or gout.

Gonorrhœal rheumatism is not unfrequently the starting-point of relapsing iritis and the other conditions named above, as well as of chronic relapsing rheumatism. Rheumatic iritis occurring for the first time with gonorrhœal rheumatism is, in my experience, more often symmetrical than other forms of arthritic iritis, or than the later attacks of iritis in the same patient; a fact which sometimes makes the distinction between rheumatic and syphilitic iritis difficult.

This statement is based on records of 104 cases of iritis with well-marked rheumatic symptoms, and 6 with gonorrhœa but no rheumatism, in all of which syphilis was, so far as possible, excluded. (a) In 34 of this series the first attack of iritis came on during, or very soon after, gonorrhœal rheumatism; and in exactly one-half of these the iritis was double. In 6 others (making 40 in all) there were iritis and gonorrhœa, but no rheumatism ("gonorrhœal iritis"), and here the proportions were the same. (b) In the remaining 70 cases the first iritis had no relation to gonorrhœa; and in the subseries the attack was single in 56 and double in, at the most, 13 (two or three being doubtful), or about one-fifth. No corresponding difference obtained in regard to relapses, the vast majority of the recurrent attacks in both subgroups (a and b) affecting only one eye at a time.

Gonorrhœal iritis.—Some cases of gonorrhœal iritis have been described, in which there is iritis due to gonorrhœa without arthritis being actually present. Probably in these cases the iritis is the first indication of gonorrhœal rheumatism. A variety of quiet conjunctivitis, not due to infection, has also been described without pain, and hardly any discharge (Despagnet and others).

Rheumatic inflammation of the conjunctival or scleral type occurring in gonorrhœa must be carefully distinguished from purulent ophthalmia due to infection with gonorrhœal pus.

In some cases of articular rheumatism in infants suffering from purulent ophthalmia the arthritis is believed to be gonorrhœal, but derived from the conjunctiva instead of the urethra.[1]

It is believed that rheumatism is the cause of some cases of non-suppurating orbital cellulitis, and of relapsing episcleritis. Rheumatism is also believed to cause some other of the ocular paralyses.

Gout.—Gouty persons are not very infrequently the subjects of recurrent iritis indistinguishable from that which occurs in rheumatism. Rheumatism and gout seem sometimes so mixed that it is not always possible to assign to each its right share in the causation of iritis; but that the subjects of true "chalk gout" are liable to relapsing iritis is undoubted. There is, on the whole, more tendency to insidious forms of iritis in gout than in rheumatism. It is also generally believed that the subjects of gout, or persons whose near relatives suffer from it, are particularly subject to glaucoma; acute glaucoma was, indeed, the "arthritic ophthalmia" of earlier authors. Hemorrhagic retinitis is also commoner in gouty persons than in others; it may be single or double, and is to be distinguished from albuminuric retinitis. It has also been observed that the children or descendants of gouty persons, without being themselves subject to gout, are liable, in early adult life, to an insidious form of irido-cyclitis, which sometimes leads to serious consequences;[2] both eyes are likely to be attacked sooner

---

[1] Clement Lucas, Brit. Med. Journ., 1885, ii. pp. 57 and 699; Fendick, ibid., p. 830; Saswornitzky, abstracted in Knapp's Archives, xv. 232 (1886). In a note with which Mr. Lucas has favored me he suggests the term "ophthalmic rheumatism" for these cases.

[2] Hutchinson, Lancet, Jan., 1873.

or later.   The cases in this group probably seem rarer than
they are, from the impossibility in many instances of getting
a full family history.

Several different clinical types may be recognized in the
large group of maladies referred to in this section under
the name of "iritis."   Besides cases of pure iritis, we meet
with examples of cyclitis, in some cases with increase, in
others with decrease, of tension ; in other groups either the
sclerotic or conjunctiva is chiefly affected, true "rheumatic
ophthalmia" without iritis ; a fourth group in which the
pain is disproportionately severe, may be spoken of as neuralgic, and the neuralgic cases are marked by sudden onset,
short duration, and great frequency.   In a large majority,
however, the iris is the headquarters of the morbid action.
All arthritic eye diseases tend strongly to relapse ; they
usually attack only one eye at a time, though both suffer
sooner or later; and they are all much influenced by conditions of weather, being commonest in spring and autumn.

The strumous condition is a fruitful source of superficial
eye diseases, which are for the most part tedious and relapsing, are often accompanied by severe irritative symptoms, but, as a rule, do not lead to serious damage.   The
best types are : (1) the different varieties of ophthalmia
tarsi ; (2) all forms of phlyctenular ophthalmia, " pustular"
or " herpetic" diseases of the cornea and conjunctiva ; (3)
many superficial relapsing ulcers of cornea in children and
adolescents, though not distinctly phlyctenular in origin,
are certainly strumous ; (4) many of the less common, but
very serious, varieties of cyclo-keratitis in adults occur in
connection with lowered health, susceptibility to cold, and
sluggish but irritable circulation, if not with decidedly
scrofulous manifestations.

Leprosy may have its seat in almost any part of the eye,
but it usually occurs first in the superficial parts, and leads
to ectropion, with exposure of the cornea, and xerosis of

the conjunctiva; or there may be a deposit of lepromata in the cornea, leading to its perforation and to panophthalmitis; iritis and cyclitis may also occur, and leprous invasion of the retina has also been seen.

Entozoa sometimes come to rest and develop in the eye or orbit. The commonest intra-ocular parasite is the *cysticercus cellulosæ;* it is excessively rare in this country, but commoner on the Continent. The cysticercus may be found either beneath the retina, in the vitreous, or upon the iris, and may sometimes be recognized in each of these positions by its movements. The parasite has been successfully extracted from the vitreous; when situated on the iris its removal involves an iridectomy. Sometimes it develops under the conjunctiva, where I have seen it set up suppurative inflammation. The *echinococcus* hydatid with multiple cysts may develop to a large size in the orbit and cause much displacement of the eyeball.

B. Eye disease, or eye symptoms, indicative of local disease at a distance.

Megrim is well known to be sometimes accompanied, or even solely manifested, by temporary disorder of sight. This generally takes the form of a flickering cloud, "flittering scotoma" of German authors, with serrated borders, which, beginning near the centre of the field, spreads eccentrically, so as to produce a large defect in the field, a sort of hemianopsia; the borders of the cloud may be brilliantly colored. It is referred to both eyes, and is visible when the lids are closed. The attack lasts only a short time, and perfect sight returns. In many patients this amblyopia is the precursor of a severe sick headache, but in others it constitutes the whole attack; it scarcely ever follows the headache. Less definite and characteristic symptoms, dimness, cloudiness, and muscæ, are complained of by some patients. Recurrent paralysis of the third nerve has several times been ascribed to megrim.

Neuralgia of the fifth nerve, especially of its first division, in a few cases precedes or accompanies failure of sight in the corresponding eye, with neuritis or atrophy of the disc. A liability to neuralgia of the face and head is not unfrequently observed in persons who subsequently suffer from glaucoma. Intense neuralgic pain in the face or head sometimes causes dimness of sight of the same eye whilst the pain lasts. The old belief that injury to branches of the fifth nerve can cause amaurosis is not borne out by modern experience,[1] injury to the optic nerve by fracture of the skull furnishing the true explanation of such cases.

Sympathetic ophthalmitis is the only known instance in which inflammation of the eyeball is caused by local disease of an independent part.

Diseases of the central nervous system may be shown in the eye either at the optic disc, papillitis and atrophy, or in the muscles, strabismus, and diplopia.

The diseases which most often cause *papillitis* are intracranial tumors, syphilitic growths, and meningitis. Abscess of the brain and softening from embolism and thrombosis less commonly cause it, and cerebral hemorrhage scarcely ever.[2] Papillitis has been found in a few cases of acute and subacute myelitis:[3] it does not occur in spinal meningitis.

In a very large proportion, Dr. Gowers thinks at least four-fifths, of all the cases of *cerebral tumor*, including syphilitic growths, optic neuritis occurs at some period. The severity and duration of the neuritis vary much, and probably depend in many cases on the rate of progress, as

[1] References to many of the earlier cases supposed to prove this relation between the fifth and optic nerves are given by Brown-Séquard in Holmes's System of Surgery, 3d ed., vol. ii. p. 206.

[2] A case by Dr. Bristowe in Trans. Ophth. Soc., vol. vi. 1886, p. 363.

[3] Gowers, loc. cit., p. 161 ; Dreschfeld, Lancet, Jan. 7, 1882 ; and Sharkey and Lawford, Trans. Ophth. Soc., vol. iv. p. 232.

well as on the character of the morbid growth. It not uncommonly sets in at no long interval before death, whilst in other cases it is very chronic. There is not much in the characters or course of the papillitis to help us in the localization of intracranial tumor ; and although a very high degree of papillitis, with signs of great obstruction to the retinal circulation, generally indicates cerebral tumor, there are many cases in which the presence of papillitis does not help us to decide the nature of the intracranial disease, whether tumor, meningitis, or syphilitic disease.

Analyzing 96 cases of fatal cerebral tumor, Edmunds and Lawford found that optic neuritis was observed in 19 of 41 cases where the disease was at or toward the convexity (or 46 per cent.); whilst it was seen in 41 of 55 cases where the disease was chiefly at the base (or 75 per cent.). In 43 cases the tumor was either in the basal ganglia or the cerebellum, and in 37 of these (= 86 per cent.) optic neuritis occurred (*Trans. of Ophth. Soc.*, 1884, vol. iv. p. 172).

Tumors also sometimes cause simple optic atrophy by pressing upon or invading some part of the optic fibres.

Intracranial syphilitic disease is a common cause of papillitis ; the disease being either a gummatous growth in the brain, or a growth or thickening beginning in the dura mater, or basilar meningitis. The prognosis is much better than in cerebral tumors if vigorous treatment be adopted early ; indeed, in all cases of papillitis where intracranial disease is diagnosed, and syphilis even remotely possible, mercury and iodide of potassium should be promptly given.

Meningitis often causes papillitis, but in this respect much depends on its position and duration. Meningitis limited to the convexity, whatever its cause, is seldom accompanied by ophthalmoscopic changes ; on the other hand, basic meningitis very often causes neuritis.

Amongst 16 cases of injury to the head ending in death Edmunds and Lawford never found optic neuritis without basic meningitis ; whilst they found no neuritis when the damage was limited to the convexity (*Ophth. Soc.*, Oct. 1886).

The neuritis in basic meningitis is probably proportionate to the duration and intensity of the intracranial mischief, being comparatively slight in acute and rapidly fatal cases, whether tubercular or not. In tubercular meningitis papillitis is very common,[1] and its occurrence seems especially related to the presence of inflammatory changes about the chiasma (Gowers); and even the neuritis occurring in cases of cerebral tumor seems often to be caused by secondary meningitis set up by the growth.[2] In a form of meningitis in young children, named by Drs. Gee and Barlow "posterior basic," optic neuritis is infrequent, though the patients often live some little time. When patients recover from meningitis the neuritis may pass into atrophy, and cause amaurosis ; such cases are well known to ophthalmic surgeons ; it is probable that some of them may be instances of recovery from tubercular meningitis. In rare cases papillitis occurs with severe head symptoms, ending in death, but without microscopic changes in the brain or membranes. Microscopical changes in the brain substance, justifying the term cerebritis, have been found in one such case by Dr. Sutton, and in another by Dr. Stephen Mackenzie.[3] It must not be forgotten that optic neuritis may be caused by various altered conditions of the blood ; and that it is occasionally seen without any evidence either of central nervous disease or of blood changes.

Hydrocephalus rarely causes papillitis, but often at a late stage causes atrophy of the optic nerves from the

---

[1] Garlick found it in 23 of 26 fatal cases, Med.-Chir. Trans., vol. lxii. Money (loc. cit.) discovered it in only 16 of 42 fatal cases. Slight papillitis is very easily overlooked in delirious or fretful children.

[2] Edmunds and Lawford, Trans. of Ophth. Soc., iii. 138, 1883.

[3] Also a case by Dr. Silk, Brit. Med. Journ., May 26, 1883.

pressure of the distended third ventricle on the chiasma.
Dr. Barlow informs me that he has several times seen a
very gross form of choroiditis ending in immense patches of
atrophy. I have recorded one such case, and seen others.

The diseases most commonly causing *atrophy not preceded by papillitis* are the chronic progressive diseases of
the spinal cord, especially locomotor ataxy. The atrophy
in these cases is slowly progressive, double, though seldom
beginning at the same time in both eyes, and it always ends
in blindness, although sometimes not until after many
years. Similar atrophy sometimes occurs in the early
stages of general paralysis of the insane, but chiefly in
cases complicated by marked ataxic symptoms. It is also,
but much more rarely, seen in lateral and in insular sclerosis. In the latter, amblyopia with slight neuritic
changes is occasionally seen, and sight may improve or
almost recover after having been defective for some time.
In cases of homonymous lateral hemianopia we find that
sometimes the blind half of the field is separated from the
seeing half by a straight line which passes through the fixation point (Fig. 93), whilst more commonly this dividing
line deviates toward the blind half in the central part of
the field, thus leaving a small central area of perfect vision.
Ferrier has suggested that in the former cases the lesion
is probably situated in the tract, and that in the latter it
lies in some part of the cortical visual centre.

Motor disorders of the eyes.—Some of the commoner
causes of ocular palsy have been already given. It may
be mentioned here that basic meningitis often causes paralysis of one or more of the ocular nerves, with squinting,
and double vision if the patient be conscious; and, further,
that the palsy in such cases often varies, or appears to
vary, from day to day.

Locomotor ataxy and general paralysis of the insane are
sometimes preceded by paralysis, usually, but not always,

temporary, of one or more of the eye muscles, causing
diplopia ; and there may for years be nothing else to attract
attention. The same disease may also be ushered in by
internal ocular paralysis. The most frequent variety is
loss of the reflex action of the pupils to sensory stimulation
of the skin and to light, whilst their associated action
remains, "reflex iridoplegia ;" when shaded and lighted
they remain absolutely motionless, but they dilate when
accommodation is relaxed and contract when it is in
action ("Argyll Robertson symptom").[1] This phenome-
non is often, though by no means always, associated with
a contracted state of the pupils, and hence the term
"spinal miosis" is often, but incorrectly, used. This reflex paralysis of the iris is one of the most valuable of the
early signs of locomotor ataxy. We do not, however, yet
know how often it may occur in healthy persons or without
eventual spinal disease; it certainly has comparatively
little significance in old persons Recent observations
show that, at least in general paralysis of the insane, loss
of reflex dilatation to sensory stimulation of the skin is
probably the earliest pupillary change [2] The complementary symptom, loss of associated, with retained reflex,
action of the pupils, has not been fully studied Any of
the other internal paralyses may also in certain cases occur
as precursors of ataxy. Paralysis of one third nerve coming
on with hemiplegia of the opposite side may, but does not
necessarily, indicate disease of the crus cerebri on the side
of the palsied third nerve.[3] Ophthalmoplegia externa has
been already mentioned ; it may here be added that cases
occur in which this condition appears to be "functional,"
in which, at any rate, the symptoms come on quickly and

[1] Argyll Robertson, Edinburgh Med. Journ., 1869, p. 703.

[2] Bevan Lewis, Trans. Ophth. Soc., vol. iii., 1883.

[3] For exceptions see Robin, Troubles Oculaires dans les Maladies de
l'Encéphale, 1880, p. 95.

pass off completely, recurring perhaps at a later period ; of these cases I have seen several in young adults.

Double ophthalmoplegia externa is the extreme type of a large and important class of ocular palsies, to which much attention has been given recently, characterized by the paralysis of certain *movements*, usually associated movements of the two eyes, not of the *muscles* supplied by a certain nerve. There may be, *e. g.*, loss of power of both eyes to look upward, both superior recti, or loss of power to look to the right, R. external and L. internal rectus ; and yet in the latter case the L. internal rectus, if differently associated, as with the R. internal during convergence, may act perfectly well. Such associated paralyses are explained by lesions, usually sclerotic, occasionally tumor, affecting the centres for certain combined movements, which are more central anatomically and higher physiologically than the centres of origin of the nerve trunks. Cases of paralysis of both third or both sixth nerves, and also of complete ophthalmoplegia, are sometimes due to symmetrical coarse disease, syphilitic gummata, for instance, of the affected nerve trunks. The symptoms in all the cases referred to in this paragraph may be temporary or permanent, acute or chronic, and caused by various fine or coarse anatomical changes ; and they are frequently associated with other and graver nervous symptoms. It is of great importance in cases of multiple and associated ocular paralysis to make out, if we can, whether the symptoms point to peripheral disease (disease of nerve trunks), or to disease of the nuclei of origin of the nerves, or to lesion of the centres for certain movements.

Insular (disseminated) sclerosis is often accompanied by nystagmus, characterized by irregularity, both of the amplitude and rapidity of the movements.

There appears to be an intimate relation between the

occurrence of *Convulsions* and the formation of lamellar cataract, this form of cataract being scarcely ever seen, except in those who have had fits in infancy. A very striking deformity of the permanent teeth is also nearly always present, depending upon an abruptly limited deficiency or absence of the enamel on the part furthest from the gum, Fig. 163 (7). The teeth affected are the first molars, incisors, and canines, of the permanent set. The dental changes are quite different from those which are pathognomonic of inherited syphilis, although mixed forms are sometimes seen. The relation between the convulsions, the cataract, and the defective dental enamel has not been satisfactorily explained. Mr. Hutchinson has collected many facts in favor of the belief that the dental defect is due to stomatitis interfering with the calcification of the enamel before the eruption of the teeth, and that mercury is the commonest cause of this stomatitis. On this hypothesis the coincidence of the dental defect and the cataract is due to mercury having been usually prescribed for the infantile convulsions from which these cataractous children suffer. It seems, however, reasonable to suppose that the defect of the crystalline lens and of the enamel, both of them epithelial structures, may be caused by some common influence; although the facts that the peculiar teeth are often seen without the cataract, and the cataract occasionally seen with perfect teeth, appear to weaken this view.[1]

Hysterical eye symptoms (see pp. 272, 378).

C. Cases in which the eye shares in a local process affecting the neighboring parts.

In **herpes zoster** of the first division of the fifth nerve the eye participates. When only the supra-orbital or

---

[1] Mr. Edgar Browne contends that in lamellar cataract without history of fits the teeth are usually good. Ophth. Review, v. 354 (1886).

supra-trochlear branches are attacked the eyeball usually
escapes or is only superficially congested. But if the
eruption occur on the parts supplied by the nasal branch,
i. e., if the spots extend down to the tip of the nose, there
is usually inflammation of the proper tissues of the eyeball,
ulceration or infiltration of cornea, and iritis; for the sensitive nerves of the cornea, iris, and choroid are derived,
through the long root of the ophthalmic ganglion, from
the nasal branch. Occasionally the eye suffers, however,
when the nasal branch escapes. The pain and swelling of
the herpetic region are often so great that the attack gets
the name of " erysipelas." In rare cases atrophy of the
optic nerve and paralysis of the third and other neighboring nerves occur with the herpes.[1]

In **paralysis of the first division of the fifth** the cornea
and conjunctiva are anæsthetic; the cornea may be touched
or rubbed without the patient feeling at all. In many
cases ulceration of the cornea, usually uncontrollable and
destructive in character, takes place. It is doubtful whether
this is due directly to paralysis or irritation of trophic fibres
running in the trunk of the fifth, or indirectly to the anæsthesia.[2] In regard to the latter, it is certain that the loss of
feeling (1) allows injuries and irritations to occur unper-
ceived, and (2) by removing the reflex effect of the sensory
nerves on the calibre of the bloodvessel, permits inflammation to go on uncontrolled.

In **paralysis of the facial nerve** the eyelids cannot be
shut and the cornea remains more or less exposed. When
a strong effort is made to close the lid the eyeball rolls
upward beneath the upper lid. Epiphora is a common

---

[1] A useful paper on facial herpes with many references by Mr.
Jessop, is published in vol. vi. of the Ophthalmological Society's
Transactions, 1886.

[2] Gowers considers it due more to irritation of the nerve than to the
anæsthesia. Diagnosis of Diseases of Brain, p. 90.

result of facial palsy. Severe ulceration of the cornea
may result from the exposure.

Paralysis of the cervical sympathetic causes some narrowing of the palpebral fissure from slight drooping of the
upper lid, apparent recession of the eye into the orbit, and
more or less miosis from paralysis of the dilator of the
pupil. No changes are observed in the calibre of the
bloodvessels of the eye or in the secretion of tears, The
pupil is said to be less contracted after division of the sympathetic trunk than when the trunk of the fifth, and with
it the oculo-sympathetic fibres, is cut, and knowledge of
this may be now and then useful in diagnosis.

In **exophthalmic goitre**, Graves's disease, the eyeballs
are too prominent, and the protrusion is almost invariably
bilateral, though not unfrequently greater on the right
side. It is often apparently increased in slight cases by an
involuntary elevation of the upper lids when looking forward, and by the lids not following the cornea as they
should do when the patient looks down.

In severe cases the proptosis may be so great as to prevent full closure of the lids, and, in these, dangerous ulceration of the cornea is to be feared. In such cases it is
beneficial to shorten the palpebral fissure by uniting the
borders of the lids at the outer canthus, or even to unite
the lids in their whole length (p. 389). No changes are
present in the fundus excepting sometimes dilatation of
arteries and spontaneous arterial pulsation. The seat of
the lesion causing this peculiar malady is not yet known.
It has been generally supposed to be due to some morbid
condition of the sympathetic, but recent speculations point
to a localized central lesion, probably in the medulla ob-
longata, as being more likely.[1]

[1] See an able paper by Dr. W. A. Fitz-Gerald in the Dublin Journ.
Med. Sci. for March and April, 1883.

Erysipelas of the face sometimes invades the deep tissues of the orbit and causes blindness by affecting the optic nerve and retina; on recovery the eye is found to be blind and the ophthalmoscope shows either simple atrophy of the disc or signs of past retinitis also. Other forms of orbital cellulitis may lead to the same result.

Note on the teeth in inherited syphilis, *with description of Fig.* 163.—None of the *first set* of teeth are characteristically altered, though the incisors frequently decay early.

In the *permanent set* only two teeth, the central upper incisors, are to be relied upon ; but the other incisors, both upper and lower, and the first molars, are often deformed from the same cause. The characteristic change in the upper central incisors appears to depend upon defective formation of the central lobe of the tooth, Fig. 163 (Nos. 2, 5, and 6). Soon after eruption of the tooth this lobe wears away, leaving at the centre of the cutting edge a vertical notch (No. 1). If the cause have acted so intensely as entirely to prevent the development of the central lobe, we find instead of the notch a narrowing and thinning of the cutting edge in comparison with the crown, and this, according to its degree, produces a resemblance to a screwdriver, or to a peg (Nos. 3 and 4). The teeth are also usually too small in every dimension, so that the incisors are often separated from one another by considerable spaces. In extreme cases all the incisors are peggy and much dwarfed. The changes are usually symmetrical, but No. 5 shows one tooth typically deformed and the other normal.

Fig. 163 (No. 7) shows in an extreme degree the changes due to absence of enamel from the permanent teeth ("mercurial," "stomatitic," "strumous," and "rickety" teeth). The change occurs in lines running horizontally across the whole set of permanent incisors and canines. When slight

20

it affects only the part near the edge, the enamel beginning as a sudden terrace or step a little distance from the edge;

FIG. 163.

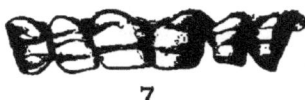

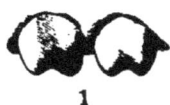

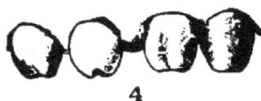

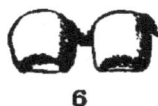

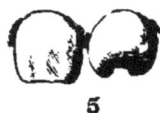

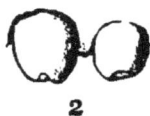

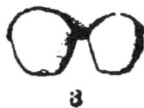

in bad cases several such "terraces" are present, and the whole tooth is rough, pitted, and discolored. The first permanent molars show a corresponding change on the grinding surface. It is this imperfection that is found present in nearly all cases of lamellar cataract, though the dental condition is common enough in persons without that or any other form of cataract.

[SUPPLEMENT.

THE PRACTICAL EXAMINATION OF RAILWAY EMPLOYÉS AS TO COLOR-BLINDNESS, ACUTENESS OF VISION AND HEARING.

BY WILLIAM THOMSON, M.D.

IN accordance with a wish expressed many months ago, that I should suggest some practical method for the examination of the employés of the Pennsylvania Railroad, as to their ability to see the colored signals by day and night used in the service, I devoted much time to the subject, in an effort to overcome the following difficulties:

1. To ascertain whether each man possesses *sight* enough to see *form* at the average distance; and *range of vision* to enable him to see near objects well enough to read written or printed orders and instructions. 2. To learn if each man has color-sense sufficient to judge promptly, by day or night, between the colors in use for signals. 3. To determine the ability of each man to hear distinctly.

The difficulties to be overcome were found in the magnitude of the task, involving the examination of thousands of men now in the service, with the necessity of extending it to all who may be hereafter employed, distributed over thousands of miles of road; and in the absence of professional experts in sufficient number, possessing enough special training to fit them to decide with precision the points at issue.

It soon became apparent that some system would be needed that could be put in force by each division superintendent, acting through an intelligent employé, under the general supervision of one or more ophthalmic surgeons of recognized skill, to whom all information collected could be transmitted, and who would be able to decide all doubtful cases, and thus protect the road from any danger arising from incapable employés, and save good and faithful men from the evil of being discharged from the company's service, or prevented from being employed on other roads on insufficient grounds.

It was believed that the facts could be collected by non-professional persons, and could be so clearly presented to the division superintendent and to the professional expert, as to enable a perfectly correct decision to be made in every case ; and that men fit for service would be recognized, whilst those deficient in sight, color-sense, or hearing, could be referred to the expert if they so desired, or transferred to places in the service where their defects, if not remediable by treatment, could do no harm either to the road or to the public.

Such a system was submitted to the general manager of the Pennsylvania Railroad, and has been perfected by the labors of a special committee of the Society of Transportation Officers in conjunction with the writer. The entire method has furthermore been submitted to a practical experimental test extending over nearly two thousand men, employed as conductors, engineers, firemen, and brakemen, and the results have satisfied the committee and myself that our object has been fully attained, and that the system proposed may now be put in force with confidence in its practical utility. As an evidence of this, I may cite two complete detailed reports, including 1383 men in all. The blanks upon which the original entries were made have all been submitted to me, and they satisfy me that the results in the summary of each of these excellent reports may be confidently accepted, and thus we have become acquainted with the fact that there were in the service of the Pennsylvania Railroad, of the 1383 men examined, 246 men deficient in the full acuteness of vision, 55 absolutely color-blind, and 21 defective in hearing.

In one of the reports, an examination, not included in the instructions from the committee, was made with colored flags and colored lights by night, and 13 men failed to be able to recognize them from a total of 24, who were color-blind to the test used for its detection, but I have little doubt whatever that the entire number of color-blind, viz., 55, would also fail under a carefully devised system of tests by the usual railroad signals.

The entire number reported as *defective* in color-sense, $4\frac{2}{10}$ per cent., is up to the average as reported by the best authorities in its percentage, but those absolutely color-blind, and hence unable to distinguish between a soiled white or gray and green, or a green and red flag, are fully 4 per cent.; and this proves that the instrument employed in this part of the examination has met our expectations fully.

As this was the point about which I had most doubt, a word or two of explanation may be proper, more especially as many good authorities declare that no examination for color-blindness should be accepted, unless made by professional specialists.

The examination for color-blindness now generally accepted and proposed by Prof. Holmgren, consists in testing the power of a person to match various colors, which are most conveniently used in the form of colored yarns. Usually about 150 tints are employed, in a confused mixture, and three test colors, viz., *light-green*, *rose* or *purple*, and *red*, are placed in the foregoing order before the person examined, who is directed to select similar colors from the mass. The examiner sits then in judgment, and decides whether the color-sense is perfect from the selections made, or from those *not* made, or from them both, and from the prompt or hesitating manner of the examined. It has been our effort to render this more simple, and to so arrange the colors that they may be identified by some number, so that an expert, although absent from the scene, would know by these numbers the exact tints selected, and thus be fully competent to declare from them the color-perception of any person whose record had been properly made. From theory based upon scientific knowledge, and from much experience, I was able to arrange an instrument that would have the real colors, and those usually confounded with them, " confusion colors," placed in such relations to each other, and so designated by numbers, as to make an examination for color-blindness possible by a non-professional person, who could conduct the testing, record it properly, and transmit it to an expert capable of deciding upon the written results. Hence there is no departure from the system of matching tints already established, the only novelty being in reducing the number of colors to those similar to the test colors, and to those usually chosen by color-blind persons, and so identifying them as to enable an absent expert or superintendent to know precisely what colors had been selected to match the test colors.

The theory of the instrument (consisting of a stick with the yarns attached, see Fig. 164), is that color-blindness is most promptly detected by using the *light-green test-skein*, and asking that it be matched in color from the yarns on the stick, which are arranged to be alternately green and confusion colors, and are numbered from one to twenty, the person being directed to select ten tints, and the examiner being required to note the numbers of the tints chosen. It will be understood that the odd numbers are the green, and the even ones the confusion colors, and that, if a person has a good color-sense, his record will exhibit none but odd numbers; whilst, if he be color-blind, the mingling of even numbers betrays his defect at a glance to the supervising expert or superintendent.

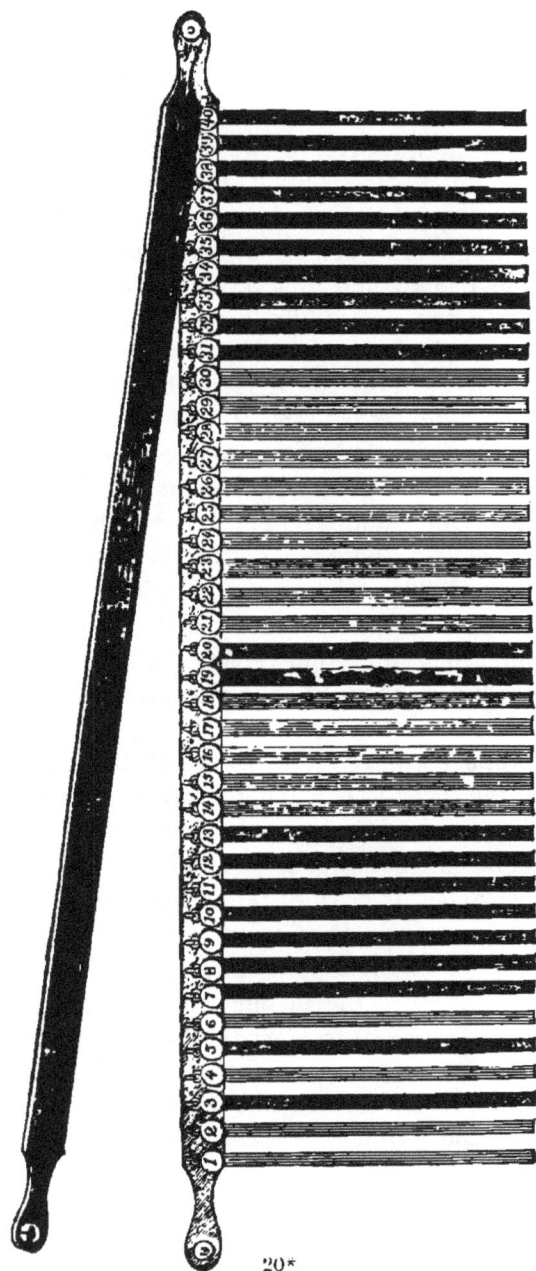

Fig. 164.

There are forty tints on the stick, and the first twenty are given to the detection of color-blindness, using the *green-test*, and if the color-sense is deficient, it will surely be revealed.

To distinguish, however, between green-blindness and red-blindness, the *rose-test* is used, and those color-blind will select indifferently, either the blues intermingled with the rose, between figures 20 and 30, or perhaps the blue-green or grays from 1 to 20, and thus reveal their defect, and establish either green- or red-blindness.

Finally, the *red-test* corroborates these results, and satisfies the most sceptical of color defect, when the "confusion tints" or even numbers between 30 and 40 are selected.

On a suitable blank these figures are placed in the order of examination, and a glance of the eye reveals the color-sense of the person examined; since, if anything but odd numbers are chosen, there is a defect; or if, with test one, anything beyond 20 is chosen; or if, with test two, anything but odd numbers between 20 and 30; or, with test three, anything but odd numbers between 30 and 40. The colors can readily be changed on the instrument, if it should be found desirable.

It is theoretically and practically a fact, that the tints as arranged in the three sets on the instrument look quite the same in color to color-blind persons, and that those having a perfect color-sense can thus form an idea of this infirmity. If, then, green and gray are indistinguishable, and green and red, when of the same depth of color, seem to be entirely the same to the color-blind, it needs no opinion from a scientific expert to convince the manager of a railroad that it would be most dangerous to place the lives of people under the guidance of an engineer who could not distinguish, if green-blind, between a soiled white and a green flag, or between a green and red flag, or other signal of these colors.

It is a fact that some of the color-blind promptly give

the proper names to the flags, and answer correctly, when asked what they would do in presence of such signals, but it must be remembered that they may see form perfectly, and have always had some perception of these colors, and do give them their conventional names, perhaps, but that they are unable to distinguish them at once and infallibly, and that it will only require a further extension of our method of testing to demonstrate the inability of persons color-blind to our examination to recognize the signals, by day or night, which are now depended upon to prevent accidents of the gravest character. This must be done by demanding that the signals be matched, and not named, and this is incorporated in the instructions herewith submitted, so that the tints which color-blind men select with the railroad signals from the instrument may hereafter be known and recorded.

My conclusions from a study of the subject in connection with the railway service are:

1. That there are many employés who have defective sight, caused either by optical defects, which are, perhaps, congenital, and which might be corrected with proper glasses, or due to the results of injuries or diseases of the eyes, remediable or not, by medical or surgical treatment.

2. That one man in twenty-five will be found color-blind to a degree to render him unfit for service where prompt recognition of signals is needed, inasmuch as color-blindness for red and green renders signals of these colors indistinguishable. It is a fact in physiological optics, however, that yellow and blue are seen by those color-blind for red and green, and that yellow-violet blindness is so rare that it might lead to the use of these yellow and blue colors, in preference to red and green, wherever possible.

3. That color-blindness, although mainly congenital and incurable, is sometimes caused by disease or injury, and that precautions might be needed to have either periodical

examinations or to insist upon it in cases where men have suffered from severe illness or injury, or when they have been addicted to the abuse of tobacco or alcohol.

4. That the method, when adopted, will enable the authorities to know exactly how many of their employés are "satisfactory in every particular" as to sight and hearing; and that the examination will have the further value of making the division superintendents acquainted with the general aptitude of the men in their divisions as to general intelligence.

5. That the entire examinations can be made at the rate of at least six men an hour; whilst that for color-sense alone can be done in a very few minutes for each man by an intelligent employé.

6. That to secure the confidence of the employés, and of competent scientific critics, as well as of the public generally, it is advisable to have some official professional specialist to whom all doubtful questions could be referred, and who should be held responsible for the accuracy of the instruments, test-cards, etc., to be put in use, and who should have a general supervision of the entire subject of sight, color-sense, and hearing.

7. That from the impossibility of subjecting the immense number of employés on our large railways to the inspection of the few medical experts available, and to secure the examination of those hereafter to be employed, some system of testing by the railway superintendents has become a necessity, and it is believed that the one proposed will answer the purpose.

PENNSYLVANIA RAILROAD COMPANY'S INSTRUCTIONS FOR
EXAMINATION OF EMPLOYÉS AS TO VISION, COLOR-
BLINDNESS, AND HEARING.

Instructions for examination as to vision, color-blindness, and hearing.—The examination will be made as to vision, color-sense, and hearing, and the following apparatus will be used:

1. A card or disk of large letters for testing distant sight. 2. A book or card of print for testing sight at a short distance. 3. An adjustable frame for supporting the print to be read, with a graduated rod attached for measuring the distance from the eye while reading. 4. A spectacle frame for obstructing the vision of either eye while testing the other. 5. An assortment of colored yarns for testing the sense of color. 6. A watch with a loud tick for testing the hearing. 7. A book or set of blanks for recording the observations. 8. A copy of an approved work on "Color-blindness."

Acuteness of vision.—For distant vision, place the test-disk or card in a good light twenty feet distant, and ascertain for each eye separately the smallest letters that can be read distinctly, and record the same by the number of that series on the card.

Range of vision.—For near vision, ascertain the least number of inches at which type D = 0.5 or 1½, can be read with each eye, and record the result.

Field of vision.—Let the examiner stand in front of the examined, at a distance of three feet, and directing the examined to fix his eyes on the right eye of the examiner, and keep them so fixed, let the examiner extend his arm laterally, and opening and shutting his hands, let him by questions satisfy himself that his hands are seen by the examined without changing the direction of the eyes; recording the result as good or defective, as the case may be.

Color-sense.—Three test-skeins—A, light-green; B, rose; C, red—will be used with the colored yarns attached to the stick; of the latter there are forty tints, numbered from 1 to 40, and arranged in three sets—a, b, and c—of which the odd numbers correspond to the colors of the test-skeins, whilst the even numbers are different or "confusion colors."

The first set is to test for color-blindness; the second to determine whether it be red or green blindness, and the third to confirm the opinion formed from the first or second test.

Place the test-skein A at a distance of not less than three feet, and, without naming the color, direct the person examined to name the color, and to select from the first twenty tints, or set (a), of the yarns on the stick, ten tints of the same color as skein A, stating that they do not match, but are different shades of the same color. Record the number of the tints so selected. Do the same with skeins B and C, using for B the tints from 21 to 30, and for C the tints from 31 to 40. If the odd numbers are selected readily, the examination may be gone over very quickly.

When color-blindness is detected, any one of the even numbers or "confusion colors" may be used as a test-skein, and the man may be directed to select similar tints, when he will most probably choose odd numbers, which should be recorded, stating the number on the stick of the "confusion color" used for a test, and then giving the numbers chosen to match it.

Then a soiled *white* flag should be shown, and the man be directed to select tints to match it, which should be recorded; next a *green*, and finally a *red* flag.

All of the particulars are to be recorded as the examination proceeds, not leaving it to memory. Use the numbers in recording. The letters indicating the set need not be used. Note whether the selection is prompt or hesitating by a distinct mark after the proper word on the blank form. When deficient color-sense is discovered, and variations in the mode of testing are made by the examiner or examined, they should be noted under remarks, or on a separate sheet to be referred to, if the blank has not room enough.

Hearing.—Note the number of feet or inches distant from each ear at which a watch, having a tick loud enough to be heard at five feet, is heard distinctly, using a watch without a tick, or a stop watch, to detect any supposed deception; and the number of feet at which ordinary conversation is heard.

Explanations.—The test-card contains letters, numbered from 20 (xx), or $D = 6$, to 200 (cc), or $D = 60$. Those measuring three-eighths of an inch, and numbered 20 (xx) or $D = 6$, are such as a good eye of ordinary power sees distinctly twenty feet or six metres distant. If a man sees distinctly only those marked C (or 100), his acuteness of vision, V., is equal to $\frac{20}{100}$ or $\frac{1}{5}$. If he sees to XX (or 20), then V. is equal to $\frac{20}{20}$ or 1, and his sight is up to the full standard. This mode of statement indicates the relative value of the sight examined, and should be used in the records. If one eye is $\frac{20}{20}$ or 1, and the other not less than $\frac{20}{55}$ or $\frac{1}{2}$x, with or without glasses, the sight may be considered satisfactory.

The power of discerning small objects at the reading distance is tested by the small print, and good sight may be assumed if one eye can see at twenty inches the matter marked $1\frac{1}{2}$ or $D = 0.5$, whilst the other distinguishes not less than $4\frac{1}{2}$ or $D = 1.5$. The small print should then be brought to the point of nearest vision for each eye, and that point mentioned in inches. A good eye should be able to read No. $1\frac{1}{2}$ at twenty inches, and have a *range of vision* up to ten inches.

The color-test will indicate whether the man is deficient in color sense. The colors are arranged in three sets, one of 20 and two of 10 each—the odd numbers are the colors similar to the test-skeins, and the even numbers are the "confusion colors," or those which the color-blind will be likely to select to match the sample skeins or colors shown him. The first 20 (*a*), numbered from 1 to 20, have green tints for the odd numbers or test-colors. In the second (*b*), 21 to 30, the test-colors are rose or purple, a combination of red and blue; and in the third (*c*), 31 to 40, they are red. Ordinarily the test will be with each set separately, but the whole 40 may be employed on any test-skein. Anything but *green* matched with *green* indicates a defect in the color sense, for which use set (*a*).

The test with the second set indicates whether red or green blindness exists. The odd numbers from 21 to 30 are purple. If either of these is matched with test-skein B, nothing is indicated, as they must appear alike to a color-blind person; but if blue is chosen, red-blindness is indicated, and if green, then green-blindness is established.

The third set (*c*) is scarcely needed, but may be used in confirmation of, or in connection with, the last, as to red or green defect.

When the numbers of the tints selected are recorded in the proper blank, color-blindness will be indicated in those instances where even numbers appear, and suspicions will arise where numbers beyond 20 are used with test-skein A, and under 21 or beyond 30 with B, and below 31 with C.

Further tests should be made of those found to be color-blind with the usual signal flags, requesting them to name each color, shown singly, and to match the colors of them from the tints on the stick, and with colored lamps; and finally to state what they understand them to mean as signals.

It will be well not to dwell on the examination of a man

found to be defective in color-sense or in vision, but to pass over each examination with the same general care, and afterwards send for those giving indications of defects, to come in singly for fuller examination. The examination should be private as far as practicable, especially excluding persons who are to be subsequently examined.

Inability to name color accurately, or to distinguish nicely as to difference in tint, is not to be taken as an evidence of color-blindness.

In testing as to hearing, if the watch used can be heard at five feet distant, and the person examined hears it only at one foot, his hearing would be 1–5, and may be so recorded in fractions. Conversation in an ordinary tone should be heard at ten feet.

It should be understood that all employés examined, failing to come up to the requirements of the above standard, shall be accorded the benefit of a professional examination. When acuteness of vision is below the standard adopted, it may be possible to restore full vision by proper glasses, when it is due to optical defects, known as near-sight, far-sight, or astigmatism, or by other medical or surgical treatment, and useful men may then be retained in the company's service.

These rules and regulations, having been approved by the Board of Managers, have been put into effect on the Pennsylvania Railroad, under the general supervision of the writer, and give entire satisfaction.]

APPENDIX.

FORMULÆ, ETC.

NITRATE OF SILVER.

1. *Mitigated Solid Nitrate of Silver* (B. P. 1885):

> Nitrate of Silver 1,
> Nitrate of Potash 2.

Fused together and run into moulds to form short, pointed sticks.

Used for granular lids and purulent ophthalmia.

The strength above given is known as No. 1, and is that which I generally use; three weaker forms are made, known as Nos. 2, 3, and 4, containing respectively 3, 3½, and 4 parts of nitrate of potash to 1 of nitrate of silver.

Pure nitrate of silver is never to be used to the conjunctiva.

2. *Solutions of Nitrate of Silver:*

> (1) Nitrate of Silver gr. x or xx,
> Distilled Water ℥j.

Used by the surgeon for purulent ophthalmia, granular lids, and chronic conjunctivitis, and some cases of ulcer of the cornea.

3. (2) Nitrate of Silver gr. j or ij,
> Distilled Water ℥j.

Used by the patient in various forms of ophthalmia; only a few drops to be used at a time, and not more than three times a day.

All solutions of nitrate of silver should be kept in glass-stoppered bottles; any trace of organic matter decomposes the salt, and a black deposit of metallic silver falls to the bottom; the action of light favors this decomposition: amber-tinted glass is said to counteract the chemical action of light. Dark-blue bottles should not be used, as they only hide the deposit of reduced silver.

SULPHATE OF COPPER.

4. A crystal of *Pure Sulphate of Copper*, smoothly pointed, may be used for touching granular lids of old standing.

5. *Lapis Divinus* :

> Sulphate of Copper 1,
> Alum 1,
> Nitrate of Potash 1.

Fused together, and camphor equal to $\frac{1}{36}$ of the whole added. The preparation is run into moulds to form sticks. It should be kept in a stoppered bottle.

Largely used for the treatment of chronic granular lids.

6. Solutions of sulphate of copper or of Lapis Divinus, gr. j in ℥j of distilled water, are also very useful for many forms of chronic conjunctivitis.

LEAD LOTION :

7.   Liquor Plumbi Subacetatis (B. P.) ʒj,
           Distilled Water Oj.
                     (1 in 160.)

Used in chronic conjunctivitis *when the cornea is sound*, and in inflammation of the eyelids and lachrymal sac.

SPIRIT LOTION :

8.   Rectified (or Methylated) Spirit ℥iv,
           Water ℥xvj.

Used as an evaporating lotion to allay or prevent inflammation of the wound after operation on the eyelids.

9. *Lead and Spirit Lotion* :

> Spirit Lotion Oj,
> Liquor Plumbi Subacetatis (B. P.) ʒij.

Used in the same cases when there is no fear that the cornea is abraded or ulcerated. A better antiphlogistic than spirit alone.

MERCURY :

10. Since the publication of Sattler's experiments on anti-septics in 1883, weak *Solutions of Perchloride of Mercury* have come largely into use for cleansing the conjunctiva, eyelids, etc.,

before, during, and after operations, this salt being, according to
that author, the best available germicide. A solution of 1 grain
in 5000 of water (common or distilled) (= gr. j in fl. ℥xij) may
be freely used for the above purposes, and a stronger one (1 to
2500) (= gr. j in fl. ℥vj) as a lotion for catarrhal ophthalmia, etc.
Some surgeons use much stronger solutions.

The Moorfields Pharmacopœia has a lotion containing 1 grain in
fl. ℥viij, or 1 in 3500.

The officinal solution (liq. hydrarg. perchlor.) contains chloride
of ammonium also, and is decomposed and rendered almost inert
if diluted with common, instead of distilled, water; but a solution
of perchloride alone in common or distilled water is stable. (Martindale's Extra Pharmacopœia.)

11. *Calomel Powder :*

Used for dusting on the cornea in some cases of ulceration. It
is flicked into the eye from a dry camel-hair brush.

12. *Yellow Oxide of Mercury* ("*Yellow Ointment,*" "*Pagenstecher's Ointment*") :

> Yellow Oxide of Mercury gr. xxiv,
> Vaseline ℥j.
>   (1 in 20.)

13. Weaker preparations, containing gr. viij or less of the
yellow oxide to ℥j (1 in 60 or less), are often better borne.

Used in many cases of corneal ulceration and recent corneal
nebulæ; a morsel as large as a hemp-seed being inserted within
the lower lid, by means of a small brush, once or twice a day. It
is also suitable for ophthalmia tarsi.

In some of the continental eye hospitals, where it is the custom
for this remedy, amongst others, to be applied by the surgeon himself, stronger preparations are used.

14. *Yellow Ointment with Atropine :*

> Yellow Oxide of Mercury gr. viij or less,
> Atropine gr. ¼,
> Vaseline ℥j.

Used in the same way as 12 and 13.

15. *Red Oxide of Mercury :*

> Red Oxide of Mercury gr. xxiv or less,
> Vaseline ℥j.

Used for ophthalmia tarsi, etc. Was formerly used for corneal ulcers and nebulæ; but the yellow oxide, which being made by precipitation is not crystalline, is now generally preferred because less irritating.[1]

16.   *Nitrate of Mercury (Citrine Ointment):*

> Unguentum Hydrargyri Nitratis (B. P.) ℨj,
> Vaseline or Prepared Lard ℥vij.

Used in the same cases as 15.

17.   *Iodoform:*

Iodoform may be used either in substance or as an ointment made with vaseline.

> Iodoform gr. x to xxx or more,
> Vaseline ℥j.

Ung. Iodoformi (B. P. 1885) :

> Iodoform gr. xlviij,
> Benzoated Lard ℥j.

18.   *Iodol*, which is odorless, may be used in the same way. The precipitated iodoform (impalpable powder) should be used in preference to the ordinary, or crystalline, form, for the eye.

SULPHATE OF ZINC :

19.   Sulphate of Zinc gr. j or ij,
            Water or Rose Water ℥j.

CHLORIDE OF ZINC :

20.   Chloride of Zinc gr. ij,
            Water ℥j.

> If there is a deposit, add of dilute hydrochloric acid just enough to make a clear solution.

---

[1] The ointment known as "Singleton's Golden Eye Ointment" appears to contain a crystalline red oxide in fine powder as its active ingredient. A sample, kindly analyzed for me by Mr. S. Plowman, contained 70 grains of the oxide to the ounce.

21. *Chloride of Zinc Paste (Caustic)*:

> (1) Chloride of Zinc 1,
> Wheat flour 2, 3, or 4.
> Water enough to make a thick paste. (St. Thomas's Hospital.)

> (2) Allow solid Chloride of Zinc to deliquesce, add a little glycerine, and make into a paste with powdered Sanguinaria. The glycerine prevents hardening on keeping. (St. Thomas's Hospital.)

> (3) Chloride of Zinc 480 grains (8),
> Wheat flour 180 grains (3),
> Water or Liquor Opii Sedativus, fl. ℥j (8). (Middlesex and Moorfields Ophthalmic Hospitals.)

> (4) Chloride of Zinc 1,
> Freshly-burned Plaster-of-Paris 2.
> Made into a paste with a few drops of water. (Druitt's " Vade Mecum," 9th ed.)

> (5) Chloride of Zinc 1,
> Oxide of Zinc 1,
> Wheat flour 2.
> Water enough to make a stiff paste, which is made into caustic points. (Squire, 13th ed.)

It would seem from the above that the exact composition of the paste is not of much importance. It would be desirable to have the point settled.

ALUM:

22. A stick of pure crystalline alum forms a very useful application for mild or long-standing cases of granular conjunctiva, and for many forms of chronic palpebral conjunctivitis. It may be used by the patient himself without the slightest risk.

23. *Lotion*:

> Alum gr. iv to gr. x,
> Water ℥j.

The above lotions are in common use in the milder forms of acute and chronic ophthalmia. The chloride of zinc occasionally irritates; it is specially used in purulent and severe catarrhal ophthalmia instead of the weak nitrate of silver lotions. The stronger alum lotion is often used in the same cases. The alum and sulphate of zinc lotions may be used unsparingly to the conjunctiva ; the chloride, even in severe cases, not more than six times a day.

CARBONATE OF SODA:

24.   Carbonate of Soda gr. x,
                   Water ℨj.

Used for softening the crusts in severe ophthalmia tarsi. A small quantity of the lotion, diluted with its own bulk of hot water, to be used for soaking the edges of the eyelids for ten or fifteen minutes night and morning.

TAR AND SODA :

25.   Carbonate of Soda ℨjss,
                   Liquor Carbonis Detergens ℨj to ℨss,
                   Water to Oj.

Used in the same cases as the last.

BORAX :

26.   Biborate of Soda gr. x to xx,
                   Water ℨj.

Used in the same cases as the last.

QUININE LOTION :

27.   Sulphate of Quinine gr. iij,
                   Acid. Sulph. dil. (B. P.) just enough to dissolve,
                   Water ℨj.
Used in diphtheritic ophthalmia.

BORIC ACID LOTION:

28.   Boric Acid 4,
                   Water 100 by weight.

Used as an antiseptic before and after operations on the eyeball, and in the treatment of suppurating ulcers of the cornea.

Boric acid in very fine powder may be used for dusting on to the cornea in cases of severe suppurating ulcer ; it causes scarcely any pain and may be applied as often as three times a day. The crystals are difficult to powder finely, but an almost impalpable amorphous powder, obtained by preventing regular crystallization, can be had.

Mr. Martindale has made for me some soluble styles containing about 60 per cent. of boric acid, for use in cases of lachrymal obstruction with much secretion of mucus.

Solutions of boric acid often tarnish steel ; instruments should therefore not be left in them.

BORIC ACID OINTMENT (B. P. 1885) :

Boric Acid gr. lxviij to ʒj of Paraffin.

CARBOLIC ACID LOTION :

29.   Absolute Phenol 5,
Water by weight 100.

Used in purulent ophthalmia. It is important to use absolutely pure carbolic acid for the conjunctiva. Severe irritation often follows if any other varieties are employed.

Lotion of *salicylic acid* is so irritating to the surface of the eye that it can seldom be used. The same objection applies to salicylic wool used for dressing the eye after operations.

30. COCAINE.

Cocaine was brought into clinical use in September, 1884, at Vienna, and in London and elsewhere early in October.

A two per cent. solution of a salt of cocaine dropped into the conjunctival sac causes smarting for about half a minute, followed by numbness, rising to complete anæsthesia of ocular conjunctiva and cornea in about two to five minutes ; in three to five minutes after the maximum is reached, feeling begins to return, but slight numbness continues for about twenty minutes. There is often a feeling of coldness as sensation is returning. Cocaine also causes widening of the palpebral fissure by retraction of the upper and lower lids, whitening of eyeball from contraction of bloodvessels, mydriasis, very slight weakness of Acc., and perhaps lowering of the eye tension. These effects last about half an hour, except the mydriasis, which remains in some degree about twenty-four hours. The pupil dilated by cocaine remains active to light and Acc. ; if atropine be added the pupil becomes larger than from either drug singly. Eserine quickly and fully overcomes the effect of cocaine. Acc. is completely paralyzed for a short time if cocaine be used every few minutes for about an hour. These effects of cocaine (except the last) are explicable on the supposition that it causes spasm of the sympathetic nerve-fibres to the eyelids, iris, and

21

superficial bloodvessels; whether a similar contraction of the arteries of the ciliary muscle, brought about by the repeated use of the drug, explains the fleeting paralysis of Acc. is open to question. Cocaine has no ascertainable action on the vessels of the retina and choroid. Cocaine is thought by some to aid the action of eserine in chronic glaucoma, when the two are used together; this is intelligible if cocaine acts by contracting the ciliary arteries.

In ophthalmology cocaine is used chiefly for anæsthesia before operations on the eyeball, and painful applications to the palpebral conjunctiva. For the former, a freshly made two per cent. solution of perfectly pure hydrochlorate of cocaine in freshly boiled distilled water is the safest preparation; but gelatine discs of the pure salt, if free from hygroscopic tendency, may be safely used. Solutions in oil or vaseline are uncleanly and not suitable for surgical purposes. Watery solutions of cocaine should be used quite fresh; even if made with boracic acid or camphor water, they often, if kept, grow fungi, and are then unsafe. Bichloride of mercury in sufficient quantity to prevent growth, sometimes, in conjunction with cocaine, causes considerable haziness of the cornea. Even cocaine alone, if too freely used, causes dryness, loosening, and even separation of the corneal epithelium: the desiccation of the corneal epithelium is said to occur in direct proportion to the frequency of use of the cocaine and of exposure of the cornea to the air, rather than to the strength of the solution employed. Not more than three applications need be made, within five minutes, before operations for cataract, etc. Cocaine has been accused of producing glaucoma, but, as far as the few recorded cases show, without much reason. For deadening granular lids, or similar conditions, a much stronger solution must be painted over the affected surface (I use a 20 per cent. solution or the solid salt). For small tumors about the lid, etc., a 4 per cent. solution is injected in different directions at the base of the growth.

LAMELLÆ COCAINÆ (B. P. 1885) $\frac{1}{200}$ gr. in each.

If the eye be congested or inflamed cocaine acts much less perfectly on the conjunctiva; but it acts as well upon an ulcerated as upon a healthy cornea. As the cocaine takes effect only on the part which it touches, the solution must be made to flow all over the cornea and conjunctiva; and as it penetrates little, if at all, it must be injected under the conjunctiva if we wish to render the later (tenotomy) stage of a squint operation painless, or to excise the eyeball under its influence. Cocaine as ordinarily used does not seem to affect the sensibility of the iris, at any rate no such action has been proved ; injection into the anterior chamber for this purpose is not practicable, even if safe.

Cocaine is used in acute iritis in conjunction with atropine, with the idea that it will assist the anodyne and mydriatic effects of the latter. My own experience does not enable me to speak strongly on this point.

For producing rapid but brief paralysis of Acc. (in ametropia) a solution containing 2 per cent. of cocaine and 2 per cent. of homatropine is recommended by Mr. Lang, and is convenient in suitable cases ; the maximum effect is gained in from 20 to 60 minutes, but soon begins to decline.

Faintness and other signs of nervous depression have been reported as due to cocaine, even when used to the eye alone. I believe that these symptoms are generally due to reaction after the mental strain attending an operation of which the patient is conscious ; for before cocaine was used we were familiar with the occurrence of faintness and vomiting from time to time when eye operations had been undergone without anæsthesia.

MYDRIATICS AND MYOTICS :

31.   (1) *Strong Atropine Drops:*

Liquor Atropinæ Sulphatis (B. P.)
(Sulphate of Atropia gr. ix,
Camphor water ℥xvjss).

Used in cases where the rapid and full local action of the drug is required. For many purposes atropine drops may be used considerably weaker than the above. Atropine (a single drop, of 2 grains to ℥j, or about 0.5 per cent.) begins to dilate the pupil in about fifteen minutes, and to paralyze the accommodation a few minutes later ; it produces wide dilatation of the pupil (8 to 9 mm.) in 30 to 40 minutes, and full paralysis of accommodation in about 2 hours. Both remain at their height for 24 hours, and the effect does not pass off entirely until from 3 to 7 days, the accommodation recovering rather sooner than the pupil. If stronger solutions be used several times, the action continues longer. The effects of atropine are only very temporarily and imperfectly overcome by eserine. Atropine slightly lowers the tension of the healthy eye, but usually increases the tension in glaucoma.

(2) *Weak Atropine Drops:*

Sulphate of Atropia gr. $\frac{1}{40}$ to $\frac{1}{4}$,
Distilled water ℥j.

Used when, for optical purposes, it is desired to keep the pupil dilated for a long time, as in immature nuclear cataract. A single drop about three times a week will generally suffice. Very weak atropine acts more on the pupil than on the accommodation.

Solutions of sulphate of atropine keep for an indefinite time; the flocculent sediment which often forms does not impair their efficiency. The mydriatics and myotics may be used in the form of ointment with vaseline or castor oil, and a smaller percentage of the drug is then necessary; the alkaloids themselves must be used, their salts not being soluble in fats and oils.

(3) *Ung. Atropinæ* (B. P. 1885):

Atropine gr. viij,
Rect. Spirit ℨss,
Benzoated Lard ℥j.

This ointment is needlessly strong for most purposes; 1 grain to 1 ounce is usually enough.

(4) *Lamellæ Atropinæ* (B. P. 1865) $\frac{1}{5000}$ gr. in each.

32. *Daturine:*

Sulphate of Daturia gr. iv,
Distilled Water ℥j.

Used as a mydriatic in cases where atropine causes conjunctival irritation.

33. *Duboisine:*

Sulphate of Duboisia gr. j.
Distilled Water ℥j.

A mydriatic, acting more quickly and powerfully, and passing off in a shorter time, than atropine. It is tolerated in cases where atropine causes conjunctivitis. To be used with caution, as well-marked toxic symptoms are sometimes caused.

Duboisine begins to act on the pupil and accommodation in less than ten minutes, produces full mydriasis in less than twenty minutes, and complete cycloplegia in about one hour. The maximum effect does not last quite so long as, and the effect passes off completely rather sooner than, that of atropine. Duboisine seldom breaks down iritic adhesions which have already resisted atropine. Its chief use seems to be for cases in which atropine causes irritation.

34. *Homatropine:*

> Hydrobromate of Homatropine, gr. iv,
> Distilled Water ʒj.

A mydriatic, acting rather more quickly and passing off much sooner than atropine; very convenient, therefore, for dilating the pupil for ophthalmoscopic examination.

Homatropine begins to act on the pupil and accommodation in from five to fifteen minutes; the greatest dilatation of pupil (usually, however, rather less than that obtained by atropine) is reached in about fifty minutes, and complete or nearly complete cycloplegia in an hour or rather less (with the solution of gr. iv to ʒj). The full effect is only maintained, however, for an hour, more or less, and both pupil and accommodation usually recover completely in twenty-four hours or less. Its action is quicker and rather more powerful if it be used with cocaine. See Cocaine.

35. *Eserine* (Physostigmine) (alkaloid of Calabar Bean):

> (1) Sulphate of Eseria gr. iv,
> Distilled Water ʒj.

Used in mydriasis and paralysis of the accommodation, whether caused by atropine or by nerve-lesions in some forms of corneal ulcer and in acute glaucoma.

> (2) A weaker solution (gr. j to ʒj) is often better borne.

Eserine begins to contract the pupil and cause spasm of the accommodation in about five minutes; its maximum effect is reached in twenty to forty-five minutes. Its full effect on the accommodation lasts only an hour or two, but the pupil does not completely recover for many hours, sometimes two or three days. A very weak solution acts more on the pupil than on the accommodation. Eserine causes pain in the eye and head, arterial ciliary congestion, and twitching of the orbicularis; the pain, sometimes severe, seldom lasts long. Eserine often lessens the tension in primary glaucoma.

> (3) *Lamellæ Physostigminæ* (B. P. 1885) $\frac{1}{1000}$ gr. in each.

All the mydriatics and myotics may be obtained in the form of small gelatine discs of known strength (made by Savory and Moore, and by Martindale), which are sometimes more convenient than the solutions. Of the mydriatics, homatropine and duboisine are much the most expensive.

36. *Belladonna Fomentation:*

> Extract of Belladonna ℥j to ij,
> Water Oj.

Warmed in a cup or small basin, and used as a hot fomentation in suppurating and serpiginous ulcers of cornea.

37. *Pilocarpine for Subcutaneous Injection:*

> Hydrochlorate of Pilocarpine gr. v,
> Distilled Water ℥j.

Dose, ℞ iij, gradually increased, to be injected daily or less often. Used in cases of retinal detachment, choroiditis, and retinitis.

38. *Pilocarpine Drops:* gr. iv to ℥j.

Pilocarpine is a myotic, like eserine, but its action is much weaker.   .

39. STRYCHNIA *for Subcutaneous Injection:*

> Liquor Strychninæ (B. P.) gr. iv to ℥j.

Dose, two minims ($\frac{1}{60}$ grain), gradually increased, for subcutaneous injection. To be injected once a day.

40. "Jequirity" seeds, obtained from a leguminous plant, are used in South America for the cure of granular lids. They can now be readily obtained in moderately fine powder. The infusion is made by soaking the powder in cold water for a couple of hours, or better, in water at 120° F., allowing it to stand till cool, and straining through muslin; it is then ready for use, but will remain active for several days. When obviously decomposed (fetid) it is no longer active. The simple powder dusted into the conjunctiva is said to be active, but two or three trials which I made with it were negative.

The action of Jequirity probably depends upon a nitrogenous ferment—not, as was for a time believed, upon a specific microbe. A substance possessing the peculiar properties of the natural seed has been separated by more than one experimenter, but does not appear to be procurable in the market; it is difficult to make, and its composition seems to vary.

As the intensity of action of Jequirity infusions of the same strength varies very much in different persons, and is sometimes very severe, it is best to use a weak preparation (1 grain of powder in 100 grains of water, or ℥j to fl.℥xijss) for all cases at first. A single prolonged application, or several applications within a few minutes, to the everted lids will suffice.

41. BANDAGES for the eyes may be of thin flannel or soft calico. A linen or cotton bandage, about ten inches long, with four tails of tape, or a loop of tape embracing the back of the head (Liebreich's bandage), is very convenient after the more serious operations. An ordinary narrow flannel bandage is better when much pressure is wanted, or if the patient be unruly. The soft, elastic, woven bandage, known as the "Leicester" bandage, is even pleasanter than flannel.

When absolute exclusion of light is desired, it is best to use a bandage made of a double fold of some thin black material.

Fine old linen is better than lint for laying next the skin in dressings after operations.

42. SHADES may be bought at the opticians' and chemists'; or may be made of thin cardboard covered with some dark material, or of stout dark-blue paper, like that used for making grocers' sugar bags. Shades of black plaited straw are also very light and convenient.

Shades, to be effectual, should extend to the temple on each side, so as to exclude all side light.

43. PROTECTIVE GLASSES.

Various patterns of glasses are made for the purpose of protecting the eyes from wind, dust, and bright light. The glasses are either flat, or hollow like a watch-glass, and are colored in various shades of blue or smoke tint. The most effectual are the ones known as "goggles;" in these the space between the glass and the edge of the orbit is filled by a carefully-fitting framework of fine wire gauze or black crape, by which side wind and light are excluded. A small air pad of thin India-rubber tubing makes the frame fit still more closely.

Other forms, known as "horseshoe" or "D," and "domed" or "hollow" glasses are also in common use.

44. TEST TYPES.

Snellen's types for testing both near and distant vision under an angle of five minutes can be obtained through Queen & Co., 924 Chestnut St., Philadelphia.

The types which I generally use for testing near vision are those used at the Moorfields Hospital, where they may be obtained. They can also be bought, conveniently mounted, of Queen & Co., 924 Chestnut St., Philadelphia. These types nearly resemble those of Jaeger, and though less correct theoretically than the corresponding type of Snellen's scale, are more convenient in practice for testing the reading power. There are several other sets of test types which it is unnecessary here to particularize.

A convenient set of tests, small enough to be carried in the pocket, can be obtained through Queen & Co., 924 Chestnut St., Philadelphia. It consists of types for near and distant vision, a pupillometer for measuring the pupil, a set of colored stuffs for color-blindness, and a small series of lenses for testing refraction. This case is intended chiefly for ward work and general medical cases. It may be also bought without the lenses.

45. OPHTHALMOSCOPES.

It is impossible to say that any ophthalmoscope is the best. When expense is not a great object, it is always better to have one of the so-called "refraction ophthalmoscopes." In these a number of small lenses are placed in a disc behind the mirror, the disc being made to revolve by finger pressure so as to bring the lenses one after another opposite the sight-hole. For medical ophthalmoscopy it is not essential to have so many lenses; about four concave and two convex will enable an erect image to be easily obtained in most cases; Liebreich's "small" ophthalmoscope and Oldham's ophthalmoscope are both very convenient forms for such use, and cost less than half as much as the refraction instruments. Every ophthalmoscope case should contain two large "objective" lenses for the indirect examination, focal illumination, and magnifying; one may be of $2\frac{1}{2}$, the other $3\frac{1}{2}$ inches focus. For the detection of incipient opacities in the lens, for direct examination without atropine, and for retinoscopy, a plane mirror is very useful

200

N
40

E
50

P N V D F L
32 25 20 16 12½ 10 3

Y P N V D F L

In addition to the ordinary concave one. It gives a weaker illumination. Such a plane mirror may be had cheaply as a separate instrument for the waistcoat pocket, but I much prefer it and the concave one for indirect examination, mounted back to back (see below).

Of the refraction ophthalmoscopes there are now a great many patterns, differing in the number and size of the lenses, the size of the mirror and lens-bearing disc, and other details. Usually the disc contains 20 to 24 lenses, and one empty circle. In the simpler forms about half the lenses are $+$ and half $-$. But in others the number of powers is immensely increased by combining lenses of different strengths, e. g., the disc may contain 24 $+$ lenses, whilst a single movable $-$ lens, rather stronger than the highest $+$, is placed behind the disc over the sight-hole; by placing it opposite the sight-hole and then bringing the various $+$ lenses over it in succession, a series of 25 $-$ powers, or 49 in all, will be obtained. In order to avoid the error caused by looking obliquely through a lens, all the better instruments (e. g., Loring's, Couper's, Morton's, and others) are so arranged that the mirror can be sufficiently inclined to receive the light, whilst the lens-bearing disc remains at right angles to the observer's line of sight. Generally speaking, the English and American instruments are much better made than the French. Of the simpler forms with only one mirror, the one introduced by Dr. Gowers is fairly efficient. Of the more expensive forms, several good ones have been derived from an early model by Mr. Laidlaw Purves, both of which may be procured from Queen & Co., 924 Chestnut Street, Philadelphia. The latest form of this instrument, made by Mr. Ferrier for myself, has three mirrors (two of them back to back in a single ring) mounted on a rotating carriage like the "nose-piece" of a microscope; it is extremely convenient and accurate. For the application of the "nose-piece" principle to the ophthalmoscope we are indebted to Mr. Lindsay Johnson. Mr. Couper's and Mr. Morton's models are very excellent and deservedly popular. In a good refraction ophthalmoscope the mirror should be thin and the sight-hole perforated; the lens-disc thin and working as close to the back of the mirror as possible; the lenses evenly mounted, centred truly, either thoroughly covered up or easily accessible for cleaning, and not less than 5 mm. in diameter.

21*

46. PERIMETERS.

The most convenient forms have an arrangement for registering the field automatically on a chart fixed behind the centre of the arc. A very complete, but complicated and expensive, one, is McHardy's; Priestley Smith's, much simpler and cheaper, is for most purposes as useful. Blix's self-registering perimeter is well spoken of by Dr. Berry. All of which may be obtained from Messrs. Queen.

47. The "CLOCK-FACE" for testing astigmatism can be had at Queen's.

48. The set of COLORED WOOLS recommended by Prof. Holmgren, of Upsala, for testing color-blindness, can be obtained for about $1.50, from Queen & Co.

In the colored plate copied by permission from Prof. Holmgren's work, *De la Cécité des Couleurs*, etc., 1877, the horizontal stripes I, IIa, and IIb, show the colors which it is, as a rule, most convenient to use as tests; and the short vertical stripes are the colors most likely to be confused with these by those affected with the ordinary forms of color-blindness. Thus, No. 1 will be confused with one or more of such buffs, pinks, etc., as Nos. 1 to 5; in slight degrees of color-defect the confusions will be limited to these pale colors.

In higher degrees of color-blindness stronger or more saturated colors will be confused; IIa, for example, or even a stronger rose color, may be confused, on the one hand, with a full blue or purple, Nos. 6 and 7; or, on the other, with a full gray or green, Nos. 8 and 9. Taking a different series of equally saturated colors, the scarlet IIb may be confidently identified with dark green or brown, Nos. 10 and 11, or with light bright green and yellow-brown, Nos. 12 and 13.

The confusion colors, Nos. 1 to 13 on the plate, are given merely as samples of the colors most commonly confused with the respective test-colors; in practice a much larger series should be employed; the more critical the patient, the larger is the number of shades and colors requisite; even markedly color-blind persons do not always match exactly the same colors with the tests. Colored worsteds are used because it is easier to obtain a very large series in this material than in any other.

The manner in which a color-blind person behaves will often ex-

I.

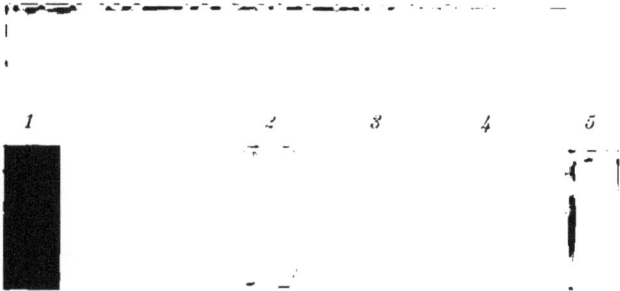

II a.

II b.

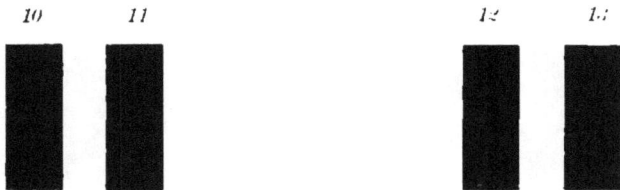

[*See page* 490]

cite suspicion of his defect.   He will perhaps place doubtfully side
by side with I, such a color as No. 2 or 5, to see whether or not
they are alike, and finally will decide that they are not quite of
the same color, though "rather alike." In such cases, and again
in others, where perhaps the patient does not understand what is
wanted, the diagnosis may often be made certain in the following
manner: Take two colors over which the patient is stumbling, or
on which he cannot express himself, say Nos. IIa and a lighter
shade of 9, add a third of the same dominant color as 9, but of a
markedly different shade, such as 10 or 12; now ask him which
pair is more alike, Nos. IIa and 9, or Nos. 9 and 10; if he says
IIa and 9 are more alike he is color-blind, and is judging of their
similarity by the *shade*, that is, the amount of white contained in
each of them, and not by their *color*. It is easy to vary this test
according to the requirements of the case.

Another good method is to tell the patient to pick out all the
skeins of one color, say green, without requiring him to match them
precisely with any test skein; if decidedly color-blind, he will confidently select not only those which are green, but a number of
others, usually gray ones. Or we may say: "Do you see any
green skeins among them?" If color-blind he will say "No," or
hesitate, or make the same mistakes as above.

A special arrangement of the wools, enabling a quick, accurate,
and uniform record of color-perception to be made, has been de-
signed by Dr. William Thomson, of Philadelphia, and is obtainable from Queen & Co.   (Supplement, page 465.)

Of the many other tests for color-blindness the following may
be mentioned :

Stilling's Tables consist of colored letters or patterns printed on
a groundwork of one of the "confusion colors." They are preferred by some to Holmgren's wool.

Donders's method determines the color-sense (or color-defect)
quantitatively by means of a light of known intensity, which
passes through apertures filled by differently colored glasses ; these
are recognized at a specified distance if the color-sense is normal.

Mr. Jeaffreson (of Newcastle) has lately constructed an ingenious
apparatus in which the colored wools, fixed in radii upon a rotating
disc, can be successively brought opposite to stationary patches of
the respective confusion colors, which are placed just beyond the
circumference of the disc : *Lancet*, July 17, 1886.

Bull (of Christiania) has introduced a quantitative test, based upon the smallest amount of color which, mixed with gray, can be recognized by the normal eye. (Obtainable from Queen & Co.) Rows of colored spots, those in each row containing a different quantity of gray, are painted in oil colors on a black background. The normal eye will distinguish the colors even in the grayest row ; the color-blind will, according to the degree of defect, confuse complementary colors in some or all of the rows. I find Bull's tables very useful, but like all painted and lithographed surfaces they reflect too much light, and thus, unless held exactly in the right position, they shine and their color is altered. Unless very carefully used, Bull's and Jeaffreson's tests are, I think, less trustworthy than a good set of wools.

An explanation of the colored plate is given on p. 490 ; it is not intended to be used as a test, but only as an illustration of the colors commonly confused.

INDEX.

www.ingramcontent.com/pod-product-compliance
Lightning Source LLC
Chambersburg PA
CBHW020856210326

41598CB00018B/1693